Contexts of Physiotherapy Practice

Contexts of Physiotherapy Practice

Joy Higgs
Megan Smith
Gillian Webb
Margot Skinner
Anne Croker

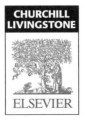

CHURCHILL
LIVINGSTONE

ELSEVIER

Sydney Edinburgh London New York Philadelphia St Louis Toronto

MT

Churchill Livingstone
is an imprint of Elsevier

Elsevier Australia. ACN 001 002 357
(a division of Reed International Books Australia Pty Ltd)
Tower 1, 475 Victoria Avenue, Chatswood, NSW 2067

ELSEVIER

National Library of Australia Cataloguing-in-Publication Data

Contexts of physiotherapy practice / editor, Joy Higgs ... [et al.]

ISBN: 9780729538862 (pbk.)

Includes index
Bibliography.

Physical therapy–Administration.
Physical therapy–Vocational guidance.
Physical therapist and patient.

Higgs, Joy.

615.82

Publisher: Heidi Allen
Developmental Editor: Samantha McCulloch
Publishing Services Manager: Helena Klijn
Editorial Coordinator: Eleanor Cant
Edited by Linda Littlemore
Proofread by Margaret Trudgeon
Internal design and typesetting by Midland Typesetters
Cover design by Lisa Petroff
Index by Mei Yen Chua
Printed by Ligare

It is the policy of Elsevier Australia to use vegetable-based inks on paper manufactured from sustainable
forests wherever possible.

6/25/09

CONTENTS

PREFACE

We have pleasure in presenting a book that captures the breadth and depth of physiotherapy professional practice in Australia and New Zealand. The book is the first of its kind and recognises an established profession that is able to reflect upon over 100 years of practice and experience. As a profession we are able to draw on our own body of knowledge to describe the context of our physiotherapy identity, scope and diversity of practice, career pathways and emerging directions.

In the book we explore contemporary physiotherapy practice, including patient-centred care, teamwork, community-based practice, clinical reasoning, research and legal and ethical obligations, evidence-based practice and cultural awareness. Threaded through the book are themes of autonomy, responsiveness to prevailing social issues, evolving models of healthcare and professional relationships. The book is divided into six content areas: the physiotherapy profession, physiotherapy practice, contexts of practice, standards and evidence for practice, working with others, and evaluation and practice management.

This book is written for beginning physiotherapy practitioners and established practitioners alike. It is intended to be a valuable resource for those working in health care practice, health policy and management and for anyone interested in understanding the context of physiotherapy practice. The majority of contributors are physiotherapists from Australia and New Zealand. The authors were chosen for their knowledge and expertise in the areas represented and their understanding of the knowledge needs of beginning practitioners. Many of the chapters include case examples that ground the content in practical applications and stimulate reflection and professional development.

We encourage readers to discuss and further develop the themes presented in this book and look forward to ongoing debate on the issues raised.

ACKNOWLEDGEMENTS

The editors acknowledge the contributions of the authors to *Contexts of Physiotherapy Practice*. We would also like to thank the peer reviewers for their comments and suggestions, Joan Rosenthal for her style and editorial guidance and the Elsevier team for their support and assistance in the production of this book.

EDITORS

Joy Higgs AM, BSc, GradDipPhty, MHPEd, PhD; The Research Institute for Professional Practice, Learning and Education and The Education for Practice Institute, Charles Sturt University, Australia

Megan Smith BAppSc(Physio), GradCertUT&L, MAppSc(CardiopulmPhysio), PhD; School of Community Health, Charles Sturt University, Australia

Gillian Webb DipPhty, GradDipEx(Rehab), MClinEd, DEd; School of Physiotherapy, The University of Melbourne, Australia

Margot A Skinner DipPhty, MPhEd, PhD; School of Physiotherapy, University of Otago, New Zealand

Anne Croker BAppSc(Physio), GradCertPubHealth; The Education for Practice Institute, Charles Sturt University, Australia

CONTRIBUTORS

Rola Ajjawi BAppSc(Physio)(Hons), PhD; The Education for Practice Institute, Charles Sturt University, Australia

Lynley Anderson DipPhysio, MHealSci, PhD; Bioethics Centre, University of Otago, New Zealand

David Baxter TD, BSc(Hons), MBA, DPhil; School of Physiotherapy, University of Otago, New Zealand

Anne Bent BAppSc, DipPhysioGradCert; Public Sector Management, James Cook University, Australia

Christine Bithell DipEd, FHEA, MCSP, MA(Education); Joint Faculty of Health and Social Care Sciences, St George's, University of London and Kingston University, London, UK

Peter Bragge LTCL, BPhysio(Hons), PhD(Physiotherapy); School of Physiotherapy, The University of Melbourne, Australia

Martin M Chadwick DipPhys, OCS(ABPTS), PGDipHS; Waikato District Health Board, Hamilton, New Zealand

Julia Coyle CSP, GradDipManipPhty, MManipPhty, GCertUniTL; School of Community Health, Charles Sturt University, Australia

Megan Davidson BAppSc(Physio) PhD; School of Physiotherapy, La Trobe University, Australia

Heather Dawson BAppSc(Physio), BEd, GradDip(ResearchMethods), School of Population Health, The University of Melbourne, Australia

Clare Delany BAppSc(Physio), MPhysio(Manip), MHlth&MedLaw, PhD; School of Physiotherapy, The University of Melbourne, Australia

Ian Edwards BAppSc(Physio), GradDipPhysio, PhD; School of Health Sciences, University of South Australia, Australia

Elizabeth Ellis GradDipPhty, MHL, PhD; Faculty of Health Sciences, The University of Sydney, Australia

Shaun Ewen BAppSc(Physio), MMIL; Onemda VicHealth Koori Health Unit, School of Population Health, The University of Melbourne, Australia

Margaret Grant BAppSc(Physio), MPrelim, MEd; Australian Physiotherapy Council, Canberra, Australia

Debra Griffiths BA, RN, LLB, LLM; School of Nursing & Midwifery, Monash University, Australia

Karen Grimmer-Somers CertHlthEc, BPhty, LMusA, MMedSc, PhD; Centre for Allied Health Evidence, University of South Australia, Australia

Miriam Grotowski BMed, DipPsychiatry(EatingDisorders), FRACGP; Marius Street Practice, Tamworth, Australia

Leigh Hale BSc(Physio), MNZCP(Neurology) MSc(Physio, Neurology), PhD; School of Physiotherapy, University of Otago, New Zealand

Peter Hamer DipPhysio, BPE(Hons), MEd, PhD, FASMF; School of Health Sciences, The University of Notre Dame Australia, Australia

Abby Haynes BA(Social Work)(Hons), GradDip(Counselling), MA(InfoKnow Man); Diversity Health, South Eastern Sydney and Illawarra Health, Australia

Cheryl Hobbs PhD; Interprofessional Learning, The University of Sydney, Australia

Jill Hummell DipOT, BA, MA, PhD; Westmead Brain Injury Rehabilitation Service, Sydney, Australia

Dale Jones BPhty; Aged and Disability Services, Katherine, Department of Health and Community Services Northern Territory, Australia

Mark Jones BSc(Psych), CertPhysTher, GradDipAdvanManipTher (ManipPhysio), MAppSc(Physio); School of Health Sciences, University of South Australia, Australia

Sue Jones BAppSc(Physio), GradDipPubSectMgt; Faculty of Health Sciences, Curtin University of Technology, Western Australia

Gwendolen Jull DipPhty, GradDipManipTher, MPhty, PhD; Division of Physiotherapy, School of Health and Rehabilitation Sciences, The University of Queensland, Australia

Jenny Keating BAppSc(Physio), GradDipManipPhysio, PhD; Department of Physiotherapy, Monash University, Australia

Peter Larmer DipMT, DipAcup, MNZSP, MPH(Hons); School of Rehabilitation and Occupation Studies, Faculty of Health and Environmental Sciences, AUT University, New Zealand

Dale Larsen BAppSc(Phty), MAppSc(ManipPhty), PhD; Macquarie St Physiotherapy Centre, Sydney, Australia; Member, Research Institute for Professional Practice, Learning and Education, Charles Sturt University, Australia

Joan McMeeken DipPhysio, BSc(Hons), MSc; Faculty of Medicine, Dentistry and Health Sciences, The University of Melbourne, Australia

Stephan Milosavljevic BAppSc(Physio), GradDipManipTher, MMPhty (Manipulative), PhD; School of Physiotherapy, University of Otago, New Zealand

Damian Mitsch GDip, MBA, ASM, FAICD; National Office, Australian Physiotherapy Association, Australia

Cathy Nall BAppSci(Physio), GradDipHealthAdmin, GradDipPhysio(Cardioth), MBA; Physiotherapy Department, Austin Health, School of Physiotherapy, University of Melbourne, Australia

David Nicholls GradDipPhys, MA; School of Physiotherapy, Auckland University of Technology, New Zealand

Narelle Patton BAppSc(Phys), MHSc(OrthopaedicManipTher); School of Community Health, Charles Sturt University, Australia

Jennifer Pynt PhD; The Education for Practice Institute, Charles Sturt University, Australia

Kathryn Refshauge DipPhty, GradDipManipTher, MBioMedE, PhD; Faculty of Health Sciences, The University of Sydney, Australia

Louisa Remedios BAppSc(Physio), GradDip(Sports), Masters(Research), PhD; School of Physiotherapy, University of Melbourne, Australia

Maggie Roe-Shaw BPhysio, GradCert(StrategicStudies), PostGradDip(Health Promotion), PostGradDip(TertiaryTeaching), MPH, PhD; Anatomy, University of Otago, New Zealand

Diane Tasker BPhty; Mountain Mobile Physiotherapy Service, Blue Mountains, Australia

Franziska Trede DipPhty, MHPEd, PhD; The Education for Practice Institute, Charles Sturt University, Australia

Bill Vicenzino BPhty, GradDipSportsPhty, MSc, PhD; School of Health and Rehabilitation Sciences, The University of Queensland, Australia

Gordon Waddington BSc, BAppSc(Phty), GradDipAppSc(ExSportsScience), MExSportsSc, MAppSc(SportsPhysio), GCHE PhD; University of Canberra, Australia

Matthew Walsh BScPT; South West Washington Medical Centre, Vancouver, Washington, USA

REVIEWERS

Yvonne R Burns AO MPhty PhD; Honorary Research Consultant (Physiotherapy), University of Queensland and Mater Health Services; Associate Professor and past Head of Physiotherapy, University of Queensland

Lucy Chipchase MAppSc DipPhysio PhD; Program Director (Physiotherapy), School of Health Sciences, University of South Australia

Maria Constantinou BPhty MPhtySt (Sports) GradCertEd FASMF APA Sports Physiotherapist; Lecturer, School of Physiotherapy and Exercise Science, Griffith University

Rosemary Corrigan BAppSc (Physiotherapy) MAppSc Doctor of Physiotherapy; Lecturer, Physiotherapy Programme, Charles Sturt University

PHYSIOTHERAPY– THE PROFESSION

PHYSIOTHERAPY IN THE 21ST CENTURY

Gillian Webb, Margot Skinner, Sue Jones, Bill Vicenzino, Cathy Nall and David Baxter

one

Key content

- The nature of the physiotherapy profession
- Physiotherapy as a major player in global health care – particularly in the fields of physical rehabilitation and health promotion
- The three key aspects of physiotherapy – education, practice and research

INTRODUCTION

Physiotherapy had its beginnings in the time of Hippocrates around the 1st century BCE. Touch, massage, hydrotherapy, exercise and rest, as recorded then, are all still fundamental components of physiotherapy practice in the 21st century. The focus of contemporary physiotherapy practice is on the provision of services to people and populations 'to develop, maintain and restore maximum movement and functional ability through the lifespan' (World Confederation for Physical Therapy (WCPT) 1999, p 28). The growth and development of these physiotherapy services requires a combination of education, research and practice. These elements are explored further in this chapter.

The professional name *physiotherapy* is synonymous with the term *physical therapy*. The titles 'physiotherapist' and 'physical therapist' are protected and are preserved for use solely by persons whose qualifications are approved by a national professional association that is a member of the WCPT (WCPT 1995a). There are currently 101 member associations of the WCPT, representing over 270,000 physiotherapists throughout the world. In Australia the national member association is the Australian Physiotherapy Association (APA) and in New Zealand it is the New Zealand Society of Physiotherapists Inc. (NZSP). The WCPT recognises that delivery and provision of physiotherapy services may vary in accordance with local cultural, socioeconomic and political circumstances; however, the principles of best practice and agreed standards of practice (WCPT 2003a) are requirements to which all physiotherapists must adhere.

The WCPT defines physiotherapy in the following way:

> Physical therapy provides services to individuals and populations to develop, maintain and restore maximum movement and functional ability throughout the lifespan. This includes providing services in circumstances where movement and function are threatened by ageing, injury, disease or environmental factors. Functional movement is central to what it means to be healthy.

Physical therapy is concerned with identifying and maximising quality of life and movement potential within the spheres of promotion, prevention, treatment/ intervention, habilitation and rehabilitation. This encompasses physical, psychological, social and emotional wellbeing. Physical therapy involves the interaction between physical therapist, patients/clients, other health professionals, families, care givers and communities in a process where movement potential is assessed and goals are agreed upon, using knowledge and skills unique to physical therapists.

The physical therapist's extensive knowledge of the body and its movement needs and potential is central to determining strategies for diagnosis and intervention. The practice setting will vary according to whether the physical therapy is concerned with health promotion, prevention, treatment/intervention, habilitation or rehabilitation.

Physical therapists act as independent practitioners, as well as members of health service provider teams, and are subject to the ethical principles of WCPT. They are able to act as first contact practitioners, and patients/clients may seek direct services without referral from another health professional.

Physical therapy is an established and regulated profession, with specific professional aspects of clinical practice and education, indicative of diversity in social, economic, cultural and political contexts. But it is clearly a single profession, and the first professional qualification, obtained in any country, represents the completion of a curriculum that qualifies a physical therapist to use the professional title and to practise as an independent professional. (WCPT 1999, p 1)

The physiotherapy profession in the 21st century is continually evolving in response to changes in health, illness and society. Global changes in technology, the increasing mobility of people and changes in lifestyle and in social practices affect us all. Changes have also occurred in the way health is perceived, moving from a biomedical model towards a biopsychosocial model that acknowledges the centrality of the person (World Health Organization (WHO) 2001). These changing views of health care are focused on community- rather than hospital-based therapy, with greater emphasis on healthy lifestyles, health promotion and injury prevention.

Global changes have also occurred in the prevalence and types of diseases, and there has been an increase in the population of elderly persons. In most countries obesity, diabetes and cardiovascular disease are major health problems, not necessarily linked to socioeconomic status. Environmental problems have become prominent (WHO 2007a). In some developing countries, the increasing use of cars and unsafe work practices are significant problems, whereas in others trauma from war or natural disasters may be important.

As different models of health care have been introduced globally, the scope and nature of physiotherapy practice have changed. There is a need for the profession to be constantly re-examining not only its role in the health care arena but also the interventions that are used by physiotherapists. The profession needs to be at the forefront of the promotion of health and wellbeing and to assist people in managing their own health to achieve their highest functional level.

In the 21st century many physiotherapists have become primary health care practitioners involved in delivering services at a population level. Physiotherapists have an important role to play as direct health care providers, as members of multiprofessional teams, as consultants to governments, nongovernment organisations (NGOs) and other relevant organisations, as developers and implementers of services, and as educators of other health care personnel.

Primary health care involves the assumption that health services should be available for all people and should be a partnership between local communities and individuals in service delivery, planning and monitoring. It should also be reflective of the local needs of the community, with practitioners remaining mindful of resources.

> Primary health care seeks to extend the first level of the health system from sick care to the development of health. It seeks to protect and promote the health of defined communities and to address individual and population health problems at an early stage. Primary health care services involve continuity of care, health promotion and education, integration of prevention with sick care, a concern for population as well as individual health, community involvement and the use of appropriate technology. (Fry & Furler 2000, p 388)

As physiotherapists we are able to provide services to people, communities and populations to develop, maintain and restore maximal movement and functional ability throughout the lifespan. Physiotherapy includes the provision of services in circumstances where the processes of ageing, injury and/or disease threaten movement and function. Full and functional movement to enable people to participate in all aspects of life and to be healthy is at the heart of physiotherapy practice. Physiotherapy is well placed to be attractive to governments, NGOs and other agencies and to be promoted because of its emphasis on nonsurgical intervention, its cost effectiveness and its growing body of evidence for treatment efficacy. Physiotherapists have a distinctive view of the body and its movement needs and potential. These factors are central to determining a diagnosis and a successful intervention strategy in every setting.

As physiotherapists it is our duty and obligation to be aware of new knowledge and new ways of thinking. We need to be able to apply this knowledge in a compassionate and professional manner. At the heart of physiotherapy is our ability to communicate effectively with our patients in order to assist them in restoring themselves to their highest functional level. This must be based on learning informed by evidence. With the status of physiotherapy changing in the 21st century there is a need for high standards of education based on the best available research evidence in order to provide appropriate and effective high quality practice.

PRACTICE

Physiotherapists are physical rehabilitation experts whose practice involves the dimensions of promotion, prevention and intervention. As physiotherapy is an autonomous profession, individual physiotherapists should have the right to exercise professional judgement in managing their patients and clients (WCPT 1995b). Autonomy also implies that physiotherapists are responsible for the management they provide and the resulting outcomes, and that they practise within the bounds of their scope of practice and within the code of ethical conduct set down by their professional organisation or regulating authority. Professional autonomy also means that physiotherapists work in an open and equal professional partnership with medical practitioners (WCPT 1995c) and other health professionals (WCPT 1995d).

As part of their ongoing professional development, physiotherapists have a responsibility to use evidence to inform their practice (WCPT 2003b). This forms the foundation of best practice in that patients, groups and communities will receive services that are based on the best evidence available. Physiotherapists should ensure that they work in an environment that embraces and promotes evidence-based practice and that they continually review and critique their practice as part of lifelong learning as well as contribute to the body of knowledge through research (WCPT 2003c).

The practice environment

Practice environments encompass the range from a hospital intensive care unit to a fitness club, workplace or individual's home (see Table 1.1). Practice may take a systems-based approach and focus on the cardiopulmonary, neurological or musculoskeletal system. However, physiotherapists have a responsibility to 'treat the whole person' as well as to provide best practice to manage a particular pathology. The physiotherapy experience for an individual may thus involve management by a variety of physiotherapists who have expertise linked to particular practice environments. For example, an unconscious patient who arrives by ambulance at a tertiary care level hospital following a car accident will initially be managed in the intensive care unit by a physiotherapist who specialises in physiotherapy in intensive care settings. As the patient improves the rehabilitation may be taken over by a physiotherapist working in the wards of an acute care setting, then a secondary care/long-term rehabilitation unit, followed by the primary or community care environment and finally by a physiotherapist specialising in workplace rehabilitation. This presents a continuum of care that takes the person back into the community and workplace, where appropriate. Physiotherapists can fulfil these roles through their specialised knowledge and use of specific skills required for cardiorespiratory care in the intensive care unit, through to functionally based exercise programs and then to appropriate design of workplaces.

Table 1.1 Range of physiotherapy environments in contemporary practice		
Tertiary care –	**Environment**	**Examples**
acute care hospital	Intensive care	Adult, paediatric
	Transplant unit	Heart, kidney
	Burns unit	Conditions involving the integumentary system
	Isolation	Severe acute respiratory syndrome (SARS)
	High dependency unit	Coronary care, neurology, postoperative
	General	Acute medical and surgical admissions
	Emergency department	Triage and acute care management of patients not necessarily to be admitted
Secondary care		
	Intermediate care rehabilitation units for people with dependency prior to community care	Traumatic brain injury, care of the elderly
	Rehabilitation	Hospital-based care

Table 1.1 Range of physiotherapy environments in contemporary practice *continued*		
Primary care –		
focus on interventions and rehabilitation	Outpatient clinics	Public or private Generalist or specialist managing a range of conditions
	Hospice	Quality care for terminal illness
	Long-term care	Individuals who are physically dependent through a congenital or acquired condition
	Rest homes	Care of the elderly
	Schools	Rehabilitation for children with special needs integrated into a school environment
	Domiciliary	Home visits
	Workplace	Rehabilitation back to work, retraining
	Sports	Management of acute injuries, physical requirements of elite athletes
	Fitness centres, health clubs	Improving exercise tolerance, weight reduction
	Community	Third phase of rehabilitation program
Primary care –		
focus on prevention and promotion of health care	Senior citizens	Community exercise, falls prevention
	Workplace	Preventive health and education
	Schools	Education, health promotion
Other		
	Management	Roles and responsibilities at physiotherapy administration level
	Postgraduate education	Formal study at an academic institute above the entry level required for practice
	Specialisation	Route to a level of expertise recognised by the profession in a particular area
	Research	Involvement in research to expand the body of knowledge in physiotherapy
	Academic	Delivery of education to physiotherapy students

Another important factor in practice in the 21st century is the shift away from the medical model to the patient- or client-centred model of health care. This places individuals and their families at the centre of the rehabilitation, giving them a key role in the management of their condition, and it also places an emphasis on community-based rehabilitation (CBR). The objective of CBR is to ensure that all people with disabilities have equal access to rehabilitation, as do all other members of society. Activities included in CBR are the prevention of causes of disabilities; promotion of positive attitudes to people with disabilities; and facilitating education, health promotion and rehabilitation (WHO 2007a).

The WHO model of International Functioning Disability and Health (ICF) (2001) is a framework that has been embraced by the WCPT and promoted for use by all physiotherapists, as it focuses on the health of individuals in relation to their function in their environment. This ICF model thus presents a framework common to all physiotherapists round the globe.

> The ICF shifts the focus to how people live with their health conditions and how these can be improved to achieve a productive fulfilling life … It changes understandings of disability to include the social aspects of disability and provides a mechanism to document the impact of the social and physical environment on a person's functioning. (WHO 2001)

CBR and the ICF have been endorsed by the WCPT (WCPT 2003c) as they empower individuals to become active participants within their communities and maximise their physical health. The need for empowerment and CBR is very evident for victims of disasters. For example, when the tsunami struck South-East Asia in December 2005, victims with physical injuries who were initially treated in nearby hospitals or in temporary setups found that their need to return home to rebuild their lives in their own communities was of primary importance to them.

The market for practice

There is a global shortage of health care workers, including physiotherapists. This shortage is most evident in rural areas and among low socioeconomic groups but is not just confined to developing nations. The situation affecting the shortage of health care workers is complex and involves a number of issues, including a rise in the need for health care workers in industrialised countries where there is an ageing population, immigration of health care workers from developing countries, demographics and underinvestment in health, and factors such as smoking and obesity, which contribute to poor health. The WCPT is an active participant in discussions initiated by the WHO on international migration (International Organisation for Migration 2006) and health workers (WHO 2007b). Such discussions include improving the opportunities for the development of physiotherapy services, educating health workers and ensuring that individuals in as many populations as possible have the right to access physiotherapy services.

The 21st century is one that demands improved health services, improved global health statistics and improved access to health services As physical rehabilitation experts, physiotherapists are well positioned to have a major impact on global health.

EDUCATION AND ADVANCING PRACTICE

The practice of physiotherapy is based on a foundation of education that meets the requirements of the WCPT that a qualification be approved by a national association and that thus allows an individual to use the title physiotherapist (WCPT 1995a). Physiotherapy practitioners acknowledge that learning and education occur on a continuous basis throughout professional life (WCPT 2003d).

Entry-level education

Guidelines for entry-level education have been agreed on by WCPT member organisations (WCPT 2007). These guidelines are also helpful to ensure that graduates from programs being developed in countries not currently within the world body, such as China, meet physiotherapy practice expectations.

Considerable diversity exists in the regional, social, economic, political, cultural and professional environments in which physiotherapy education is conducted across the world. There is wide variation in the duration, type and location of physiotherapy programs. WCPT recommends that entry-level programs be based on university study over a minimum of four years, which results in the preparation of graduates who are autonomous practitioners. In addition, programs should demonstrate achievement of professional recognition standards and registration requirements through external accreditation (WCPT 2003d). Although there is variation in the methods used to achieve entry-level qualification, graduates should attain the appropriate level of knowledge, skills, abilities and attributes defined for entry-level physiotherapy practice, regardless of the type of qualification and mode of delivery.

Through their physiotherapy education, graduates must not only learn the tools of current physiotherapy practice but be equipped to advance the clinical, educational and research practice of physiotherapy in the future (Threlkeld 2007). Although clinical practice is the major role for physiotherapists, educational programs provide vehicles for professional change through a combination of research, education and practice.

Entry-level physiotherapy education programs are typically conducted in colleges and universities. The program structures vary widely. Although the WCPT guideline states that entry-level programs should be the equivalent of four years' full-time study at university level (WCPT 2007), the educational frameworks for preparing physiotherapy graduates are diverse. They range from diplomas and advanced diplomas in colleges through to four-year baccalaureate degrees, three-year baccalaureate degrees with honours (Bithell 2006), two-year graduate entry masters degrees (McMeeken 2006, Redenbach & Bainbridge 2006) and graduate entry professional doctoral degrees (McMeeken 2006, Threlkeld & Paschal 2007) in the university sector.

As applications for entry to physiotherapy programs far exceed available places, entry is usually competitive. Applicants are selected on the basis of academic merit and/or interview, depending upon institutional philosophies (Bithell 2006, McMeeken 2006, Redenbach & Bainbridge 2006, Threlkeld & Paschal 2007). The increasing numbers of physiotherapy programs have resulted in student populations becoming increasingly diverse with respect to age, ethnicity and prior qualifications (McMeeken et al 2005).

In Australia in 1976 physiotherapists were granted the right to autonomous practice. This had a profound effect on the educational programs for physiotherapists. Changes in curricula needed to be made to embrace this new status. A physiotherapist had to be able to make independent clinical decisions, to reason effectively and to base decisions on available evidence.

Physiotherapy curricula incorporate two main teaching and learning elements: academic and clinical education. Members of academic staff assume responsibility for curriculum design, implementation, monitoring and evaluation, whereas clinical education is often delivered in partnership with experienced clinical educators with oversight by the academic institution. A strong foundation of biomedical, behavioural and physiotherapy sciences underpins the development of clinical skills, evidence-based practice and clinical reasoning. Particular emphasis is placed on the expertise required for primary contact practitioners to effectively assess and treat clients across the life span, in a range of settings, using a variety of models of care. Professional skills of communication, legal and ethical practice, reflective practice, patient education and commitments to continuous quality improvement and lifelong learning are also developed.

Clinical education programs provide authentic and engaging learning experiences for students, as well as opportunities for them to demonstrate their achievement of physiotherapy competencies within a wide range of clinical settings under the supervision of experienced physiotherapists. Early exposure to the clinical setting helps students to integrate and apply their knowledge and skills and to experience interdisciplinary team approaches to the delivery of health care in a variety of practice settings. The traditional focus on acute, inpatient and subspecialty care has shifted to self-management, ambulatory care and population health initiatives, and clinical education programs are designed to reflect these trends (WCPT 2007).

Rapid expansion in the numbers of physiotherapy programs in recent years without a concomitant increase in health care workers and services has placed increasing pressure on the number of clinical education opportunities available, leading to innovations to meet clinical education demands. The model of a 1:1 student to supervisor ratio is often not sustainable in accommodating increasing numbers of students and is not necessarily educationally the most appropriate. Different models of clinical education have been developed, including 1:2, 1:4 and 1:6 models of supervision incorporating peer coaching. These models have been shown to provide superior clinical reasoning outcomes without compromising the efficiency of service delivery (Ladyshewsky 2002, Ladyshewsky et al 1998).

In areas of acute care, and where patient safety is of concern, low- and high-fidelity simulation is increasingly used to decrease the burden on clinical education and reduce the risk of adverse events, helping students to develop skills and decision making in a safe environment (Blackstock & Jull 2007). Other forms of virtual learning, such as online simulation role plays, are also used to enhance clinical decision making, student engagement and authenticity of learning experiences.

Entry-level physiotherapy programs are charged with the responsibility of ensuring that graduates have the appropriate knowledge, skills and abilities to practise safely, effectively and independently in a range of settings. For the most part, physiotherapy programs are required to demonstrate that they meet relevant accreditation requirements in terms of course structure, design, delivery and outcomes, and that their graduates meet the relevant physiotherapy standards. Typically the program includes academic, practical and clinical education components of sufficient breadth and depth to ensure development of beginning level practitioner competencies. For example, in Australia, all entry-level physiotherapy programs must be accredited by the Australian Physiotherapy Council (APC) according to its accreditation standards (APC 2006). As part of the accreditation process, providers must demonstrate that their graduates are able to meet the Australian Standards for Physiotherapy (APC 2006). Similarly in New Zealand, entry-level programs must meet the competencies set by the New Zealand Physiotherapy Board (1999).

Physiotherapy graduates need to be effectively prepared to cope with future demands. Thus, in the development of expertise, the design and delivery of physiotherapy education needs to facilitate evidence-based practice so that students learn to solve complex problems at the individual, group and community level and within a global context. Nine standards of practice are defined by the APC, covering key outcome areas for entry-level physiotherapists. They include:

- demonstration of professional behaviour appropriate to physiotherapy
- effective communication skills
- the ability to access, interpret and apply information to continuously improve practice
- assessment of clients; interpretation and analysis of assessment findings
- development of physiotherapy intervention plans
- implementation of safe and effective physiotherapy interventions
- evaluation of the effectiveness and efficiency of physiotherapy interventions
- the ability to operate effectively across a range of settings (APC 2006).

Given the exponential growth and rate of change of knowledge over the last decade, physiotherapy education programs can no longer attempt to teach students everything they need to know. Programs are therefore moving from teacher-centred or didactic approaches towards student-centred and problem-based or case-based learning, which focus on students knowing *how* to learn rather than knowing everything there is to learn (WHO 2006). This change entails a shift away from heavily content-based curricula with high workloads and assessments, which are more likely to encourage students to adopt a surface approach to learning, to helping students to develop an in-depth approach to their study (Lizzio et al 2002).

Many of today's students have grown up as 'digital natives', whose worlds are surrounded by technology, and who are active in social networking through the use of chat rooms, blogs, wikis and mobile phones (Sandars & Morrison 2007). The challenge for physiotherapy educators is to provide engaging learning experiences that not only capture multimedia rich environments, but actively engage students in their learning and provide rich feedback on their performance, utilise group work to capitalise on social learning opportunities, and provide opportunities for interaction with teaching staff.

Postgraduate education

With the introduction of primary contact practitioner status in 1976 came increased responsibilities for physiotherapists. This led to the development of postgraduate education to support the advanced knowledge and skills required for practice. Postgraduate programs, usually in the format of a postgraduate diploma or coursework masters degree, commenced in the musculoskeletal area (manipulative physiotherapy and sports physiotherapy) and are now offered in a wide range of specialty areas (e.g. neurology, continence and women's health, cardiorespiratory, neurodevelopmental paediatrics, aged care, occupational health, hand therapy and acupuncture) in several countries including Australia, New Zealand and the United Kingdom (UK) (Bithell 2006, McMeeken 2006). Most recently, clinical doctorates offering advanced practice subjects in a specific clinical area have been developed. As described shortly, these opportunities may satisfy the requirements for clinical specialisation in countries such as Australia.

Although there have been concerns about the financial viability of some post-graduate programs, linked primarily to the relatively small numbers involved (e.g. in specialised areas such as cardiorespiratory care), many providers of physiotherapy programs have recognised their importance and continue to provide such courses. Given current and future developments in advanced practice and specialisation it is likely that the number of physiotherapists with advanced postgraduate qualifications will continue to grow, resulting (along with the developments in entry-level education) in an increasingly highly educated and skilled workforce, with a profile more in common with medicine than with other allied health professions.

A wide variety of research programs at the masters or doctoral level are also available in universities. These programs offer the opportunity to undertake an individual supervised research project with submission of a thesis upon completion. Research programs are offered in a wide range of specialty areas and provide an intense intellectual challenge through investment of considerable effort. Research in a specialty area results in deep understanding of the area, and graduates of these programs often become national and international leaders in their area. Furthermore, in parallel with the development and expansion in education there has been a concomitant development in research capabilities and capacity within the profession (e.g. the number of physiotherapists with PhDs), leading to increased research volume and output and a greater focus on evidence-based practice.

The process of physiotherapy specialisation

For many years, Australian and New Zealand physiotherapists have had the opportunity to undertake a pathway to specialisation through colleges associated with their respective professional bodies. In Australia, the title 'Specialist' can be awarded by the Australian College of Physiotherapists (ACP), an entity of the APA. This level of title was deliberately established to be rigorous, to give it significance and a high profile. Along with the title of Specialist comes membership of the ACP, the title of 'Fellow' and the right to use the letters FACP (Fellow of the Australian College of Physiotherapists). The use of the title 'Specialist' by members other than FACPs has been a breach of the APA code of conduct; however, the title is being used in an informal sense quite widely to describe the skills and experience required to undertake particular roles.

Fellowship of the ACP is awarded following one of two pathways, monograph or clinical specialist, the latter pathway also giving the Fellow the right to use the title 'Clinical Specialist'. Until recently there was little interest in embarking on the specialisation process. Those who undertook the process were senior physiotherapists, held in the highest esteem by the profession. These Fellows comprised the ACP. In recent years, however, steadily growing demand came from APA members to finalise an integrated structure for specialisation. The debate around the nature of specialisation has been current in the profession for a number of years and was to some extent precipitated by an excellent editorial in the *Australian Journal of Physiotherapy* (Robertson et al 2003). This editorial proposed that the title Specialist be awarded to physiotherapists who have achieved Level 2 or titled membership of a national group.

The national groups of the APA (NGs) have the right to award 'titled' or Level 2 membership to their members on completion of either an accredited university postgraduate qualification or an alternative pathway comprising a number of components, both clinical and theoretical, that are completed outside the university system. By 2007, some 800 physiotherapists had achieved the status of titled membership as awarded by the NGs, largely from the sports and musculoskeletal NGs. This level of titling is now required for affiliation of sports physiotherapists with Olympic or Commonwealth Games sports teams. In other specialties and areas, the requirement of a certain level of further education in order to undertake particular types of work is gaining currency. Primary contact roles in the public sector are an example of this.

While the development of routes to specialisation was significant to the profession in Australia (and was widely applauded), there was also widespread recognition of the need to review existing arrangements. At least one NG, through its clinical academic standards committee, commenced preliminary work on Level 3 membership, to create a pathway for its members to use the title of Specialist. The lack of integration of the NG processes with those of the ACP, perceived inconsistencies across NGs in respect of accreditation processes for titled membership, the low uptake of the ACP specialisation process, and the strong demand from members to rationalise and streamline the process, resulted in the APA Board of Directors in 2005 prioritising the development of an integrated framework for specialisation. This initiative was also stimulated by developments in the UK, which have resulted in the title of Specialist being quite commonly available. As a result, the APA agreed in 2006 on a new framework for specialisation within the physiotherapy profession in Australia (see Fig 1.1).

Various benefits were anticipated from the new specialisation framework. In the public sector these included:

- linking of specialist qualifications to the establishment of particular positions, where appropriate. Thus, when a new physiotherapy department is being established, the stream leaders/subdepartment heads for key areas should have specialist qualifications. Similarly, a new orthopaedic service would not be established without the appointment of an orthopaedic surgeon. The same thinking will also set benchmarks for new programs.

In the private sector these included:

- facilitating second opinion and consultancy arrangements
- providing better structure for mentorship arrangements.

In relation to the recognition of the physiotherapy profession in the wider health care community these included:

- helping to improve salary levels, once recognition of specialist qualifications was built into industrial frameworks, i.e., public sector award structures or enterprise agreements
- driving differential rebates for specialists from third party payers and potentially also insurers such as Medicare
- helping to underpin current proposals for physiotherapists to be able to refer directly to specialists
- improving choice for patients and referrers
- encouraging uptake of university Clinical Masters and Clinical Doctorate courses, contributing to the sustainability and viability of these programs, particularly for smaller specialties such as cardiorespiratory, neurological and paediatric physiotherapy.

It was recognised by the APA that the success of these developments would be contingent upon getting a critical number of specialists in place. Thus the APA decided as part of its implementation plan to fast-track the opportunity to achieve specialist status for many of the existing expert and experienced clinicians within Australia. As a result of this, in 2007 some 35 physiotherapists completed the necessary clinical examinations and were awarded fellowships. The fast-track process will be concluded in 2009, after which a new process will begin. The new specialists will then provide the

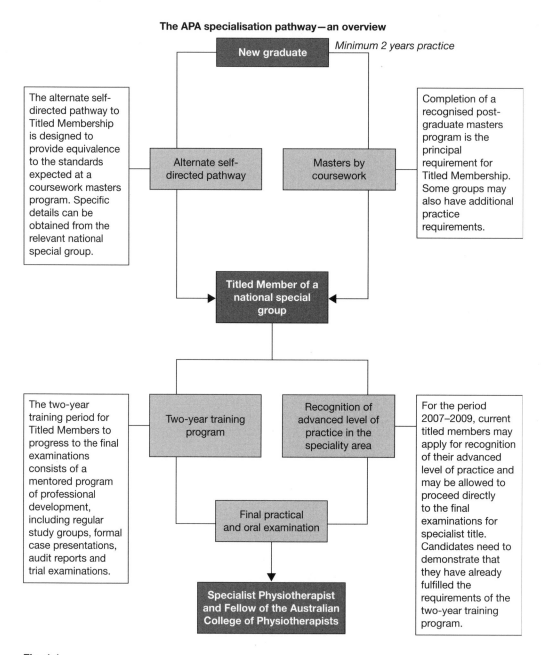

Fig. 1.1

Reproduced from *Standards for accreditation of physiotherapy programs at the level of higher education awards*, 2006, Australian Physiotherapy Council

support for physiotherapists wishing to undertake specialisation. It is also anticipated that, by that time, the requisite critical mass of specialists will be in place and many of the benefits outlined here will be realised.

Specialties that have been included to date are cardiorespiratory, occupational health physiotherapy, musculoskeletal, neurological, paediatrics and sports. Emerging clinical specialist areas, such as primary care physiotherapy (which includes rural health, emergency department physiotherapy and generalist physiotherapy) and oncology, may well also become specialist areas once the necessary educational frameworks have been established and there is a critical mass of physiotherapists seeking specialist recognition.

Where to from here for education and practice?

Physiotherapists of the 21st century require a much greater capacity to work in an interprofessional context to ensure effective management of clients with increasingly complex and chronic problems. Skills and intervention strategies relevant to working with various populations in community-based settings are essential to the provision of care to greater numbers of patients but with a relative level of decline in resources. Rapid advances in health care and knowledge bases mean that physiotherapists of the future must be adept at locating, critically appraising and developing new knowledge to ensure that they remain at the cutting edge of clinical practice. The advanced knowledge and skills of physiotherapists undertaking postgraduate and specialist education will provide them with opportunities to undertake advanced scope of practice roles within the health care system. Such roles are discussed further in Chapter 2.

RESEARCH

Research into physiotherapy, as well as in the cognate basic and applied sciences, is increasingly informing all facets of physiotherapy, from education of entry-level practitioners and from everyday professional practice through to professional development and specialisation. A review of publications in a major physical therapy journal in 1995 revealed a predominance of clinical or craft-based knowledge publications (Robertson 1995). Since then there has been a focus on developing ways to move to a more research-centred profession.

Research and education

Evidence shows that the inclusion of research-based courses in entry-level curricula reduces the major identified barrier to research (knowledge of research literature) and leads to improvements in understanding research literature and its importance in the clinical context (Connolly et al 2001). Transfer of the application of evidence-based knowledge to clinical practice appears not to be reinforced by clinical practice in the new physiotherapist one year out from graduation (Connolly et al 2001), indicating the need for ongoing attention to the implementation of evidence-based practice in education and professional development programs.

Research careers in physiotherapy

Academic physiotherapy staff positions reflect the shift in emphasis to a more research informed curriculum with a minimum requirement for most appointments at universities being a PhD or a track record commensurate with such research training. Not surprisingly, the entry-level health care professional's attitude to being involved in research appears to be related to academic staff profile (Delin 1994). Although this exposure leads to an increased utilisation of research literature by students (Delin 1994), there is also the effect of enthusing a number of physiotherapy graduates and postgraduate physiotherapists so that they consider research as a career. As a result a small but growing number of physiotherapists are taking on research roles as their sole expression of professional practice or as a significant part of a mix of research and clinical physiotherapy practice. For example, in Australia there has been a move to increase the number of research-only positions within most universities, with many developing conjoint positions with industry (e.g. state health departments, institutes of sport) through a range of funding mechanisms (e.g. inter-institutional collaborative joint ventures, Australian Research Council Industry Linkage grants, postdoctoral fellowships and research career development awards).

EDUCATION, RESEARCH AND THE 'THEORY–PRACTICE GAP'

An international trend has been the development of joint roles or appointments between academic and clinical institutions (typically larger teaching hospitals). Appointees are called lecturer/practitioners in the UK (similar to the terminology used in nursing) and such roles were primarily designed to strengthen the links between academia and clinical practice (to redress the gap that developed in some cases with the transfer of preregistration education into universities) (Stevenson et al 2004). Joint appointments are becoming more common in Australia and New Zealand, and the establishment of such roles on a wider scale could be an important development for the profession, providing a closer link between the clinical and academic professions and helping to realise some of the benefits already identified for specialist and extended scope roles (e.g. in terms of career opportunities for physiotherapists).

Measures of research activity/engagement by the profession and the community

Physiotherapy associations in several countries have recognised the need for research informed education and practice by commencing and supporting charitable trusts to fund research activities. Some examples are the Foundation for Physical Therapy of the American Physical Therapy Association (established 1979), the Physiotherapy Research Foundations of the Chartered Society of Physiotherapists in the UK (established 1980) and initiatives of the APA (established 1988). Although still relatively recent developments, these research foundations signify a maturation of the profession as well as highlighting the significance placed on research by the profession. In recent times, physiotherapists and physiotherapy research has been increasingly funded through competitive national and international schemes. For example, during the period 2000–07 there was a 16-fold increase in the amount of funding allocated to researchers under the 'Rehabilitation and Therapy: Occupation and Physical' research fields, courses and disciplines classification (RFCD) of the National Health and Medical Research Council of Australia. This would likely include a majority of physiotherapy research but does not account for other RFCD codes under which physiotherapy research would appear. There are a number of ways in which the increase in physiotherapy-related research may be demonstrated. For example, if we consider the long held association between physiotherapy and sports, during the period 2000–07, 30% of all National Health and Medical Research Council of Australia funding for sports-related projects and personal research support was awarded to physiotherapists. Notwithstanding these changes, the funding provided for physiotherapy related research in relevant health care areas is still but a small proportion of the national agenda (<1%), underlining the need for a continued effort in consolidating research within physiotherapy practice as well as increased advocacy.

Translation of research to practice

The actual impact of this expanding body of research on the physiotherapy profession, and on its position in the health care system, is yet to fully emerge. A qualitative study by Wiles and Barnard (2001) showed that senior physiotherapists in the National Health Service (NHS) in the UK felt that the emergence of evidence-based practice would threaten professional autonomy but, perhaps surprisingly, senior and junior physiotherapists viewed it as an opportunity to strengthen the profession. A recent review of four major journals of physiotherapy (*Australian Journal of Physiotherapy, Physical Therapy, Physiotherapy, Canadian Journal of Physiotherapy*) revealed that, although there has been an increase in the number of original research-based publications, there was still a dearth of publications with direct application to patient care (Miller et al 2003). Research in physiotherapy is an evolving construct, increasingly becoming part of the fabric of contemporary physiotherapy, with a base of significant contributions to the general scientific literature by rehabilitation research (Tate 2006).

SUMMARY

The physiotherapy profession in the 21st century is well situated in the broad framework of the health workforce to meet the challenges of the future. It has established educational programs of excellence, it has embraced research as the underpinning of practice, and it has positioned itself as a primary health care profession in health promotion and injury prevention, with the ability to provide services to people and populations to develop, maintain and restore maximum movement and functional ability throughout the life span.

Reflective questions

- What are the key factors that are influencing the evolution of the profession in the 21st century?
- What are the challenges that face the physiotherapy profession in your area of practice?

References

Australian Physiotherapy Council 2006 Standards for accreditation of physiotherapy programs at the level of higher education awards. Australian Physiotherapy Council, Canberra

Bithell C 2006 Entry-level physiotherapy education in the United Kingdom: governance and curriculum. Physical Therapy Reviews 11:145–155

Blackstock F, Jull G 2007 High-fidelity patient simulation in physiotherapy education. Australian Journal of Physiotherapy 53:3–5

Connolly B H, Lupinnaci N S, Bush A J 2001 Changes in attitudes and perceptions about research in physical therapy among professional physical therapist students and new graduates. Physical Therapy 81(5):1127–1136

Delin C R 1994 Research attitudes and involvement among medical-students and students of allied health occupations. Medical Teacher 16:183–196

Fry D, Furler J 2000 General practice, primary health care and population health interface. In: General practice in Australia: 2000. Commonwealth Department of Health and Aged Care, Canberra, p 388

International Organisation for Migration 2006 International dialogue on migration, summary report, May 2006. Available: http://www.iom.int/jahia/jsp/index.jsp 24 Nov 2007

Ladyshewsky R 2002 A quasi-experimental study of the differences in performance and clinical reasoning using individual learning versus reciprocal peer coaching. Physiotherapy Theory and Practice 18: 17–31

Ladyshewsky R, Barrie S, Drake V M 1998 A comparison of productivity and learning outcome in individual and cooperative physical therapy clinical education models. Physical Therapy 78(12):1288–1298

Lizzio A, Wilson K, Simons R 2002 University students' perceptions of the learning environment and academic outcomes: implications for theory and practice. Studies in Higher Education 27(1):27–52

McMeeken J 2006 Physiotherapy education in Australia. Physical Therapy Reviews 11:83–91

McMeeken J, Webb G, Krause K L et al 2005 Learning outcomes and curriculum development in Australian physiotherapy education. AUTC Project Report. Available: http://www.physiotherapy. edu.au/physiotherapy/go/home/pid/125 24 Nov 2007

Miller P A, McKibbon K A, Haynes R B 2003 A quantitative analysis of research publications in physical therapy journals. Physical Therapy 83(2):123–131

New Zealand Physiotherapy Board 1999 Registration requirements competencies and learning objectives, 2nd edn. Physiotherapy Board, Wellington

Redenbach D, Bainbridge L 2006 Canadian physiotherapy education: the University of British Columbia example. Physical Therapy Reviews 11:92–104

Robertson V J 1995 A quantitative analysis of research in physical therapy. Physical Therapy 75(4): 313–322

Robertson V J, Oldmeadow L B, Cromie J E et al 2003 Taking charge of change: a new career structure in physiotherapy. Editorial Australian Journal of Physiotherapy 49(4):229–231

Sandars J, Morrison C 2007 What is the Net Generation? The challenge for future medical education. Medical Teacher 29:85–88

Stevenson K, Chadwick A V, Hunter S M 2004 National survey of lecturer/practitioners in physiotherapy. Physiotherapy 90:139–144

Tate D G 2006 The state of rehabilitation research: art or science? Archives of Physical Medicine and Rehabilitation 87(2):160–166

Threlkeld A J 2007 Guest editorial: world physical therapist education. Physical Therapy Reviews 12: 82–83

Threlkeld A J, Paschal K A 2007 Entry-level physical therapist education in the United States of America. Physical Therapy Reviews 11:156–162

WCPT 1995a Protection of title. Declarations of principle and position statements approved at the 13th general meeting of WCPT, June 1995. Available: http://www.wcpt.org/ 24 Nov 2007

WCPT 1995b Autonomy. Declarations of principle and position statements approved at the 13th general meeting of WCPT, June 1995. Available: http://www.wcpt.org/ 24 Nov 2007

WCPT 1995c Relationships with medical practitioners. Declarations of principle and position statements approved at the 13th general meeting of WCPT, June 1995. Available: http://www.wcpt.org/ 24 Nov 2007

WCPT 1995d Relationships with other health professionals. Declarations of principle and position statements approved at the 13th general meeting of WCPT, June 1995. Available: http://www.wcpt. org/ 24 Nov 2007

WCPT 1999 Description of physical therapy. Declarations of principle and position statements approved at the 14th general meeting of WCPT, May 1999. Available: http://www.wcpt.org/ 20 Sep 2007

WCPT 2003a Standards of physical therapy practice. Declarations of principle and position statements approved at the 15th general meeting of WCPT, June 2003. Available: http://www.wcpt.org/ 24 Nov 2007

WCPT 2003b Research. Declarations of principle and position statements approved at the 15th general meeting of WCPT, June 2003. Available: http://www.wcpt.org/ 24 Nov 2007

WCPT 2003c Community based rehabilitation. Declarations of principle and position statements approved at the 15th general meeting of WCPT, June 2003. Available: http://www.wcpt.org/ 24 Nov 2007

WCPT 2003d Education. Declarations of principle and position statements approved at the 13th general meeting and revised at the 15th General Meeting of WCPT, June 2003. Available: http://www.wcpt. org/ 24 Nov 2007

WCPT 2007 Guidelines for physical therapist professional entry-level education. Approved at the 16th general meeting of WCPT, June 2007. Available: http://www.wcpt.org/ 24 Nov 2007

Wiles R, Barnard S 2001 Physiotherapists and evidence based practice: an opportunity or threat to the profession? Sociological Research Online 6. Available: http://www.socresonline.org.uk/6/1/wiles. html 21 Dec 2007

WHO 2001 International functioning disability and health (ICF), accepted at the fifty-fourth World Health Assembly, 22 May 2001. Available: http://www.who/int/en 18 Dec 2007

WHO 2006 The world health report 2006 – working together for health. Available: http://www.who. int/whr/2006/en/index.html 24 Nov 2007

WHO 2007a Data and statistics. Available: http://www.who.int/research/en/ 18 Dec 2007

WHO 2007b First global forum on human resources for health. Available: http://www.who.int/ mediacentre/events/meetings/hr_forum/en/ 8 Feb 2008

CURRENT TRENDS IN PHYSIOTHERAPY PRACTICE

David Baxter and Cathy Nall

two

Key content

- Factors influencing current trends in physiotherapy practice
- The context of modern health care
- Multidisciplinary approaches to health care delivery
- Three main influences on physiotherapy practice – education, increasing professional autonomy and clinical specialisation
- Advances in specialist and extended scope roles for physiotherapists

---

INTRODUCTION

Physiotherapy is a dynamic and rapidly evolving profession that has progressed from a repertoire of a limited range of techniques and modalities under medical prescription to fully autonomous practice in a range of specialist areas, each characterised by high levels of clinical reasoning, expertise and skills. Current and recent trends in the development of physiotherapy practice are underpinned by a range of factors, the most salient of which are considered in this chapter. They include external drivers, such as the context within which modern health care is delivered and the changing nature of health care, as well as drivers from within the profession, such as increasing levels of education (entry-level and postgraduate), professional autonomy and clinical specialisation. Perhaps the most significant and exciting trend within professional practice is the development of specialist and extended scope roles for physiotherapists, leading to enhanced, cost effective care for patients.

MODERN HEALTH CARE

When reviewing current trends and developments within physiotherapy practice it is important to consider some aspects of the wider context of modern health care, in terms of three main areas: the costs of health care, the health care workforce, and patients' expectations.

Health care costs

The costs of providing health care have risen markedly in the 'developed' nations over the last five decades, and particularly over the last 20 years. In the USA, the world's largest economy, health care costs have consistently risen at a faster rate than the growth in the economy; the proportion of gross domestic product (in effect the nation's output) spent on health care rose from 5% in 1960 to 16% in 2005, and is estimated to top 20% by 2016 (Henry J Kaiser Family Foundation 2007).

Various factors have been identified as driving such change, including increases in the wealth of some nations (wealthier nations – and individuals – can afford to spend more on new health care products, technologies and services), changes in population demographics (e.g. populations in developed countries are ageing and therefore health care costs are rising) and changes in disease prevalence (in particular, increasing levels of diabetes that are linked to obesity) (Henry J Kaiser Family Foundation 2007). In industrialised nations, rising levels of obesity are recognised as a more significant health issue than ageing populations (Mills & Mills 2007). Rennie and Jebb (2005) recently reported that the prevalence of adult obesity in the UK has almost trebled in just over two decades; in 2002, 23% of men and 25% of women were obese. Perhaps of greater concern is that, although it is somewhat lower in children than in adults, the prevalence of obesity in children is increasing at a similar rate to that in adults (Rennie & Jebb 2005). There is also an association between obesity levels and other health problems. In particular, for the first time in history levels of obesity (previously associated with affluence and abundance in many cultures) are now higher in low socioeconomic groups and in minority groups and some indigenous populations.

Managing health care expenditure, which is rising steadily in response to these new demands, has become a major concern for most national and state governments, and has led to an increasing focus on such areas as managed care, clinical governance, evidence-based practice and cost effectiveness of clinical services. However, the effectiveness of measures such as the promotion of evidence-based practice through national clinical guidelines (e.g. for the management of acute low back pain) and the establishment of bodies to oversee best practice based upon evidence (e.g. the UK National Institute of Clinical Excellence) on limiting health care spending is debatable. Indeed, the implementation of new 'well evidenced' approaches or treatments may actually increase costs. Alternatively, many governments have sought to increase the efficiency of health care delivery, for example by restructuring provision through devolution or de-medicalising certain roles and tasks (e.g. nurse prescribing). Linked to this has been an increasing focus on measures aimed at disease prevention and tackling inequalities in health across socioeconomic groups and geographical regions.

Trends in the physiotherapy profession associated with these developments include widening the scope and areas of practice (e.g. within health promotion and community health care teams) and increasing the opportunities for the development of specialist roles such as the consultant physiotherapist positions within the UK's National Health Service (NHS). Conversely, attempts to manage or contain health care costs, such as the use of physiotherapy treatment profiles by New Zealand's Accident Compensation Corporation (ACC) or limitations on the number of treatments provided as has occurred in the UK NHS, have caused tensions within the professional community and some patient groups. Less contentiously, the promotion of clinical guidelines to underpin evidence-based decision making and practice has become a characteristic feature of clinical practice; however, the extent to which such guidelines have influenced clinical practice is variable. For example, although the benefit of interventions such as exercise are well recognised and increasingly promoted as cost effective forms of treatment in the guidelines for many conditions (not least those associated with obesity, such as hypertension), the extent to which individual practitioners have changed their practice in response to these recommendations is debatable.

In Australia, a further barrier to the uptake of cost effective evidence-based interventions provided by physiotherapists is the structure of the Commonwealth Medicare Benefits Schedule. This uncapped fee-for-service funding model pays a rebate for health services provided by health professionals; however, most items are for services provided by medical practitioners and there is only one item providing a rebate for physiotherapy intervention.

This item is part of the Enhanced Primary Care program in which general practitioners (GPs) can refer patients with chronic and complex conditions to physiotherapists for a maximum of five visits per year (across all required allied health professions). This model precludes many patients with conditions amenable to physiotherapy intervention from accessing the care they need and results in perverse incentives to use expensive medical care over more cost effective physiotherapy care. The condition of stress incontinence is a prime example of this problem. It has been demonstrated that one episode of physiotherapy intervention focusing on re-education of pelvic floor muscles at a cost of some $300 can cure 80% of women with this problem. However, the only intervention reimbursed through the Medicare system for the majority of patients is surgical intervention, at a cost of $4000–6000 and with all the attendant risks and loss of work time associated with such surgery (Neumann et al 2005).

For patients who can afford to pay for private physiotherapy, this is not an issue. But the many patients who cannot afford to pay must either try to access the very limited public services, go without intervention, or opt for surgical intervention with its attendant risks, downtime and far greater cost to the taxpayer.

Health care workforce

Current and projected health workforce shortages represent a global concern in both the developed and developing nations. Estimates by the World Health Organization (WHO) indicate a global shortage of some four million health care workers across all levels and professional areas (WHO 2006). Within many countries, workforce planning strategies have been devised in an attempt to meet the need for health care workers. Strategies have included measures to increase recruitment to the health care professions (such as providing subsidised or supported training opportunities), to enhance retention of the existing workforce, and to encourage return to practise for those who had previously changed careers. However, such attempts to manage the health care workforce have led to particular problems in some areas. For example, discrepancies between training places provided under workforce plans and funding for new positions in the NHS have led to large numbers of unemployed new graduate physiotherapists in the UK. Additionally, this is an increasingly global market place, with a significant 'transfer market' in a number of areas, ranging from nurses and assistants to consultant surgeons.

Within New Zealand, it has been projected that there will be a shortage of between 40,000 and 70,000 health care and disability workers over the next 20 years (Ministry of Health (MoH) 2004, MoH and DHBNZ Workforce Group 2007). In response to the situation, a career framework has recently been proposed to improve recruitment and retention across the entire health care workforce in New Zealand, ranging from foundation workers to specialist clinical posts (MoH and DHBNZ Workforce Group 2007). This important and timely initiative is based upon a model of continuing professional and career development for all workers within the health care system in the country. In terms of physiotherapy, it also represents a useful model and framework to support the progression of physiotherapists within the public health care sector and the development of specialist physiotherapist roles as currently proposed by a joint working group of the New Zealand College of Physiotherapy and the New Zealand Society of Physiotherapists Inc. (NZSP) (Mueller et al 2007).

The situation in Australia is no less alarming. As a result, the Council of Australian Governments (COAG) commissioned the Productivity Commission to undertake a review of the health workforce. Released in January 2006, this review recommended that the health workforce needed to work more effectively to meet this challenge; suggestions for how to do this included establishing a national registration and accreditation scheme, cultivating an evidence-based approach to an expansion in Medicare funding, and developing more responsive education and training arrangements (Australian Government Productivity Commission 2005). The majority of these recommendations have now been taken up to some extent. One important initiative resulting from the review is the establishment of the National Health Workforce Taskforce to action the COAG requirements and act as the primary vehicle for driving reform in this area.

Patients' expectations

Perhaps one of the most salient characteristics of the contemporary health care environment is the prevalence of empowered or activated patients, who increasingly expect to be treated as equal partners in their care and have a voice in health policy. They are informed consumers with expectations of choice rather than prescription. For example, they expect to be offered complementary or alternative treatments as well as orthodox treatments (Mullan 2002).

One element of this increasing empowerment is the ready availability of health care information through the internet: the latest medical knowledge is now as easily accessible to patients as it is to health care professionals. In such an information-rich environment, where textbooks, articles and dedicated websites are available to all, there is no longer any exclusivity to professional knowledge. However, although the internet may well provide a useful gateway to relevant medical knowledge for the average patient, it is important to recognise that advice available online is often contradictory and that there is no independent verification of the accuracy of such information. Under these circumstances it is often difficult for patients to determine which advice is credible, for example in terms of the best treatment option for their condition.

Health care professionals therefore have an increasingly important role to play in providing patients with informed guidance on health care knowledge and treatment options, helping to enhance patient understanding and, in turn, patient choice. In these circumstances, the roles of health care practitioners have evolved from simply providing expert advice (as an informed professional instructing the 'lay' patient) to guiding patients through the various treatment options available, as well as the contesting advice and information (Baxter 2003a, 2003b).

THE EVOLUTION OF PHYSIOTHERAPY PRACTICE

Physiotherapy practice has changed dramatically since the inception of the profession in the late 19th century. Changes have been particularly evident over the last several decades. The most salient developments are changes in education, professional autonomy, developments in the scope of practice, and changes in clinical specialisation.

Professional autonomy

Physiotherapy has steadily evolved from a profession based upon the provision of a limited range of (doctor-) prescribed physical modalities and exercise to one centred on autonomous practitioners with the skills to see patients as agents of first contact, complete a comprehensive examination, make a diagnosis, devise a treatment plan, instigate and provide appropriate treatment, monitor treatment and refer to other health care professions. Although this list represents more of an aspiration than a reality in some of its member organisations, professional autonomy is recognised by the World Confederation for Physical Therapy (WCPT 2007).

Realisation of this degree of professional autonomy has been a major achievement for the profession, and has underpinned the development and widening of roles for physiotherapists both within and outside the public health sector, including private practice and community and rural health services. Taken together with current changes within the wider health care arena (as discussed above), the breadth of physiotherapy practice has expanded considerably, and is likely to continue to do so in the future. As part of this expansion, and particularly in some countries where autonomous practice is already well established, development of specialist and extended scope roles for physiotherapists represents a logical evolution for the profession.

In Australia, first contact practice has been an accepted ethical practice for physiotherapists since the late 1970s. This radical shift in the profession was built on arguments presented by Galley and others, who had a vision for the future of physiotherapy that encompassed physiotherapists working as independent practitioners with or without medical referral (Galley 1975, 1976). Since then, primary contact practice has grown considerably. It is estimated that each year some eight million physiotherapy attendances in Australia occur in this way (Australian Physiotherapy Association (APA) 2005).

However, despite its widespread acceptance in the *private* sector, primary contact physiotherapy has been established within Australia's *public* sector only in the last few years. Primary contact practice in the public sector first developed among physiotherapists assessing patients who had been referred by GPs to orthopaedic surgeons and neurosurgery outpatient departments. This development was based on the success of similar models in the UK (Daker-White et al 1999, Hattam & Smeatham 1999, Hockin & Bannister 1994, Hourigan & Weatherley 1994, Weale & Bannister 1995), where physiotherapists have undertaken the primary role in case management, including triaging patients referred by GPs to see medical consultants (principally in orthopaedics and rheumatology), ordering and interpreting diagnostic tests, performing injections (e.g. joint injections), then either listing those requiring surgery or managing those appropriate for physiotherapy intervention.

In Australia, as in the UK, the establishment of primary contact practice was driven by long waiting times for first outpatient appointments and the fact that, due to the funding structure of the Australian health care system and other access issues, many patients who had conditions amenable to physiotherapy interventions were not given the opportunity to receive them.

Scope of practice and clinical specialisation

The scope of physiotherapy practice has developed significantly over the history of the profession, and continues to expand. Although musculoskeletal and orthopaedic, neurological and cardiorespiratory physiotherapy may still be regarded as the three main areas of practice, at least in terms of regulatory authorities and entry-level curricula, the breadth and scope of current physiotherapy practice is better reflected in the range of specialist or clinical interest groups represented within national professional bodies. For example, within the NZSP (with a membership of around 3000) there are currently 10 such groups, with interests in acupuncture, cardiothoracic or cardiorespiratory physiotherapy, hand therapy, manipulative physiotherapy, neurology, occupational health, older adults, paediatrics, sports and orthopaedics. Other national bodies have groups devoted to women's health, hydrotherapy, animal physiotherapy and electrotherapies, as well as education and research (see Ch 6). Apart from such recognised subgroups within each professional body, there are also well established groups based upon advanced teaching, practice or skills, with governance structures outside the profession (e.g. the McKenzie Institute (http://www.mckenziemdt.org/ accessed 19 Dec 2007) and the Mulligan Concept (http://www.bmulligan.com/ accessed 19 Dec 2007)). In many ways, these groups have become the central strength of the profession (in terms of professional networks, developing advanced competencies, and continuing professional development opportunities), and they will continue to develop nationally and indeed internationally (e.g. with groups such as the International Federation of Orthopaedic Manipulative Therapists and the International Acupuncture Association of Physical Therapists).

It is important to stress that such developments are not unique to the physiotherapy profession, and need to be seen within the wider context of well established and increasing specialisation within other health care professions (including medicine and nursing). Continuing changes and developments in the nature of health care provision have provided a powerful driver to increasing specialisation, and will do so for the foreseeable future.

CONTEMPORARY PRACTICE: TRENDS IN HEALTH CARE DELIVERY

Wider trends and developments in health care delivery have affected physiotherapy practice in a variety of ways. The most salient of these in terms of relevance to current physiotherapy practice are the following.

Multidisciplinary teams. For many complex and chronic conditions (e.g. brain injuries and chronic musculoskeletal pain) it is recognised that clinical effectiveness is dependent upon a coherent multiprofessional approach to management. Within contemporary health care, multidisciplinary teams (including medical staff, nurses, occupational therapists, physiotherapists, and speech and language therapists) have become the central element for the management of many conditions. In such cases, it is important that health care professionals can work competently and effectively within a multidisciplinary team, while recognising the specialist skills of other professionals in the team (see Ch 20).

Passive to active. There has been increasing recognition of the value of exercise and activity as an effective intervention in health care, especially given concerns about the health care problems associated with sedentary lifestyles and the alarming rise in obesity levels worldwide (as discussed above). The widespread promotion of exercise equipment in the media and government initiatives that encourage people to stay active (e.g. through Sport and Recreation New Zealand) point to a greater recognition of the importance of exercise (or, perhaps more accurately, lack of exercise) in health promotion. This represents an important challenge and opportunity for the physiotherapy profession. On one hand, exercise therapy and prescription have long been considered central elements in physiotherapy treatment and practice, and represent some of the best-supported physiotherapy interventions in terms of published evidence. However, it is also regarded as a component of the role of other professionals, such as exercise physiologists, and quasi-professionals, such as personal fitness trainers, who have been quick to realise the potential opportunities in targeting the wider health care rather than the more limited fitness market.

Self-management. Another important trend, particularly in the management of chronic disease, has been the recognition of the key role of patients in the management of their conditions (Lorig et al 2005). Based on the principles of enabling patients to understand and take control of their conditions, this approach is now espoused by many health professionals as a way to both improve patient engagement in therapy and enhanced quality of life and deal in a cost effective manner with the growing number of people with chronic disease.

Home-based care. The provision of care in people's homes or within the community setting has become an increasingly important component of contemporary health care. Notable initiatives include legislation to underpin care in the community in the UK (*National Health Service and Community Care Act 1990*), which was designed to shift the focus for many services from hospitals and other institutions to the person's community. Health care professionals have embraced this change in emphasis through the development of community-based working initiatives, principally through team-based working. For physiotherapists, this has included the development of positions for community physiotherapists, who are essentially primary care and generalist in their focus, and neurorehabilitation physiotherapists, who support or provide rehabilitation for patients with stroke in the community.

Several state health jurisdictions in Australia have adopted 'Casemix' funding for acute care, in which episodes of care are funded according to the diagnosis related group (DRG) into which they are classified. This has resulted in an incentive to discharge patients as early as possible. Consequently, home-based care programs have been developed to ensure that early discharge is undertaken safely. Programs such as Hospital in the Home and Post Acute Care support patients at home until they are fully independent.

ADVANCED PRACTICE IN AUSTRALIA AND NEW ZEALAND

As indicated in Chapter 1, there have been significant developments in physiotherapy education over the last several decades. In common with several other countries, entrance to physiotherapy education in Australia and New Zealand is competitive and available to only the highest academic achievers. Courses are rigorous and focus on extensive periods of supervised clinical practice, resulting in a workforce with extensive clinical knowledge and skill levels that has the potential to contribute more to health care advances.

This has created a strong impetus for physiotherapists to take on new roles. This impetus has also arisen from the wider issues in health care identified above (including workforce shortages), which are responsible for the common occurrence, particularly in outer urban and rural areas, of physiotherapists being faced with patients who cannot access appropriate health care in a timely way. In addition, when patients are able to access care, the care provided by a physiotherapist who has additional training may optimise the quality of care the patient receives.

Pilot projects already undertaken in Australia (Oldmeadow et al 2007) have replicated findings from the UK that show that only a minority of patients referred to orthopaedic surgery departments actually require the services of a surgeon. In the majority of cases, such referrals can be just as effectively managed by an advanced practice or specialist physiotherapist practitioner. Furthermore, there were high levels of satisfaction with the physiotherapy service among patients and doctors, including GPs and consultants (e.g. Byles & Ling 1989; Hattam & Smeatham 1999, Hockin & Bannister 1994, Hourigan & Weatherley 1994). The benefits associated with this model of specialist physiotherapy practice have contributed to the Queensland Government's decision to introduce a $4.3 million initiative to roll out this model across metropolitan and rural Queensland (Robertson 2007).

Physiotherapists have also been appointed to emergency departments to manage soft tissue injuries. These physiotherapists manage patients directly from the triage screen, alleviating the need for such patients to see a medical practitioner if not required. This leaves emergency doctors free to undertake more acute emergency work and, thus, significantly reduces the waiting time for triage category 4 and 5 patients. The Department of Human Services Victoria has recently acknowledged the value of primary contact physiotherapy practice in emergency departments by including it as a key strategy to reduce waiting times under its 2007/08 Models of Care Funding Initiative.

In New Zealand, similar initiatives have focused on employing physiotherapists with expanded roles (see Mueller et al 2007). These include a dedicated back pain program within the Auckland Regional Pain Service, based upon early intervention offered by a senior physiotherapist who provides a comprehensive clinical assessment and education for the patient. The primary driver for the establishment of this program, as with similar initiatives in the UK and Australia, was the long waiting time for patients to see an orthopaedic surgeon. The success of the program (e.g. 101 referrals taken from the waiting list in one year) is evidenced by its development into a physiotherapist-led First Specialist Assessment Clinic for individuals with nonspecific back pain not requiring spinal surgery.

Another initiative at Christchurch Hospital, *Front Door Physio*, has seen the establishment of a full-time position for a physiotherapist, based within the hospital's emergency department. This physiotherapist can offer an immediate physiotherapy assessment to those presenting to the department, along with advice, treatment and, where indicated, the issue of appropriate equipment.

EXTENDED SCOPE PRACTICE

Alongside the establishment of advanced practice roles, there has also been a move within the profession towards the establishment of what are known as extended scope practice positions. The title or designation for physiotherapists with advanced clinical skills and expertise has been a matter of some debate and confusion, with terms such as *practitioner* (cf nurse practitioner), *extended scope physiotherapist*, *enhanced scope physiotherapist*, and *physiotherapy specialist* all being adopted at various stages, in some instances to describe a single role (Gardiner & Wagstaff 2001).

Although there is undoubtedly some degree of overlap between the roles of advanced practice or specialist physiotherapists and extended scope practitioners (see Fig. 2.1), the latter has come to be used to describe new, primary contact roles within the public sector that are currently outside the legislative scope of practice. Indeed, in Australia, the APA National Advisory Council at its May 2006 meeting decided that the Association would confine use of the term *extended scope practice* to activity currently outside legislative scope in Australia. Similarly, in New Zealand, current recommendations from the Society and College support the restricted use of the term *extended scope* to those already specialised physiotherapists who take on roles that are outside the currently recognised scope of practice.

This is a potentially exciting development for physiotherapists, and has been recognised as of strategic importance for the future of the profession. In its *Vision 2020* document (APA 2005), the APA stated that the scope of physiotherapy practice in Australia would expand over the coming years. Specific areas identified as part of this expansion included:

- substantially increased roles for physiotherapists in presurgery preparation and postsurgical rehabilitation, as well as in triage, emergency and intensive care
- limited prescribing rights, that is, prescription of a limited range of pharmaceuticals by some physiotherapists. This is in keeping with initiatives in a number of countries to de-medicalise prescription rights. In Australia, the new National Health Workforce Principal Committee (which has come out of the recommendations of the Australian Productivity Commission) has specifically identified nonmedical prescribing as a key priority
- limited injecting rights for some physiotherapists, including joint injection (as already occurs in the UK) and injection of botulinum toxin. In particular, in many Australian health jurisdictions discussions are already under way to determine how legislative change might be implemented so that, for instance, neurological physiotherapists who work in movement disorder clinics will be able to inject botulinum toxin like their colleagues in the UK
- increased use of diagnostic imaging technology such as ultrasound scanners.

These examples are in keeping with similar developments in the UK and with developments currently under consideration in New Zealand. In establishing such roles there are a number of associated challenges that need to be recognised, not least of which are the legislative and funding frameworks for physiotherapy in Australia and New Zealand.

In Australia, the majority of new *advanced practice* or specialist roles are already regulated by (mostly state-/territory-based) Acts of Parliament, such as the various Physiotherapists' Registration Acts and Poisons Acts. Although other proposed new

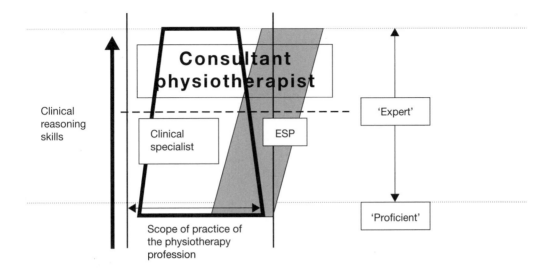

Fig. 2.1 Profile of clinical specialist and ESP and their relationship to consultant AHP. Reproduced from *Specialisms and Specialists: Guidance for Developing the Clinical Specialist Role*, 2001, The Chartered Society of Physiotherapy, p 3, with permission

This schematic illustrates the relative overlap in terms currently used to describe 'advanced' or 'expert practice'. The x-axis represents the breadth or scope of health care, with the current scope of practice clearly delineated. The area beyond the right hand line is outside the current scope of physiotherapy practice, and therefore an individual practising 'beyond' this line is 'extending scope'. The y-axis represents increasing levels of clinical reasoning and skills, with the lowest (dotted) line indicating the extent of 'proficient' practice (e.g. a well-qualified physiotherapist with several years post-qualification experience). At a certain level (denoted by the dashed line), increased levels of clinical skills and reasoning are recognised as 'expert' practice. The clinical specialist's role becomes more focused (specialised), but still sits within the original scope of practice of physiotherapy (e.g. clinical specialist in orthopaedics). In contrast, the role of the extended scope practitioner (ESP) has crossed outside the current scope of practice (e.g. into joint injection, limited prescribing, etc). The area marked by the upper box represents the breadth and level of skills of the recognised position of 'Consultant Therapist' (established within the NHS in the UK). It is interesting to note that the scope of practice is temporal in nature: the boundaries on scope will – inevitably – change over time.

roles, such as ordering more extensive investigations (e.g. CT and MR scans) and specialist referral (physiotherapist-to-specialist and specialist-to-physiotherapist) are within current legislative scope, they are determined (or restricted) by the structure of funding under the Medicare Benefits Schedule.

Over the next few years, changes to legislation to enable physiotherapists to undertake additional roles currently outside the legislative scope of practice in Australia will be dependent upon continued negotiations between the physiotherapy profession and the appropriate state or territory health jurisdictions that have responsibility for the development and review of health practitioner legislation. In the longer term, this will become the responsibility of the proposed new national health practitioner registration system, flagged for development by the Council of Australian Governments (2006) in response to the recommendations of the Australian Government Productivity Commission's review of the health workforce (2005). However, it is expected that any changes that occur prior to the implementation of this new system will help inform the final structure of the national legislation.

Educational implications of specialist and extended scope practice

Development of the type of specialist or extended scope roles described above depends upon the establishment of appropriate education, training and credentialling arrangements for physiotherapists.

In the UK, credentialling of specialist or extended scope roles has become the responsibility of the institution or facility in which the physiotherapist practises. In effect, the establishment of a specialist or consultant therapist position is service driven. For example, a consultant physiotherapist position might be created to fulfil the particular requirements for such a position within a chronic pain service. Although this approach may have the advantage of being service- or needs-led, it is unnecessarily duplicative, as recognition of individual therapists (and thus their advanced skills and experience) is not portable between facilities. Thus the title of Consultant Physiotherapist is in effect limited to a position in a particular Hospital Trust or National Health Service facility, rather than being applicable to the physiotherapist.

In contrast, within Australia and New Zealand, the relevant professional bodies and colleges are currently considering a range of possible options for credentialling that would ensure appropriate competencies and standards of practice, but also allow the physiotherapist (not the position) to be recognised across health jurisdictions and settings.

Benefits for health care delivery of specialisation and extended scope

The potential benefits to the patient, health care system and wider community associated with these new roles for physiotherapists are largely self-evident, and include the following.

More effective deployment of medical practitioners. The available evidence indicates that, where specialist or extended scope practitioner roles have been introduced, senior medical personnel have been more effectively deployed. For example, consultant orthopaedic surgeons can concentrate their efforts on more serious cases requiring surgery, rather than performing triage on referrals from GPs. In the UK, the introduction of these specialist practitioner roles has led to more effective delivery in both primary and secondary care musculoskeletal services.

Decreased cost by reducing unneeded GP visits. There are obvious advantages in providing direct access to specialist or extended scope practitioners as first contact agents, rather than the patient's GP acting as referral agent or gatekeeper, not least in terms of the cost of an unneeded visit.

Faster access to services. Direct contact with specialist or extended scope practitioners enables patients to have faster access to appropriate services, assessment and treatment.

Enhanced clinical outcomes. As indicated above, research has shown that treatment provided by physiotherapists working as specialists or extended scope practitioners was highly effective and cost effective.

Patient satisfaction. Given the benefits already articulated above, it is perhaps not surprising that research in the UK has shown that levels of patient satisfaction with the services provided by specialist or extended scope physiotherapists are consistently as high as (or even higher than) those for similar services provided by medical practitioners (Byles & Ling 1989, Daker-White et al 1999, Langridge & Moran 1984). A more recent study in Australia has reported similar results (Oldmeadow et al 2007).

Better utilisation of a highly trained sector of the health workforce. Physiotherapists are highly educated and skilled workers within the modern health care workforce, and are therefore well placed to take on specialist or extended roles.

As well as the above, there are other clear benefits to the physiotherapy profession, including the following.

Reduced attrition of clinicians. Development of specialist and extended roles enhances retention within the profession due to opportunities for the most highly qualified to undertake more satisfying and challenging work

Enhanced career paths and opportunities. Such roles also provide individual therapists with enhanced career opportunities.

SUMMARY

The changing needs of health care provision in the 21st century, while presenting many challenges, have also presented the physiotherapy profession with unique opportunities to undertake new directions. Role innovation, specialisation and new educational structures are key examples of these and are already resulting in a professional workforce that is more responsive and flexible. For example, developments in preregistration and postgraduate training have provided physiotherapists with the requisite skills to use the evidence base underpinning physiotherapy practice to provide effective, high quality health care. With the increasing costs of health care (due in part to rising levels of diseases linked to inactivity and obesity), coupled with increasing pressures on the health care workforce, there are opportunities for further diversification of physiotherapy practice. It is important that the profession continues to play a proactive role in such development if it is to continue to take a leading role in providing cost effective, high quality health care.

Reflective questions

- What are some of the new directions for physiotherapy practice?
- How will the opportunities for specialisation benefit the community and the profession?

References

Australian Government Productivity Commission 2005 Australia's health workforce. Research Report, Canberra

APA 2005 Australian Physiotherapy Association Vision 2020. APA, Canberra

Baxter D 2003a The changing face of professional education. Physical Therapy Reviews 8(2):55–56

Baxter D 2003b Responding to the complex nature of modern healthcare? Physical Therapy Reviews 8(3):111–112

Byles S E, Ling R S M 1989 Orthopaedic out-patients – a fresh approach. Physiotherapy 75(7):435–437

Council of Australian Governments Communiqué 2006 COAG Response to the Productivity Commission Report on Australia's Health Workforce. Available: http://www.coag.gov.au/meetings/140706/docs/attachment_a_response_pc_health_workforce.rtf 8 Jan 2008

Daker-White G, Carr A J, Harvey I et al 1999 A randomised controlled trial: shifting the boundaries of doctors and physiotherapists in orthopaedic outpatient departments. Journal of Epidemiology and Community Health 53:643–650

Galley P 1975 Ethical principles and patient referral. Australian Journal of Physiotherapy 21(3):97–100

Galley P 1976 Patient referral and the physiotherapist. Australian Journal of Physiotherapy 22(3):117–120

Gardiner J, Wagstaff S 2001 Extended scope physiotherapy: the way towards consultant physiotherapists? Physiotherapy 87(1):2–3

Hattam P, Smeatham A 1999 Evaluation of an orthopaedic screening service in primary care. Clinical Performance and Quality Health Care 7(3):121–124

Henry J Kaiser Family Foundation 2007 Health care costs: a primer. Henry J Kaiser Family Foundation, Washington

Hockin J, Bannister G 1994 The extended role of a physiotherapist in an outpatient orthopaedic clinic. Physiotherapy 80(5):281–284

Hourigan P, Weatherley C 1994 Initial assessment and follow-up by a physiotherapist of patients with back pain referred to a spinal clinic. Journal of the Royal Society of Medicine 87(4):213–214

Langridge J C, Moran C J 1984 A comparison of two methods of managing patients suffering from rheumatoid arthritis. Physiotherapy 70(3):109–113

Lorig K, Ritter P L, Plant, K 2005 A disease-specific self-help program compared with a generalized chronic disease self-help program for arthritis patients. Arthritis Care and Research 53(6):950–957

Mills P, Mills J 2007 Fighting globesity: a practical guide to personal health and sustainability. Random House New Zealand, Auckland

MoH 2004 Ageing New Zealand and health and disability services: demand projections and workforce implications, 2001–2021. Discussion document. Ministry of Health, Wellington

MoH and DHBNZ Workforce Group 2007 A career framework for the health and disability workforce in New Zealand. Ministry of Health and District Health Boards New Zealand, Wellington

Mueller J, Taylor L, Copeland J et al 2007 Advanced Practitioner Working Party: a consultation document. New Zealand Society of Physiotherapists and New Zealand College of Physiotherapy, Wellington

Mullan F 2002 Time-capsule thinking: the health care workforce, past and future. Health Affairs 21:112–122

National Health Service and Community Care Act 1990. Available: http://www.opsi.gov.uk/acts/acts1990/Ukpga_19900019_en_1 13 Jan 2008

Neumann P B, Grimmer K A, Grant R E et al 2005 Physiotherapy for female stress urinary incontinence: a multicentre observational study. Australian and New Zealand Journal of Obstetrics and Gynaecology 45(3):226–232

Oldmeadow L B, Bedi H S, Burch H T et al 2007 Experienced physiotherapists as gatekeepers to hospital orthopaedic outpatient care. Medical Journal of Australia 186(12):625–628

Rennie K L, Jebb S A 2005 Prevalence of obesity in Great Britain. Obesity Reviews 6(1):11–12

Robertson S 2007 Smart physio initiative improves waiting lists. Queensland Government Ministerial media statement. Available: http://cabinet.qld.gov.au/MMS/StatementDisplaySingle.aspx?id=54032 7 Jan 2008

WCPT 2007 Declaration of principle: autonomy. Declarations of principle and position statements approved at the 13th general meeting of WCPT, June 1995 and revised and re-approved at the 16th general meeting of WCPT, June 2007. Available: http://www.wcpt.org/ 24 May 2008

Weale A, Bannister G 1995 Who should see orthopaedic outpatients, physiotherapists or surgeons? Annals of the Royal College of Surgeons of England 77(suppl):71–73

WHO 2006 The world health report 2006 – working together for health. World Health Organization. Available: http://www.who.int/whr/2006/en/ 26 Dec 2007

HISTORICAL PHASES IN PHYSIOTHERAPY

Jenny Pynt, Dale Larsen, David Nicholls and Joy Higgs

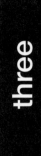

Key content
- The historical emergence of physiotherapy
- Physiotherapy practice eras

INTRODUCTION

In a book for physiotherapists in the 21st century what is the place of history? In this chapter we present the evolution of the practice and the profession of physiotherapy so that those entering and working in this profession will appreciate that:

- entering and working in a profession means becoming part of the history of that profession
- an understanding of the sociocultural and historical evolution of the profession comes from studying its history
- the practice of physiotherapy today is informed by its historical contextualisation
- today's practice creates its future history
- the knowledge underpinning current physiotherapy practice is part of the ongoing history of ideas.

Having this historical appreciation and insight into the nature and emergence of current practice and knowledge allows physiotherapists to contribute to the quality and development of both their practice and their profession.

To address these issues and goals we present three main historical frames of reference in this chapter. The first recognises the earliest origins of physiotherapy, in ancient history. Readers will see how in the medical practices of ancient Egyptian, Greek and Chinese civilisations the origins of today's physiotherapy practices gave birth to practices that were developed during the 17th and subsequent centuries. The second phase of physiotherapy practice commenced when physiotherapy gained an identity as an occupation. In this context we present the changing foci of physiotherapy practice in response to various historical and sociocultural trends and events. The importance of this section lies in the explanation it provides for the evolution of physiotherapy practice and the lessons that can be learned from past eras in shaping new directions as a response to contextual dynamics and, conversely, as an instigator of change (e.g. in the services physiotherapy can provide and the wellbeing of the communities physiotherapists serve). Our third segment looks at physiotherapy as an organised profession that emerged during the last century. We draw together the evolving practices of physiotherapy and the public recognition physiotherapy has gained as an important and respected contributor to the health care system and the wellbeing of people and society.

THE EMERGENCE OF PRACTICES IN ANCIENT TIMES AS FORERUNNERS OF PHYSIOTHERAPY PRACTICES

Therapeutic practices from past medical traditions pre-empted modern physiotherapy practices, in some instances by millennia. Many of these treatments were grounded in careful observation of signs and symptoms and reactions to treatment, and demonstrate the role of experiential knowledge in the formation of current practices. Other regimens reflected the impact of sociocultural concepts of the day.

Ancient Egypt

As far back as ancient Egyptian times there were medical practices that have connections with today's physiotherapy practice. The oldest extant medical treatise, known today as the Edwin Smith papyrus, dates to 1700 BCE and is a copy of a text thought to have originated around 2500 BCE in ancient Egypt. In a time when mankind considered disease to be retribution from the gods this text is unique in that it is almost devoid of magico-religious incantations. It is considered to be both the first medical textbook and the oldest example of inductive process in the history of medicine (Breasted 1930). The treatise addresses issues of joint and muscle injury, and neurological and respiratory illness. It describes the examination of 48 case presentations, including the history of the injury, examination of movements, palpation, diagnosis, consideration of contraindication to treatment and, in one instance, logical alternative treatment depending on predicted treatment reactions. The papyrus is of interest to physiotherapists in that it contains the first written evidence of the use of manipulation to reduce dislocation of the mandible, positioning with scapular retraction to realign displaced fracture of the clavicle, realignment and plaster splinting for fractures, and poultices for sprained joints and tendons. The papyrus is incomplete, finishing tantalisingly before the treatment for low back pain is described.

Ancient Greece

Significant medical knowledge that was to inform health care in subsequent centuries was acquired in ancient Greece under the auspices of the legendary Greek physician, Hippocrates (Porter 1997). This knowledge and the practices of ancient Greek medicine from the 5th century BCE are preserved in a collection of books known as the *Hippocratic Corpus*. From these texts we know that Hippocratic medicine was based on the 'understanding, empirical and rational, of the workings of the body in its natural environment' and that medical knowledge grew from careful observation and experience (Porter 1997, p 56). This ethos is demonstrated in *On Articulations* (Hippocrates Vol. VIII), one book of the *Corpus*. This historical record contains evidence that, for some presentations of kypho-scoliosis, ancient Greek physicians followed a therapeutic regimen that pre-empted modern-day approaches by 2500 years. Treatments consisting of mobilisation, traction using a wheel and axle apparatus, positioning the lumbar spine into extension and attempts at the use of a lumbar roll are all described for correction of kypho-scoliosis. This regimen encapsulates the ancient Greek philosophy that treatment should correspond with the laws of nature in opposing deformity and restoring normal postural harmony.

Ancient Greek medicine also stressed the importance of diet and exercise in the prevention of illness and maintenance of harmony within the body. The introduction of gymnasiums, with a variety of weight resistance equipment, personal trainers and masseurs, can be traced to ancient Greece. The idea of 'a healthy mind in a healthy body', which was to underscore the return of mass exercise in the 19th century, originated in Hippocratic times.

Ancient China

Ancient Chinese medicine was akin to Hippocratic medicine in that it was grounded in a hypothesis emphasising the importance of balance and harmony of the body within itself and with the external world. In the 3rd century CE during the Han dynasty there was a physician, Hua Tho, whose exercise regimen was underpinned by the Taoist belief that harmony prevented illness. The great Chinese historian Joseph Needham wrote of Hua Tho: 'Chinese physicians trace back to him the great developments of medical gymnastics, massage and physiotherapy' (Needham et al 2000, p 52). Hua Tho developed a routine of exercises combined with deep breathing and massage. This regimen aimed to improve digestion and circulation, prevent stasis and stiffness and restore harmony. Although Hua Tho's rationale arose from a different epistemology, it is interesting to note in evidence-based literature the importance accorded to movement and correct breathing in the maintenance of health.

The West 1600–1900

As the West emerged from the Middle Ages the philosophy that illness was a punishment from God began to fade. A passionate desire to return to the glories of ancient Greece pervaded many facets of human endeavour, including medicine (Porter 1997). Thus in the 17th century the practice of Hippocratic medicine continued, juxtaposed with daring and innovative thinking. During the Age of Enlightenment the transition from Hippocratic medicine to empirico-analytical inquiry laid the foundations of biomechanics (Borelli 1680), orthopaedics (Andry 1743) and occupational health (Ramazzini 1713). Medicine was now based on an understanding of the function and structure of the body from an engineering perspective, and illness was considered a breakdown of mechanics. In his treatise *Diseases of workers*, Ramazzini proposed from his observations that the workplace, work postures and lack of exercise were detrimental to the health of workers. By the 18th century orthopaedic medicine focused on preventive and corrective treatment of idiopathic scoliosis. Traction re-emerged as a treatment. The school of thought fostered by Andry regarding the treatment of scoliosis thrived and continued into the 19th century. Children and adults were subjected to prolonged treatment using traction, extension exercises and posture correction in specialised institutions.

The increased interest in exercise in the 19th century re-introduced the concept of mass physical education first practised by the ancient Greeks. The remedial gymnastics regimen developed by Swedish military gymnastics instructor Per Ling stimulated great interest in mass exercise classes throughout Europe. Needham (1956) has suggested that Ling was influenced by ancient Chinese medicine. During the 17th and 18th centuries in the West, coinciding with the inception of the East India trading companies, interest arose in many aspects of Chinese culture. Jesuit priests were sent to China to exchange medical and religious ideas. Stimulated by this exchange of knowledge, the Jesuit priest Amiot wrote a treatise on a Chinese breathing and exercise regimen, which he referred to as Cong-Fou (Amiot 1779). These exercises were based on the concept that gentleness developed strength and that, in the pursuit of harmony, the body should not be punished by exercise. Ling, however, changed the manner in which exercises were performed to accord with his philosophy that health is strength. Thus exercise in the West was revolutionised. It now reflected the prevailing Victorian sociocultural concept that harmony could be achieved by subordinating the body to the will and that character could be strengthened by exercises demanding willpower. Exercise for the masses was promoted by governments as a method of sociocultural rehabilitation, to improve waning national willpower and identity. This particular use of exercise flagged the importance of sociocultural factors in the evolution of physiotherapy practice.

PHYSIOTHERAPY PRACTICE ERAS: A HISTORY OF SCIENTIFIC EVOLUTION AND SERVICE TO A CHANGING SOCIETY

The development of Western physiotherapy can be divided into four eras according to the prevailing focus of clinical practice at the time. In each of these eras there was a progressive and at times dramatic advance in the scientific basis for physiotherapy practice, a shift in practice focus in response to prevailing sociocultural conditions, and a response to the needs of society in relation to key historical events or circumstances (e.g. epidemics). Through each stage there was an expansion of practice scope and contribution to health care, along with an evolution in the strength of physiotherapy as a credible profession.

The first era, identified as the 'massage era', corresponds to the time frame 1880–1913. The second era, the 'peripheral neuromusculoskeletal dysfunction era' (1914–1945) was significantly influenced by World War I and by poliomyelitis epidemics. Both events required a response from the profession to assist in the treatment and management of patients who presented mainly with peripheral neuromusculoskeletal dysfunction.

The third era, the 'neurological era', encompassed the period 1946–1980. At the beginning of this era rehabilitation practice gained impetus, as physiotherapists were required to assist in the management of World War II casualties. Existing areas of practice such as orthopaedics expanded and new areas emerged, including plastic surgery and spinal cord injury rehabilitation (e.g. the development of the National Spinal Injuries Unit at Stoke Mandeville in England) (Barclay 1994). The main clinical focus during this era was the management of patients who were affected by dysfunction of the central nervous system (CNS) (Sahrmann 2002).

The fourth era, the 'movement era' (1981–present) reflects the core of contemporary physiotherapy practice, which identifies movement dysfunction as the primary problem addressed by its intervention (Sahrmann 2002). The emphasis on movement dysfunction encompasses consideration of the musculoskeletal, neurological, cardiopulmonary and metabolic systems of the human body. This emphasis is replicated in contemporary definitions of physiotherapy such as that of the World Confederation for Physical Therapy (WCPT 1999), described in Chapter 1.

The massage era: 1880–1913 (pre-World War I)

Prior to World War I, 'medical massage' therapy in the Commonwealth countries developed following the British model, with education in anatomy, physiology and the basic sciences being provided by doctors. Massage training in the form of an apprenticeship, for example as stipulated by the Australasian Massage Association rules and regulations for the state of New South Wales 1905 (Bentley 2006), was provided by senior massage therapists in hospitals. The Commonwealth countries followed their British counterpart by incorporating other treatment modalities such as medical gymnastics and electrotherapy into their practice. The Australasian Massage Association quickly developed a unique two-year diploma program in association with universities within Australia. A similar program began at the University of Otago in New Zealand in 1913 (Taylor 1988). Early American physiotherapy was also based on the practice of massage, but the profession in that country did not emerge until 1917 when the Americans entered World War I and introduced 'reconstruction aide' programs to respond to the need to rehabilitate wounded soldiers (Murphy 1995).

The peripheral neuromusculoskeletal dysfunction era: 1914–1945

In the aftermath of World War I physiotherapists in the Commonwealth countries and the USA needed to undertake management of the war wounded, many of whom had orthopaedic and peripheral nerve injuries (Le Vay 1990). As a consequence there was an expansion of physiotherapy practice within orthopaedics, and other new treatments including hydrotherapy and electrotherapy were developed to meet the rehabilitation requirements of returning soldiers (Barclay 1994, Murphy 1995). There was also a shift in practice from passive therapy in the form of massage to active exercise. In the United Kingdom, Dr James Mennell (Snr) had begun teaching physiotherapists manipulative techniques at St Thomas' Hospital in London as early as 1914, and many of these physiotherapists became adept in this practice during World War I (Barclay 1994). Physiotherapists such as the Australian Geoff Maitland (who was to become a prominent manual therapist in subsequent years) were influenced by the writings and teachings of Mennell.

With the outbreak of poliomyelitis epidemics physiotherapists in Australia, the UK, Canada, the USA and New Zealand became involved in the development of diagnostic muscle testing procedures and therapeutic muscle re-education programs (Barclay 1994).

The neurological era: 1946–1980

During this era improved health care enabled many patients with injuries to the CNS to survive, and they became the predominant patient populations requiring physiotherapy once the use of the Salk vaccine eradicated poliomyelitis (Murphy 1995). Throughout this period many eclectic treatment approaches (e.g. neurodevelopmental treatment, proprioceptive neuromuscular facilitation and a motor relearning program) evolved for patients with CNS dysfunction (e.g. stroke, head injury, cerebral palsy) where the specific pathophysiology of the disorder was unknown (Sahrmann 2002).

Alongside the emphasis on neurological physiotherapy in this era, manual therapy began to emerge as an important aspect of hospital and private practice based physiotherapy. Physiotherapists were increasingly attracted to courses such as those conducted by Dr James Cyriax (Barclay 1994), who was Mennell's successor at St Thomas' Hospital. Many physiotherapists, such as Grieve, Kaltenborn, Maitland and McKenzie, went on to create conceptual frameworks for manual therapy practice.

These men were influential in developing and disseminating their particular manual therapy knowledge and skills worldwide. The focus of these teaching programs was on skill acquisition and the precise application of passive movement techniques to address vertebral and peripheral joint dysfunction. Collectively, these courses provided a rationale for physical treatment that concentrated on joint structure and biomechanics as an explanation for the presumed cause–effect relationships observed in patients' signs and symptoms and the passive treatment protocols.

During this era physiotherapy educators in all countries, including Australia, were intent on enhancing existing educational programs by raising them to degree standard, at the same time providing postgraduate education opportunities (Bentley, 2006). The moves towards specialisation and emphasis on research were evident in the development of the Association of Chartered Physiotherapists in Research in the UK in 1977. Similar organisations developed in other countries over the next two decades (Barclay 1994, Bentley 2006).

The movement era: 1981–present

From the 1980s, originating in manual therapy practice, the terms *examination*, *evaluation*, *diagnosis*, *prognosis*, *intervention*, *re-examination*, and *assessment of outcomes* have become standard terminology guiding practice. An emphasis on evidence-based practice has been prevalent in Western countries since the 1990s, and the current specialised areas of practice include cardiorespiratory, musculoskeletal, neurological, occupational health, paediatric and sports physiotherapy, as well as women's health and gerontology.

In the 21st century physiotherapists are required to define, evaluate and demonstrate quality service delivery and outcomes. High quality physiotherapy care involves appropriate classification of presenting problems, risk management, treatment decision making and evidence-based practice strategies and outcome measures that reflect stakeholders' needs and the cost implications of service delivery (Grimmer et al 2000).

Dividing the evolution of physiotherapy practice into eras facilitates an understanding of the vast growth of the profession since its inception. We now revisit the massage era, to understand the intriguing factors that led to the formation of the profession.

THE EMERGENCE OF PHYSIOTHERAPY AS A PROFESSION

The profession of physiotherapy today in the West owes much of its existence to the conscientious actions of four young nurses and midwives who, in the summer of 1894, formed a professional organisation to counter the massage scandals enveloping Victorian London (Nicholls & Cheek 2006). Their actions were provoked by an article in the *British Medical Journal* (1894) that called massage parlours 'pandemoniums of vice'. Legitimate massage, it seems, had become a convenient way for brothels to avoid prosecution, and the lack of regulation of advertising inflamed the situation to the point where no-one knew who was a legitimate therapist and who was a prostitute. Legitimate masseuses around the country were drawn into the scandal, and a campaign was launched by Ernest Hart, the pioneering editor of the *British Medical Journal*, to bring about change (*British Medical Journal* 1894). Hart called for the formation of a professional body to take charge of the education and registration of masseuses. In response, the four women founders created the Society of Trained Masseuses (STM) to show that massage could be legitimised. The actions of the founders, under the leadership of Rosalind Paget, represent some of the most elegant tactics used by the many professions that emerged at the end of the 19th century to establish their legitimacy (see box below). Those same tactics continue to have an enduring influence on physiotherapy today.

The most significant steps taken by the founders of the STM

1. Define strict rules of professional conduct
2. Court medical patronage
3. Establish examination systems
4. Create an agency to manage doctors' referrals
5. Adopt biomechanics as the profession's underlying philosophy

---

The Society's rules (STM 1895) stated that the STM would offer training only to women (hence the Society of Trained *Masseuses* and not *Masseurs*). The rules forbade masseuses from massaging men unless specifically directed by a doctor, and only then in 'nursing' cases. The founders encouraged doctors to regard the profession favourably by instigating such measures, but also by gaining the patronage of eminent doctors who became signatories to the STM's enterprise (Incorporated Society of Trained Masseuses c.1912).

Adherence to the STM's principles was maintained via an examination system that assessed not only the students' knowledge but also their personal suitability and their attitude to professionalism (Nicholls & Cheek 2006). Upon registration, graduates were included within the STM and provided with patients through the referral agency that continued to monitor standards of practice, quality of treatment, pay rates and the expansion of the profession. These measures were important in convincing the general public and the medical profession that the STM was the only legitimate response to the massage scandals of 1894. In addition, these measures had an enduring effect upon the practices of physiotherapists around the globe, particularly in the post-colonial countries of Australia, Canada, India, New Zealand and South Africa, where the legacy of the English system of massage can still be seen today.

It is important to remember that physiotherapy was not born of a particular invention (like the radiography profession, for instance). Nor did the profession form around a concern for a particular region of the body (like dentistry or podiatry). Instead, physiotherapy as an organised and self-regulated profession was formed to legitimate and regulate therapeutic touch and, in so doing, 'colonised' a health care territory that had existed for many years before: massage, remedial exercise and electrotherapy.

The STM, arising in the late 19th and early 20th centuries, had to contend with English Victorian values, and had to adopt a view of the body that removed all sensual elements from treatments that involved touch. Denying men access to the society promoted the idea that the STM was a legitimate organisation. As Grafton (1934, p 229) argued, the founder's quest was to 'make massage a safe, clean and honourable profession, and it shall be a profession for British women'. The fledgling physiotherapy profession was also able to gain respectability by adopting a strategy of association with the medical profession (Barclay 1994, Taylor 1988). This stance implied a choice to be closely associated with orthodoxy and to accept medical dominance and supervision, with its inherent subordination to doctors (Katavich 1996). Although this strategy had political advantages (such as recognition by orthodox medicine), it delayed the development of the profession's own professional competence, knowledge base and political awareness, all of which did not emerge in their own right until the mid-1960s (Miles-Tapping 1989).

Possibly one of the most profound influences upon the profession's development came from the adoption of a biomechanical view of the body as the basis of its practice (Nicholls & Cheek 2006). It was important that students could be trained to touch people without any hint of sensuality. Masseuses needed to be desensitised to the aesthetic qualities of massage, and the most effective way to do this was to treat the patient's body as a machine. Through its publications and examinations, the STM began the process of regulating the curricula of massage training institutions throughout England and strictly defining how 'correct' massage should be practised (Palmer 1901).

A biomechanical view was embodied in the anatomy, kinesiology and physical training of the students, and it appeared throughout numerous massage manuals as a detached, depersonalised approach to the body of the patient. Massage was taught as a technique and physiological effect, rather than as a vehicle for pleasure, comfort or intimacy. A biomechanical perspective allowed the masseuse to view the body as a machine: to remove its aesthetic qualities; to touch the patient's thigh and not think of it as a sensual act, to think instead of the origins and insertions of muscles and the structures being massaged (Mennell 1920). Vitally, it brought the 'legitimate' massage profession closer to the medical and, most especially, the surgical profession, and it showed the public the professional face of massage practice.

In the years following World War I, the STM consolidated its position as *the* legitimate English massage profession and began to export its systems throughout the Commonwealth. Welfare reforms in the 1930s brought fresh opportunities for expansion of the profession. The polio, influenza and tuberculosis epidemics and the casualties from the War gave masseuses ample opportunity to develop new skills, and the creation of the welfare state in England, Australia, New Zealand and elsewhere created a secure environment in which the profession could flourish. New physiotherapy departments were created, new forms of profession-specific legislation were drafted (such as the *New Zealand Physiotherapy Act 1949*), and new professional subspecialties emerged.

During the middle of the 20th century, following World War II, there was considerable expansion in the practices of physiotherapy. Around the world the profession (in its various regional practice approaches) had created subdivisions based on the same body system differentiation seen in medicine generally. Physiotherapy was divided into branches, the largest being respiratory, musculoskeletal and neurological. Each branch played its part in the state's response to what Beveridge (1942) called the *five giants*, the five greatest threats to the health, wealth and happiness of the population: want, disease, idleness, ignorance and squalor. However, unlike the other great orthodox health professions, physiotherapy took a different approach to the health of the nation. Where other health professions targeted public health in the population as a whole, physiotherapists focused upon the dysfunctions present in the body of the individual patient.

During the second half of the 20th century changes both within and outside the profession led to an expansion of the perspectives of physiotherapy. The formation of the WCPT and its first congress in London in 1953 promoted the exchange of ideas and coincided with the development of educational programs, raising them to degree status, at the same time facilitating postgraduate education opportunities. Expanding opportunities for travel, education and communication resulted in a challenge to the local orientations of practice and to the predominantly biomedical frameworks of education. These challenges came particularly from physiotherapists who brought back new teachings and practices from their work overseas.

Attainment of degree status of the educational programs for physiotherapy in the latter decades of the 20th century required the inclusion of behavioural sciences as well as biomedical sciences. These subjects were increasingly taught by scientists in these fields rather than physiotherapists. Curricula placed increased emphasis on subjects such as sociology and psychology, applied physiology and biomechanics, in addition to the traditional kinesiology and therapeutic methods. Research methods also gained an important place in curricula. As a consequence physiotherapists began to look more widely and critically at their practice and their potential contributions to health care both in scope (beyond individual clients) and appraisal of decision making rationales. The idea of the professional as a responsible, autonomous decision maker rather than a skilled therapist gained prominence. Around this time the introduction of legislation and the WCPT's endorsement of the first contact (non-referral) practitioner status of physiotherapists occurred. This change in policy occurred in Australia in 1976 (Twomey & Cole 1985) and subsequently in New Zealand, the USA, Canada, and then the UK. Today direct referral by physiotherapists is being considered for MRI, CT scans and specialist consultation. Under the umbrella term of 'extended scope' physiotherapy, discussed more widely in Chapter 2, practice is expected to expand into other new roles (see box below).

Anticipated new roles for 'extended scope' practice
- A substantially increased role in presurgery preparation and postsurgical rehabilitation, and in triage, emergency and intensive care
- Prescription of a limited number of pharmaceuticals by some physiotherapists
- Limited injecting rights for some physiotherapists
- Minor surgery

Changes in legislation to enable physiotherapists to undertake these additional roles, which currently fall outside the legislative scope of practice, will require negotiation with the appropriate health jurisdictions. Negotiations are expected to occur over the next few years.

Today, we see multiple influences upon the profession. The need for a legitimate, orthodox health profession that is trusted and understood by the general public and the medical profession is no less pressing than it was more than a century ago. It is clear, however, that we are moving into an era where health care is becoming increasingly expensive and problematic to fund and provide. Physiotherapists are faced with patients who cannot access appropriate medical care in a timely fashion due to workforce shortages, particularly in rural areas. The population is ageing and bringing with it the challenges of addressing complex health care problems such as multiple co-morbidities and chronic ill health. What models of health care in general and physiotherapy in particular will suitably address these needs? Will physiotherapy, as it is today, meet the needs of a population that is demanding more from health care and increasingly turning to information technology, self-help and complementary medicine for solutions? These and other questions regarding future trends are pursued in other chapters.

SUMMARY

In this chapter we have stressed the importance of history in identifying whence the profession of physiotherapy has come and the lessons that can be learned from that journey. The study of history teaches the need to be critical of trends, both past and present. It reminds us that today's knowledge and challenges are the history of the future.

Reflective questions

- What have you learned from the history of physiotherapy that can enhance your understanding of physiotherapy practice today?
- How will you be shaping tomorrow's history?

References

Amiot J M 1779 Notice du Cong-Fou des Bonzes Tao-sée. In: Batteaux C et al (eds) Mémoires concernant l'histoire, les sciences, les arts, les moeurs, les usages, etc. des Chinois, par les Missionaires de Pekin, vol 4. Chez Nyon, Libraire, Paris

Andry N 1743 Orthopaedica: or, the art of correcting and preventing deformities in children, vol 1. Classics of Medicine Library, Birmingham

Barclay J 1994 In good hands: the history of the Chartered Society of Physiotherapy 1894–1994. Butterworth-Heinemann, Oxford

Bentley P 2006 The path to professionalism: physiotherapy in Australia to the 1980s. Australian Physiotherapy Association, Melbourne

Beveridge W 1942 Social insurance and allied services. HMSO, London

Borelli G A 1680 On the movement of animals (trans Maquet P 1989). Springer-Verlag, Berlin

Breasted J H 1930 Edwin Smith surgical papyrus. University of Chicago Press, Chicago

British Medical Journal 1894 Astounding revelations concerning supposed massage houses or pandemoniums of vice, frequented by both sexes, being a complete exposé of the ways of professed masseurs and masseuses. Wellcome Institute Library, London, Ref SA/CSP/P.1/2: British Medical Association

Grafton S A 1934 The history of the Chartered Society of Massage and Medical Gymnastics. Journal of the Chartered Society of Massage and Medical Gymnastics, March, 229

Grimmer K, Beard M, Bell A et al 2000 On the constructs of quality physiotherapy. Australian Journal of Physiotherapy 46(1):3–7

Hippocrates Vol. VIII (trans and ed Potter P 1995). Harvard University Press, Cambridge

Incorporated Society of Trained Masseuses c. 1912 Prospectus of the Incorporated Society of Trained Masseuses, Wellcome Institute Archive: SA/CSP/P.1/3. Wellcome Institute Library, London

Katavich L 1996 Physiotherapy in the new health system in New Zealand. New Zealand Journal of Physiotherapy 24(2):11–13

Le Vay D 1990 The history of orthopaedics: an account of the study and practice of orthopaedics from the earliest times to the modern era. The Parthenon Publishing Group, Canforth

Mennell J P 1920 Massage: its principles and practice, 2nd edn. P. Blakiston's, Philadelphia

Miles-Tapping C 1989 Sponsorship and sacrifice in the historical development of Canadian physiotherapy. Physiotherapy Canada 41(2):72–80

Murphy W 1995 Healing the generations: a history of physical therapy and the American Physical Therapy Association. Greenwich Publishing Group, Lyme, CT

Needham J 1956 History of scientific thought. Cambridge University Press, Cambridge

Needham J, Gwei-Djen L, Sivin N 2000 Science and civilisation in China: biology and biological technology. Cambridge University Press, Cambridge

Nicholls D A, Cheek J 2006 Physiotherapy and the shadow of prostitution: the Society of Trained Masseuses and the massage scandals of 1894. Social Science and Medicine 62(9):2336–2348

Palmer M D 1901 Lessons in massage. Balliere, Tindall and Cox, London

Porter R 1997 The greatest benefit to mankind. Harper Collins, London

Ramazzini B 1713 De morbis artificum (Diseases of workers) (trans Wright W C 1964). Hafner, New York

Sahrmann S A 2002 Diagnosis and treatment of movement impairment syndromes. Mosby, St. Louis, MO

Society of Trained Masseuses 1895 Minutes of committee meeting. Unpublished manuscript. Wellcome Institute Library, London, Ref SA/CSP/B.1/1/1

Taylor L A 1988 Dunedin school of massage: the first ten years of physiotherapy training in New Zealand. University of Otago, Dunedin

Twomey L T, Cole J 1985 The changing face of physiotherapy practice. Physiotherapy Practice 1:77–85

WCPT 1999 Description of physical therapy. 14th General Meeting of the World Confederation for Physical Therapy, London

THE PHYSIOTHERAPY WORKFORCE

Margaret Grant and Joan McMeeken

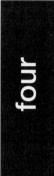

Key content
- Nature of the physiotherapy workforce
- Factors influencing the physiotherapy workforce

INTRODUCTION

The physiotherapy workforce of the 21st century will be influenced by extrinsic factors such as changing population demographics, emerging health conditions, globalisation and technology. The physiotherapy profession is well placed to adapt to these factors through its proven capacity as a flexible, innovative and cost effective workforce (The Chartered Society of Physiotherapy 2006a). Although the physiotherapy workforce of the future will be shaped by its adaptation to extrinsic factors, the profession and individual practitioners have the intrinsic potential to mould the workforce from within by creating and maximising opportunities in this dynamic environment. This chapter provides descriptive information about the physiotherapy workforce in Australia and overseas and identifies some of the factors that will influence the shape of the workforce as well as those that have the potential to do so.

THE PHYSIOTHERAPY WORKFORCE IN AUSTRALIA

Brief history

In Australia 'physiotherapists' have been reported in the workforce as health care practitioners since the time of the gold rushes in the 1850s (Bentley 2006). These practitioners treated their patients with exercises, electrotherapy and massage. A review of longitudinal population data and accounts of the history of physiotherapy in Australia indicates that there has long been a relationship between population numbers, demand for physiotherapy services and the education of practitioners to meet workforce needs. Because of the gold rush over 49% of the Australian population in 1861 was located in Victoria (ABS 2006). It was also around that time that physiotherapy university education began in Australia. In the late 19th century, Eliza McCauley studied anatomy, including dissection, at the University of Melbourne, Victoria. Following completion of her clinical studies at the Melbourne Hospital, McCauley began teaching her students (Bentley 2006). The Australasian Massage Association was founded in 1905, and a year later it formalised the program that had been established by McCauley at the

University of Melbourne. Interstate programs followed rapidly, with one established in 1907 at the University of Sydney, New South Wales, and another in 1908 at the University of Adelaide in South Australia (Chipchase et al 2006).

As the Australian population grew, the demand for physiotherapists in other states increased. Physiotherapy programs began at the University of Queensland in 1938 and in Western Australia in 1951.

Estimating the physiotherapy workforce

It is difficult to accurately identify the number of practising physiotherapists in Australia. One useful indicator is the number of registered physiotherapists in Australia. Registration of the physiotherapy workforce was considered an important requirement by the early physiotherapists in order to protect the community and maintain professional standards. Registration through government legislation was first achieved in Victoria in 1922 and was subsequently introduced in all states (Bentley 2006). A physiotherapist must be registered to legally practise physiotherapy in each state or territory in Australia. However, until a national system of registration is implemented in Australia, physiotherapists must register separately with each state or territory in which they practise. Consequently, a single practitioner may be registered in two or more jurisdictions. It is also common for physiotherapists working in nonclinical positions such as research or management to maintain their registration. Therefore the total number of registered physiotherapists may not accurately reflect the physiotherapy workforce in Australia. From time to time, workforce data are also collected by government agencies such as the Australian Institute of Health and Welfare (AIHW), the Australian Bureau of Statistics (ABS) and the various state government health departments. Combining the registration data and the various sources of workforce data provides reasonable estimates of the characteristics of and changes in the physiotherapy workforce in Australia.

Schofield & Fletcher (2007) reported that in 1986 there were 5928 people in the Australian community who identified themselves as physiotherapists in clinical practice, and by 2001 the number of clinical physiotherapists had risen by nearly 70% to 10,039. Data from the AIHW (2006) indicate that with the inclusion of academics and administrators there were about 15,400 registered physiotherapists in 2002, with a female to male ratio of about 70:30. By 2007 the total number of registered physiotherapists in Australia had increased by a further 27% to 19,607 (Australian Physiotherapy Council 2007). On the basis of data from the AIHW (2006), it is estimated that the total number of registered physiotherapists may include up to 5% of multiple registrations.

The geographical distribution of registered physiotherapists varies across Australia, as shown in Table 4.1. If only about two-thirds of registered physiotherapists are practising, as the recent data from Schofield and Fletcher (2007) would suggest, it is estimated that, at the time of publication, there would be an average of 62 practising physiotherapists per 100,000 of the population.

Table 4.1 Estimated number of registered physiotherapists per 100,000 of the population for each Australian state/territory in 2007

	Population ('000), June 2007*	Registered PTs, 2007[#]	Estimated PTs/100,000 population
ACT	339	378	112
SA	1584	1652	104
WA	2105	2086	99
NSW	6889	6713	97
Vic	5205	4775	92
Qld	4182	3506	84
NT	202	141	70
Tas	493	356	72
Total	21 017	19 607	93

PTs: physiotherapists
*Data from the Australian Bureau of Statistics (2007)
[#]Data from the Australian Physiotherapy Council (2007)

PHYSIOTHERAPY WORKFORCE SHORTAGES

Physiotherapy workforce shortages occur when the supply of physiotherapists does not meet the demand for physiotherapy services. Physiotherapy workforce shortages have been frequently identified, particularly following World Wars I and II and during the poliomyelitis epidemics of the 1930s and 1950s (Bolwell, personal communication). In Australia, the Department of Employment and Workplace Relations (DEWR) has demonstrated that there were insufficient numbers of physiotherapists in the health workforce for 20 of the past 25 years and 12 of the past 13 years (DEWR 2007, Human Capital Alliance 2005), with growing pressures for more physiotherapists.

Supplying the physiotherapy workforce in Australia

One strategy to address workforce shortages is to increase the supply of physiotherapists. Since the mid-1990s when there were six physiotherapy programs at baccalaureate level, there has been a rapid expansion in both the number of physiotherapy programs in Australia and the student intake into the programs. This has occurred partly in response to the critical workforce shortages in physiotherapy in Australia. In 2007 there were 19 entry-level physiotherapy programs with graduates entering the profession at baccalaureate, masters and doctoral levels. The masters and doctoral degrees are termed graduate entry programs. This type of program accelerates the attainment of a physiotherapy qualification for graduates of cognate degrees and is another strategy to increase the supply of physiotherapists to the workforce.

After a period of relative stability of about 775 graduates a year in the 1990s, by 2003 there were 836 physiotherapy graduates. In 2006 about 1100 graduates completed physiotherapy degrees, and in 2007 this number was likely to increase to 1283 (McMeeken et al 2008). Further increases in the number of graduates were projected, as more than 1350 students commenced physiotherapy programs in Australia in 2007. Despite the increase in physiotherapy programs and student numbers, by the end of 2007 shortages of physiotherapists were identified in all states and territories except South Australia (DEWR 2007).

In the mid-1990s the ratio of male to female physiotherapy students was approximately 50:50. More recently, in common with the general Australian university undergraduate population, the proportion of female students has increased to about two-thirds. The ratio of about 50:50 males to females still exists in the graduate entry programs (McMeeken et al 2008). Students from rural areas and students born outside Australia are well represented among physiotherapy graduates, but Indigenous Australians and those from low socioeconomic backgrounds are underrepresented in proportion to their numbers in the population (McMeeken et al 2005).

Generally, women have been more likely to have time out of the workforce and to work part-time, although there is an increasing tendency for men also to work shorter hours (Schofield & Fletcher 2007). Thus the current numbers of graduates may not be sufficient to replace those either temporarily or permanently out of the physiotherapy clinical workforce. This is of major concern when there are particularly critical shortages in cardiorespiratory physiotherapy, paediatrics, critical care, oncology and aged care, and in the public sector more generally in outer metropolitan, rural, regional and remote areas.

In addition to graduates from Australian universities, the physiotherapy workforce in Australia is supplied by physiotherapists who have completed qualifications in another country. These are referred to in this chapter as international physiotherapy graduates. To be recognised for migration to Australia, and to register to practise as a physiotherapist, an international physiotherapy graduate (other than New Zealand registered physiotherapists) must successfully complete an assessment process administered by the Australian Physiotherapy Council. In response to the shortages reported by DEWR, physiotherapy is classified by the Department of Immigration and Citizenship (DIAC) as an occupation in demand. Consequently, international physiotherapy graduates have preferential migration status through a variety of skilled migration visa categories (DIAC 2007). The Australian Physiotherapy Council has reported a subsequent increase in the number of international physiotherapy graduates completing the assessment process, from 24 in 2003 to 81 in 2007. Table 4.2 provides a breakdown of the countries of education of the international physiotherapy graduates.

It is clear that increasing numbers of physiotherapists from India and England are entering the physiotherapy workforce in Australia. The Australian Physiotherapy Council reported further increases in the number of applications received from international physiotherapy graduates in 2007. Future projections indicate that more than 100 international physiotherapy graduates will complete the assessment process per year.

International students who graduate from entry-level physiotherapy programs at Australian universities can also apply for migration to Australia as physiotherapists. In this chapter we refer to these physiotherapists as international undergraduate students. Following completion of their physiotherapy studies, international undergraduate students are also entitled to preferential migration status through the classification of physiotherapy as an occupation in demand for migration purposes. Immediately after completion of a physiotherapy degree at an Australian university, international undergraduate students can apply to migrate to Australia and register to practise physiotherapy. This is likely to be a contributing factor to the growing numbers of international undergraduate students undertaking physiotherapy programs at Australian universities. A recent study commissioned by DIAC demonstrated a threefold increase

Table 4.2 Countries of education of international physiotherapy graduates completing the recognition process in Australia in 2003 and 2007 (Personal communication, Australian Physiotherapy Council)

Country of education	2003	2007
Argentina	1	0
Brazil	0	2
Egypt	1	0
England	7	22
Germany	3	4
Hong Kong	0	1
Hungary	0	2
India	5	31
Korea	1	0
Lebanon	0	1
Netherlands	2	7
Nigeria	0	1
Philippines	1	1
Singapore	1	1
South Africa	0	4
Taiwan	1	1
Thailand	0	1
United States	1	1
Zimbabwe	0	1
TOTAL	24	81

in international physiotherapy undergraduate students from 79 in 1996 to 239 in 2004 (Birrell et al 2006). The Australian Physiotherapy Council reported that between 2003 and 2007 the number of applications for assessment for migration purposes by international undergraduate students following graduation more than doubled from 24 to over 50 per year. The different educational and cultural backgrounds of the physiotherapy graduates working in Australia have the potential to influence the physiotherapy workforce through emergence of new practices.

Entry-level graduates and the physiotherapy workforce

In the latter half of the 20th century many new graduates began professional practice in public hospitals. The increased numbers of physiotherapy graduates and factors within the rapidly changing health system, including decreased length of stay of patients in hospital, expanded community care services, and increased use of technology, have led to a relative decrease in the number of positions in public hospitals. As a result, an increasing proportion of new graduates enter practice in public and private community settings. This is likely to be another factor that will shape the physiotherapy workforce because future career options and choices are often influenced by a practitioner's early experiences in the profession.

Postgraduate physiotherapy education and the workforce

Learning to be a physiotherapist is a lifelong process, beginning with admission to an accredited physiotherapy program and ending with retirement from active practice (European Region of World Confederation for Physical Therapy 2007). Lifelong learning and participation in continuing professional education is an expectation of the physiotherapy profession in Australia (Australian Physiotherapy Council 2006). In addition to self-directed learning and attendance at professional development courses and conferences, it is common for physiotherapists to continue to undertake additional postgraduate study at a university.

Australian physiotherapists were pioneers in the development of specialist skills and knowledge. The first postgraduate course in muscle re-education in Australia was organised in 1932 by Vera Carter and Charles Hembrow (Bentley 2006). The first postgraduate certificate course in manipulative (musculoskeletal) physiotherapy was established in 1965 by Geoffrey Maitland in South Australia. By 1974, this course had been extended to a 12-month postgraduate diploma program and was conducted in both South Australia and Western Australia. Since then, universities have also offered specialist physiotherapy programs in paediatrics, cardiorespiratory, neurology, women's health, gerontology and sports physiotherapy. In 1971 the Australian College of Physiotherapy was inaugurated, providing formal recognition for specialist physiotherapists in cardiorespiratory, musculoskeletal, neurological, occupational health, paediatric and sports physiotherapy (Bentley 2006). At the time of writing, completion of a university-based masters qualification is an important first stage of specialisation. Extensive clinical experience in the area of practice as well as postgraduate clinical doctorates provide further options for individual physiotherapists to gain recognition as specialists and contribute particular knowledge and skills to the workforce.

About one-half of physiotherapists describe their regular clinical work as 'generalist', and the others work in specialist areas. The Physiotherapy Labour Force Survey (Department of Human Services 2006) currently recognises as specialist areas of clinical physiotherapy practice: cardiorespiratory, occupational health, gerontology/geriatrics, musculoskeletal, neurological, paediatrics, women's health, orthopaedic, rehabilitation and sports physiotherapy. Additionally, many physiotherapists are employed in non-clinical areas, including administration or management and health promotion, and others work as academics and researchers. There are further opportunities for physiotherapy graduates in federal and state heath departments, in public health work and project work.

FACTORS INFLUENCING THE PHYSIOTHERAPY WORKFORCE

Ageing populations, changing technology and increasing community expectations are combining to place significant pressure on health systems. The World Health Report (2006) now estimates a shortage of about 4.3 million health workers, including physiotherapists.

Changing population demographics

Physiotherapy practice encompasses all body systems and illness and disease from acute to chronic and across the life span. However, physiotherapists have particularly valuable contributions to make to the health of communities as the proportion of older people increases. This demographic change adds to the burden of chronic diseases such as arthritis, cardiovascular disease, respiratory compromise, diabetes, obesity and dementia. As the proportion of the population aged over 65 years increases, so too the demand for physiotherapy services by this sector of the community grows. It has been reported that physiotherapy consultations by people 65 years and over grew by 43% between 2001 and 2004/5 (AIHW 2006). Additionally almost two million people aged 25–64 years were estimated to be living with a disability in Australia in 2003, with the most common group of disabling conditions affecting mobility (AIHW 2004).

Health funding

Australia has a dual-funded health system, with public facilities available to all through the Medicare Benefits Scheme (MBS) (Australian Government Medicare 2007). Physiotherapy is most commonly available at no direct cost in publicly funded facilities or through payment in a private practice. In the latter, clients pay directly or through their private health insurance scheme, or the physiotherapist is reimbursed through a third party payer such as a worker's compensation or motor accident insurance scheme. Some patients with chronic conditions may receive a limited number of treatments in a private practice through the MBS.

A higher percentage of women work in public sector physiotherapy, whereas men are more likely to work in private practice (AIHW 2006). Anderson and colleagues (2005) studied 2002 workforce data from the New South Wales (NSW) Physiotherapists Registration Board. They indicated a reduced workforce growth rate in the public sector from 50% in 1987 to 41.4% in 2002. Similar public sector percentages are reported across the country (AIHW 2006, Department of Human Services 2006). Long-term tracking of work patterns in NSW also demonstrates that a higher proportion of physiotherapists (39.4%) were working part-time (under 30 hours per week) in 2000 compared to 26.8% in 1975 (Anderson et al 2005).

Emerging health conditions

Physiotherapists increasingly have important and expanding roles to play in health promotion and the maintenance of optimal physical function and mental health. These roles are likely to grow as a result of the changes in population demographics but also as a result of deteriorating physical environments and the fragmenting of social structures. Emerging diseases such as severe acute respiratory syndrome (SARS), the ongoing devastation of human immunodeficiency virus (HIV) and acquired immunodeficiency syndrome (AIDS), and the re-emergence of killers such as tuberculosis will present both challenges and opportunities for future physiotherapists (McMeeken 2007).

Changes in technology

There is a strong focus on research evidence for practice in Australia. As a result there has been a reduction in the use of some treatment approaches such as electrotherapy where levels of research have been only modest (Herbert et al 2001). Nevertheless there is increasing opportunity to use sophisticated measurement tools including computer aided movement analyses such as Vicon® or Gaitrite®. Quantifiable feedback to patients on their performance in exercise or functional activities can be obtained via electromyography, pressure sensors and rapid feedback through digital photography or video recording. Electronic technology for patient self-management, such as transcutaneous electrical nerve stimulators or electromyography, requires patient education to ensure safety and effectiveness away from the direct guidance of the physiotherapist. Most recently there have been developments in low bandwidth telemedicine in physiotherapy assessment, diagnosis and management (Russell et al 2006).

Globalisation

Australian physiotherapists have long had a reputation for international mobility, although generally to English-speaking countries (Bentley 2006). The regulation and practice of physiotherapy, and therefore the characteristics of the workforce, vary considerably throughout the world. Key influences on the profession and the workforce include health care funding and systems, population demographics, cultural factors and political regimes. Cultural competence is a critical issue in working abroad, especially in less well resourced countries. Overseas electives during university study provide an opportunity for students to experience some of these issues first hand while working in another country and culture.

In most developed countries physiotherapy is recognised within the health care system and is funded either through the health system administered by the government, through health insurance agencies, through direct payment by the user or through a combination of these sources.

Carroll and McMeeken (2000) demonstrated continued high levels of global mobility of Australian qualified physiotherapists within the first two years after graduation. Their expectations of autonomous practice, to which they are accustomed in Australia, are not always fulfilled. Autonomy of practice commenced in Australia in 1976, and the World Confederation for Physical Therapy (WCPT) accepted a controversial proposal in 1978 by the Australian Physiotherapy Association and agreed that primary contact practice would be interpreted in each country according to its own standards (Bentley 2006). Three decades later, physiotherapists in many countries are still permitted to treat patients only following referral by a medical practitioner.

Table 4.3 summarises the key differences in education, regulation and autonomous practice in several countries, as well as the reported incidence of workforce shortage. A workforce shortage occurs in a country when the demand for physiotherapists exceeds supply. Variations among countries in both the number of physiotherapists and the size and demographics of the population create considerable differences in the demand for and supply of physiotherapists and, therefore, in reported workforce shortages (WCPT 2005).

Government strategies to address workforce shortages are normally developed in response to an existing shortage. It is not uncommon for there to be a delay between the reporting of workforce shortages and the development and implementation of strategies to increase supply – for example by increased allocation of funding for student places or by the education of physiotherapy assistants to facilitate more effective use of physiotherapists' knowledge and skills. As implementation of such strategies may also occur within workforce environments with different levels of demand, there is a risk of creating an oversupply of practitioners and subsequent unemployment. This

Table 4.3 Comparison by country of education, regulation and autonomous practice of physiotherapists and reported incidence of workforce shortages

Country	Educational program accreditation*	Registration or license to practise*	Examination for registration*	Autonomous practice*	Workforce shortage*,#
Australia	Yes – Australian Physiotherapy Council (APC)	Yes – mutual recognition of registration between states	Graduates of national universities – no, international graduates – yes	Yes	Yes
New Zealand	Yes – Physiotherapy Board of New Zealand	Yes	Graduates of national universities – no, international graduates – yes, for some only	Yes	Yes
Canada	Yes	Yes credentialling/ licensing with provincial college	Graduates of national universities and international graduates – yes	Yes	Yes
United States of America	Yes	Yes – state-based	Graduates of national universities and international graduates – yes	Limited	Yes
United Kingdom	Yes – multiple regulators	Yes	Graduates of national universities – no, international graduates – yes	Yes	Not for new graduates
Ireland	Yes	Yes	Graduates of national universities – no, international graduates – yes	Yes	Yes, but not for new graduates
Sweden	Yes	Yes		Yes	EU mobility
Japan		Registration in prefecture	Graduates of national universities and international graduates – yes	No	

Table 4.3 Comparison by country of education, regulation and autonomous practice of physiotherapists and reported incidence of workforce shortages *continued*				
Taiwan	Guidelines	Yes	Graduates of national universities and international graduates – yes	No

* Personal communication, Australian Physiotherapy Council
# World Confederation for Physical Therapy (2005)

has been reported in the United Kingdom where, in 2006, 70% of new graduate physiotherapists were unemployed (The Chartered Society of Physiotherapy 2006b).

WORKFORCE OPPORTUNITIES FOR PHYSIOTHERAPISTS

Expanding and extending the role of physiotherapists in the health workforce

Although physiotherapists in Australia have been autonomous primary contact practitioners since 1976, those working in publicly funded hospitals have continued to have less autonomy and primary contact status than their private sector colleagues. This has meant that, for many years, the valuable knowledge and skills of physiotherapists in the public health workforce have not been fully utilised, and the scope of practice of physiotherapists working within publicly funded hospitals has not reflected that of physiotherapists in private practice settings. For example, for a football player who injured his ankle during a weekend match and attended the emergency department at a hospital the initial assessment and treatment would be undertaken by a doctor, whereas if he attended a private physiotherapy practice the initial assessment and treatment would be undertaken by a physiotherapist.

In recent years, however, there has been greater recognition of the capacity of physiotherapists to work as autonomous primary contact practitioners in publicly funded hospitals. In orthopaedic and neurosurgery outpatient clinics, physiotherapists are making decisions regarding the need for surgical consultation or physiotherapy, and in emergency departments they are undertaking musculoskeletal injury triage and management. Physiotherapists are taking responsibility for falls assessment, managing paediatric orthopaedic and movement disorder clinics, and non-invasive ventilation services, and are offering urology/continence management (Nall 2006). These activities are within the normal realm of physiotherapy practice in the wider community but represent an expansion of the scope of physiotherapy practice within the public health sector. If the supply of physiotherapists is to meet the demands of expanded and extended roles within the health workforce there will be a need for other practitioners to assist physiotherapists with tasks that are low risk and repetitive in nature. This will require physiotherapists to engage with changes in roles and to optimise the new opportunities for physiotherapists within the health workforce. The inclusion of interprofessional education within entry-level physiotherapy programs and formal recognition of physiotherapy assistant programs within the Australian Qualifications Training Framework are both key elements for the restructuring of the physiotherapy workforce in Australia.

In 2000, an editorial in the *British Medical Journal* indicated changes that were considered essential in the UK to reconstruct the working relationship between doctors and other health professionals (Davies 2000). The changes would allow the relatively expensive (and frequently scarce) skills of medical practitioners to be better deployed, with less role overlap, and would allow other health professionals to undertake additional roles. Research supports the contention that such replacement maintains and often improves quality of care, does not lead to increased organisational costs and, in fact, is often more cost effective (Buchan & Dal Poz 2002). Increasingly, evidence from the UK and project reports from physiotherapy in Australia, such as those concerning physiotherapists undertaking assessments in general practice, indicate that there is extensive scope for physiotherapists to undertake primary care roles in the public sector and to extend their professional activities into additional areas. Physiotherapy interventions for certain conditions are more appropriate than medical care, and there is significant and growing research evidence demonstrating the clinical effectiveness and cost efficiency of physiotherapy. For example, the Physiotherapy Evidence Database (PEDro) website includes more than 6000 randomised controlled trials, systematic reviews and evidence-based clinical practice guidelines in physiotherapy. Despite this evidence, physiotherapists within the public sector are generally unable to provide many of these services without the approval of medical practitioners. Many patients with musculoskeletal conditions who wait for long periods for consultations with medical specialists could be assessed by physiotherapists and triaged as required into urgent consultation, physiotherapy management or discharge.

Concurrent with the expansion of roles in the public sector to better utilise the knowledge and skills of physiotherapists, there has been recognition of logical extensions of the scope of autonomous practice in some areas of physiotherapy to enable practitioners to provide a more seamless service to their patients. Postgraduate clinical doctorate programs are providing the education required for additional extended physiotherapy roles, with more pharmacology and clinical therapeutics and advanced radiology in their curricula (e.g. The University of Melbourne 2007). Physiotherapists who complete education in these extended areas and commence practice will be pioneers of the profession in Australia in terms of shaping the future roles of physiotherapists in the health workforce. Physiotherapy-led arrangements are becoming increasingly common in the UK for orthopaedic waiting lists and outpatient services (Hattam & Smeatham 1999, Weatherley & Hourigan 1998). A randomised controlled trial by Daker-White et al (1999) demonstrated that orthopaedic physiotherapy specialists are as effective as post-fellowship and assistant orthopaedic surgeons in assessing and managing general practitioner referrals to orthopaedic outpatient departments. Patients were more satisfied with their physiotherapy specialists, and it was reported that physiotherapists ordered fewer radiographs and were more cost effective. Similar results have been reported by Childs et al (2005) in a study in the USA, in which randomly selected physiotherapists and student physiotherapists undertook a standardised examination that assessed knowledge in managing musculoskeletal conditions. Medical students, interns, residents and a range of medical specialists had previously been assessed by the same examination. Higher levels of knowledge for managing musculoskeletal conditions were demonstrated by experienced physiotherapists than by medical staff at all levels except for orthopaedic surgeons.

Physiotherapists in the broader workforce

Physiotherapists are well placed to apply many of their skills in other areas of the workforce. Interactions with clients and the cycle of assessment, diagnosis, intervention and reassessment often result in the development of highly refined interpersonal and problem-solving skills by physiotherapists. The application of clinical reasoning and evidence-based practice often gives physiotherapists the capacity to think more strategically and globally. Many physiotherapists successfully translate these skills to nonclinical contexts and may further enhance their workforce opportunities by completion of postgraduate studies in non-physiotherapy disciplines including law, management and public health.

SUMMARY

The roles of physiotherapists in the health workforce will continue to evolve within a dynamic environment. Although local and global factors will create challenges for the profession, they will also create tremendous opportunities. The roles of physiotherapists in the future will be shaped not only by these extrinsic influences but by the preparedness of practitioners to adapt to change within the health workforce and by commitment within the profession to advocate for a strong and sustainable workforce that ensures high standards of physiotherapy for the Australian community in the 21st century.

Reflective questions

- What are the recruitment and retention issues facing the physiotherapy profession in your country and region?
- What are the factors that support a strong and sustainable profession? What are your responsibilities in relation to this matter?

References

Anderson G, Ellis E, Williams V et al 2005 Profile of the physiotherapy profession in New South Wales (1975–2002). Australian Journal of Physiotherapy 51:109–116

ABS 2006. Available: http://www.abs.gov.au/AUSSTATS/abs@.nsf/mf/ 3105.0.65.001 12 Dec 2007

ABS 2007. Available: http://www.abs.gov.au/ausstats/abs@.nsf/mf/3101.0/ 12 Dec 2007

Australian Government Medicare 2007. Available: http://www.medicareaustralia.gov.au/ 12 Dec 2007

AIHW 2004 Disability and its relationship to health conditions and other factors. Available: http://www.aihw.gov.au/publications/index.cfm/title/10082 12 Dec 2007

AIHW 2006 Physiotherapy labour force 2002. AIHW cat. no. HWL 37. Health and Labour Force Series no. 36, AIHW, Canberra

Australian Physiotherapy Council 2006 Australian Standards for Physiotherapy. Australian Physiotherapy Council, Canberra

Australian Physiotherapy Council 2007 Australian Physiotherapy Council Annual Report 2006–2007. Available: http://www.physiocouncil.com.au 12 Dec 2007

Bentley P 2006 The path to professionalism: Physiotherapy in Australia to the 1980s. Australian Physiotherapy Association, Melbourne

Birrell B, Hawthorne L, Richardson S 2006 Evaluation of the general skilled migration categories. Available: http://www.immi.gov.au/media/publications/research/gsm-report/index.htm 18 Dec 2007

Buchan J, Dal Poz M R 2002 Skill mix in the health care workforce: reviewing the evidence. Bulletin of the World Health Organization 80(7):575–580

Carroll S, McMeeken J M 2000 Establishing the value of rural clinical placements during undergraduate allied health education. Coordinating Unit for Rural Health Education in Victoria, Melbourne

Childs J D, Whitman J M, Sizer P S et al 2005 A description of physical therapists' knowledge in managing musculoskeletal conditions. BMC Musculoskeletal Disorders 6:32. Available: http://www.pubmedcentral.nih.gov 12 Dec 2007

Chipchase L S, Galley P, Jull G et al 2006 Looking back at 100 years of physiotherapy education in Australia. Australian Journal of Physiotherapy 52:3–7

Daker-White G, Carr A J, Harvey I et al 1999 A randomised controlled trial: shifting boundaries of doctors and physiotherapists in orthopaedic outpatient departments. Journal of Epidemiology and Community Health 53(10):643–650

Davies C 2000 Getting health professionals to work together. British Medical Journal 320:1021–1022

DEWR 2007 National state skills shortage list. Available: http://jobguide.thegoodguides.com.au/text/skillsShortages.cfm 12 Dec 2007

Department of Human Services 2006 Physiotherapy labour force Victoria 2003–04. Victorian Government Department of Human Services, Melbourne

DIAC 2007. Available: http://www.immi.gov.au/skilled/general-skilled-migration/skilled-occupations/occupations-in-demand.html 12 Dec 2007

European Region of World Confederation for Physical Therapy 2007. Available: http:/www. physio-europe.org 12 Dec 2007

Hattam P, Smeatham A 1999 Evaluation of an orthopaedic screening service in primary care. British Journal of Clinical Governance 4(2):45–49

Herbert R D, Maher C G, Moseley A M et al 2001 Effective physiotherapy. British Medical Journal 323:788–790

Human Capital Alliance 2005 Recruitment and retention of allied health professionals in Victoria – a literature review. (Report to the Victorian Government Department of Human Services) Human Capital Alliance, Melbourne

McMeeken J M 2007 Physiotherapy education in Australia. Physical Therapy Reviews 12:83–91

McMeeken J M, Grant R, Webb G et al 2008 Australian physiotherapy student intake is increasing and attrition remains lower than the university average: a demographic study. Journal of Physiotherapy 54(1):65–71

McMeeken J M, Webb G, Krause K L et al 2005 Learning outcomes and curriculum development in Australian physiotherapy education. Available: http://www.physiotherapy.edu.au/physiotherapy/go 12 Dec 2007

Nall C 2006 Australian Physiotherapy Association submission to the Productivity Commission. Available: http://www.apa.advsol.com.au/independent/documents/ submissions/HealthfundingrepsApr06.pdf 10 Dec 2006

Russell T G, Theodoros D G, Wootton R 2006 Assessing the risk of falls in the elderly via low-bandwidth telemedicine. Journal of Telemedicine and Telecare 12(suppl 1):113–4

Schofield D J, Fletcher S L 2007 The physiotherapy workforce is ageing, becoming more masculinised, and is working longer hours: a demographic study. Australian Journal of Physiotherapy 53:121–126

The Chartered Society of Physiotherapy 2006a Response to the workforce review team provisional recommendations for NHS physiotherapy workforce for England 2007/08. Available: http://www.csp.org.uk/director/newsandevents/physioalerts.cfm?item_id=DAD4B100C348785389C9080D970D6D14 18 Dec 2007

The Chartered Society of Physiotherapy 2006b Urgent action needed to secure jobs for newly qualified physios. 7 out of 10 still out of work, says CSP. Available: http://www.csp.org.uk/director/newsandevents/news.cfm?item_id=95BD9AB500AC0B04CB2C380167B8603A 12 Dec 2007

The University of Melbourne 2007 Doctor of Clinical Physiotherapy overview 2007 Available: www.physioth.unimelb.edu.au/programs/pgrad/progs/coursework/dcp/ 12 Dec 2007

The World Health Report 2006 Working together for health 2006. Available: http://http://www.who.int/whr/2006/en/index.html 12 Dec 2007

WCPT 2005. Available: http://www.wcpt.org/ 12 Oct 2007

Weatherley C R, Hourigan P G 1998 Triage of back pain by physiotherapists in orthopaedic clinics. Journal of the Royal Society of Medicine 91:377–379

BECOMING A MEMBER OF A HEALTH PROFESSION: A JOURNEY OF SOCIALISATION

five

Joy Higgs, Jill Hummell and Maggie Roe-Shaw

Key content

- Joining the profession
- Professional socialisation

INTRODUCTION

Joining the physiotherapy profession is at the same time the end point of completing a professional entry degree program, the starting point of a career in physiotherapy, and part of an ongoing journey of becoming a member of this health profession. Membership of the physiotherapy profession begins with joining the profession, becoming registered through a physiotherapy regulatory authority or registration board, and (often) choosing to join a professional association. It involves a commitment throughout one's career to meet the expectations set for health professionals by society, the workplace and the profession, and to recognise that the privileged place in society accorded to professionals comes with the obligation and responsibility to meet those expectations.

In this chapter we report on our collaborations in doctoral research (Hummell 2007, Roe-Shaw 2004) that examined the nature of professions and the processes involved in becoming a health professional, particularly a physiotherapist, and the influences of education, the workplace and mentors on this process. And we look at the experiences that may be encountered during the process of professional socialisation.

WHAT IS A PROFESSION?

A *profession* is a self-regulated occupational group having a body of knowledge, an inherent culture and a recognised role in serving society. Professions operate under continual scrutiny and development, and are self-regulated, accountable and guided by a code of ethical conduct in practice decisions and actions. Membership of a profession requires completion of an appropriate (commonly degree-based) intensive educational program. Professionalisation is the transformation of an occupational group into a profession, producing a distinguishable professional group and culture.

The term *professional* can be used to refer to a member of a profession. It can also describe a standard of conduct expected of members of a profession. Professional behaviour (or *professionalism*) comprises those actions, standards and considerations of ethical and humanistic conduct expected by society and by professional associations from members of professions. Being a member of a *health profession* such as physiotherapy brings additional challenges. Physiotherapists provide services to members of society and have a duty of care towards them. Moreover, their clients are often (not always) vulnerable through illness, pain and disability. To enhance people's wellbeing is the prime objective.

PROFESSIONAL SOCIALISATION AND DEVELOPING A PROFESSIONAL IDENTITY

Professional socialisation refers to the acculturation process (that occurs through entry education, reflection, professional development and engagement in professional work interactions) by which an individual develops both the expected capabilities of the profession and a sense of professional identity and responsibility.

During professional socialisation, emerging members of a profession become immersed in the culture of their profession and workplaces, and through this acculturation they develop an understanding of:

- professional codes of conduct and boundaries delineating the acceptable from the (professional) taboo, along with the professional, legal and ethical sanctions associated with transgressions from professional conduct
- the roles and responsibilities of members of the profession and the role relationship between practitioners and other professionals (of the same and related professions), the public and other people encountered during their work
- the professional work context, including the goals, roles and procedures of that system (Cant & Higgs 1999).

The attributes, capabilities and behaviours acquired during professional socialisation (Cant & Higgs 1999) include:

- values and behaviour patterns that enable individuals to fulfil the role society expects of members of that profession (Ewan 1988). This includes having a community-oriented rather than self-oriented interest, and behaviour that reflects a duty of care
- an attitude and behaviour consistent with professionalism, comprising learned value sets and codes of behaviour and an occupational morality
- an identity as a member of a particular profession
- 'a self-image which permits feelings of personal adequacy and satisfaction in the performance of the expected role' (Ewan 1988, p 85)
- the technical ability to perform the roles inherent in the profession, based on the acquisition of a body of esoteric knowledge and technical skills
- the ability to use generic skills such as communication skills as part of performing responsibly and competently as a professional and as a graduate of higher education
- a commitment to maintaining competence and the provision of high quality health care services.

Professional socialisation is not a single event, nor does it occur in a particular context or period; it is a continuing process because the information base of the profession changes and because the work context and professional culture are continually evolving (Cant & Higgs 1999). It involves anticipatory socialisation or the formulation of expectations about one's future professional role, it occurs during university education (both on and off campus) and in workplace settings, it is a key element of the experience of newly qualified professionals, and it reflects the ongoing evolution of the practitioner's professional identity and capabilities that continues to occur across his or her career.

PROFESSIONAL SOCIALISATION IN THE PRE-GRADUATION YEARS

Today there are many educational paths to entry into the physiotherapy profession: undergraduate, masters entry and doctoral entry degrees. In each case students may have completed a previous degree in a range of fields from arts to science, education, biomedical science or closely related programs such as exercise and sports sciences and human movement sciences. Students' backgrounds can vary considerably in relation to their life experiences and roles, past health and physiotherapy encounters and work experience. All of these learning situations bring different entry abilities, interests and understandings, upon which physiotherapy education builds.

A number of challenges are faced by teachers, curriculum developers, clinical educators, professional role models and learners during the pre-graduation years of professional socialisation. In Chapter 9 the authors discuss the notion and nature of communities of practice and the impact of these learning contexts on promoting learning that is situated or contextualised within the cultures of physiotherapy and health care. In essence, each practice community and practice preparation community (including the professional entry curriculum environment) shapes students' learning, their sense of what a physiotherapist and a health professional should be and what is expected of them in their workplaces and work roles. When students graduate from these programs they should have acquired a professional identity, the expected practice competencies (as a minimal expectation) as determined by their professional bodies (e.g. the Australian Physiotherapy Association), the capacity to critique and develop themselves as physiotherapy professionals, and relevant generic competencies. These generic competencies include the ability to apply theoretical knowledge in practice situations, provide rationales for clinical decisions, communicate effectively with clients and staff and have a lifelong learning approach to their careers (Adamson et al 1996).

Professional entry programs have a responsibility to prepare students for entry-level physiotherapy practice as beginning practitioners. The workplace contributes to this professional entry education, primarily through the provision of student clinical placements, and then shares in the professional development responsibility of graduates. Clinical placements (whether in blocks or a final clinical year) provide an induction and *practice run* for dealing with workplace realities. Placements help to frame students' expectations and perceptions of a variety of physiotherapy workplaces (e.g. private practice, hospitals, community settings). In these contexts students become socialised into their profession. They assess and treat clients and, although their supervisor retains the legal responsibility for overall client care and observes client outcomes, what they do *really matters* (Roe-Shaw 2004). Students also develop working relationships with other physiotherapists and team members from a range of professions.

There are often gaps between the taught expectations of the workplace (generated in professional entry program curricula) and practice expectations after graduation. To some extent these gaps are unavoidable because the consequences of actions in classroom simulations with fellow students are not as great as with ill or disabled clients in clinical settings (Roe-Shaw 2004). Sometimes these gaps arise from avoidable educational deficiencies, such as the isolation of academics from the real world, lack of clinical or teaching expertise of clinical educators, inadequate resourcing or patient access in clinical settings, and clinical systems that are unprepared for or unsupportive of student education (Roe-Shaw 2004). Addressing such barriers to quality clinical education is the responsibility of educators and health care providers, both of whom have a role in producing competent future health care employees. Students also have an important role in ensuring the quality of their clinical education experience and outcomes. They should be active agents in their education, self-directed learners and self-evaluators, and these are roles they should carry forward into their professional lives.

Physiotherapists' educational preparation is influential in shaping their experiences of early employment. The participants in Hummel's (2007) study of allied health graduates' first year of employment highly valued their clinical placements and the university subjects with high professional relevance and direct clinical application because these assisted their successful integration into the workplace, particularly their adjustment transition. Australian physiotherapists participating in the research of Hunt et al (1998, 1999) and Hummell (2007) believed that their professional entry courses adequately prepared them for the core components of their initial jobs. This preparation contributed to their ability to provide quality client services commensurate with their knowledge, skills and experience, to use clinical reasoning, reflection, problem-solving and self-directed learning skills, to use evidence from a range of sources and to adopt an evaluative approach to client service provision (Hummell 2007). However, new graduates perceived themselves as inadequately prepared for the complex lived realities of their work roles and the work stressors they experienced (Hummell 2007, Roe-Shaw 2004).

Clinical educators, with their expertise in physiotherapy and teaching, are commonly highly influential in shaping the quality of student learning during clinical placements. Clinical educators organise the placement program and access to patients; they facilitate students' learning and supervise their practice (including patient assessment, treatment and management), provide constructive feedback and assess students' performance. Finding appropriate patients for individual students is a key role for clinical educators. All students benefit from a progression from familiar and easy clients to more difficult and unfamiliar clients and from light to heavy client caseloads. Not only does this facilitate their learning in a structured learning environment, it also prepares them progressively for graduate workload levels. Lack of such grading in learning and preparation has been identified as contributing to reality shock in the workplace. Roe-Shaw's (2004) New Zealand study of the professional socialisation of physiotherapists found the greatest level of reality shock was reported by graduates who had not experienced increasing workload levels and complexity during student placements. They entered the workforce expecting high levels of support from experienced physiotherapists, light caseloads and a limited level of responsibility. They were shocked to discover that workplace reality involved high direct client caseloads with limited supervision or mentoring and complex non-client work tasks such as meetings, ward rounds, patient note writing, team meetings and family meetings. Hummell (2007) found that clinical placements incorporating a graded increase in client workloads, responsibility and accountability and a graded reduction in direct supervision, in combination with effective supervision and support, contributed to graduates' smooth transition into the workplace and a reduced level of reality shock. Participants in her research also reported that, particularly in the final year of the course, university subjects that addressed the realities of initial employment, including the complexity of work roles, managing work stressors and seeking supervision/mentoring, reduced their reality shock and facilitated their initial workplace transition.

BECOMING A MEMBER OF A HEALTH PROFESSION – THE IMPORTANT FIRST YEAR AFTER GRADUATION

The commitment and skill of practitioners in the workplace have been shown to be influenced by the systems and resources available to support them (Southon 1994). Within each workplace, individuals build competency in their professional role. In the physiotherapy profession, workplaces set expectations of their workers in relation to responsibilities and privileges. Workplace system rules, restrictions, norms and expectations are important in the professional socialisation process in the context of workplace learning. The literature on workplace learning focuses on improving performance for the benefit of the organisation and improving learning for the benefit of the employee (Boud 1998). Each workplace is different, and systems can vary considerably. Some workplaces have strongly supportive cultures and are rich in technology and equipment available for physiotherapy practice, whereas others lack such cultures and resources. For New Zealand physiotherapists Roe-Shaw (2004) identified the impact of the variations in workplace system rules, restrictions, norms and expectations on new graduates' professional socialisation experiences. Factors that could positively influence these physiotherapists' socialisation included effective support and mentoring systems, adequate professional development opportunities, and resources. Factors that could negatively influence these experiences included limited formal and informal support and mentoring systems, hospital hierarchy and bureaucracy, rotation difficulties (including lack of choice), on-call dilemmas, lack of professional development opportunities and limited resources such as email, internet and libraries (Roe-Shaw 2004).

Hummell's doctoral research (2007) examined Australian physiotherapy graduates' first year of work experience and produced a *model of workplace integration of allied health graduates in the first year of employment* (see Fig. 5.1). In this model, the integration of new graduates into the workforce and workplaces is interpreted as a multi-dimensional process. The dimensions are (a) graduates' experiences, (b) professional entry education, (c) workplace influences, and (d) graduate factors such as the ability to cope with stress. Each of these dimensions influences the quality of graduates' experiences, their workplace transitions and the outcomes for workplaces and graduates. The model also identifies the complex relationships between these influences and outcomes, and recognises the crucial importance of supportive workplace environments in promoting graduates' successful workplace and workforce integration, and positive graduate and workplace outcomes. It clearly identifies that the quality of graduates' educational preparation (see above), the workplace environment, and graduates' abilities and attributes can facilitate or impair their workplace transitions, outcomes, workplace and workforce integration and professional socialisation.

Hummell (2007) found that allied health graduates in their first year of employment successfully socialised into their professions and achieved the following outcomes when they worked in highly supportive workplace environments: successful transitions to higher levels of performance during the first year, enhanced skill development, confidence, job satisfaction, stress management skills and the capacity to provide quality

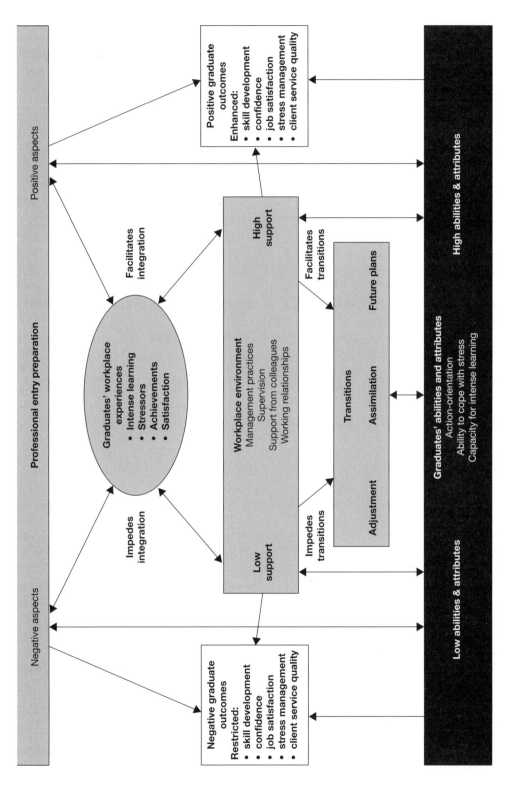

Fig. 5.1 Model of workplace integration of allied health graduates in the first year of employment. Reproduced from *Allied health graduates' first year of employment*, 2007, by J Hummell, Unpublished PhD thesis, The University of Sydney, p 195

client services commensurate with their knowledge, skills and experience. In contrast, unsupportive workplace environments were found to impair graduates' professional socialisation, transitions and graduate attributes and satisfaction; these graduates perceived themselves as providing client services of limited quality and seriously considered resigning from the workplace and potentially leaving their profession. Roe-Shaw's (2004) New Zealand participants experienced dissatisfaction with their career choices more frequently than those in Hummell's (2007) Australian study.

Hummell (2007) identified three transitions experienced by graduates in their first year of employment. These were (a) adjustment to the workplace and work role, which tended to occur in the first 6 months, (b) assimilation into the workplace and workforce, which tended to occur in the second 6 months, and (c) future workforce planning, which occurred towards the end of the first year in the workforce. Key indicators of a successful (first) *adjustment* transition were identified as: completing core client and non-client duties with confidence and competence, lower levels of stress and fatigue than in the early months of employment, a sense of belonging to the physiotherapy profession and workplace, and self-assurance about when to seek assistance from supervisors and when to be autonomous. Key indicators of a successful *assimilation* were identified as acceptance and respect as integral team members by physiotherapy and multidisciplinary colleagues and a perception of themselves as confident and competent professionals who made clear contributions to client service provision. Key indicators of a successful *future workforce planning* transition were identified as an enthusiasm for physiotherapy's contribution to client services and broad or specific plans to continue working as a physiotherapist.

The first year of employment for physiotherapists is characterised by intense learning, work stressors and satisfaction (Hummell 2007, Solomon & Miller 2005). For Australian (Hummell 2007) and Canadian (Solomon & Miller 2005) physiotherapists, the positive aspects of their work most commonly exceeded the negative aspects. In contrast, Roe-Shaw (2004) found that recently graduated physiotherapists in New Zealand were disappointed in the lack of professional status accorded to them in hospital settings. A common theme was a lack of awareness in medical and other allied health professions of the role and professional entry education of physiotherapists. A key part of the professional socialisation of new graduates is recognition of their role by those in the workplace. This adds to a person's sense of professional identity and job satisfaction (Wright 1997). Lack of recognition by workplace colleagues can result in job dissatisfaction, burnout and premature exit from the profession.

A key feature of physiotherapists' initial employment is the wide range of work stressors encountered and the high level of stress experienced (Hummell 2007, Tryssenaar & Perkins 2001). Key sources of stress are the graduates' limited knowledge, skills and experience, the life and death issues experienced in intensive care units during night rotations (Hummell 2007), role issues (Miller et al 2005), and conflict with other team members or clients (Roe-Shaw 2004). The steep learning curve and high level of work stress tend to be more marked in the early months of the initial job (Hummell 2007, Solomon & Miller 2005). Physiotherapists' initial workplace experiences are also characterised by a steady although uneven growth in confidence in their work role and job satisfaction gained from a range of sources, but most importantly from observing and contributing to client progress (Hummell 2007, Solomon & Miller 2005). Hummell (2007) found that recently graduated physiotherapists perceived that they provided quality client services within the limitations of their knowledge, skills and experience.

Roe-Shaw's (2004) study of recent physiotherapy graduates in New Zealand produced a model of the experience of professional socialisation (see Table 5.1). The model encompassed two sets of themes. The first related to *experiences of professional socialisation*, including the dynamic workplace interactions of seeking, searching, coping and developing. The second set of themes related to the *context of professional socialisation* and included systemic, personal and professional barriers and enablers to professional socialisation in each individual participant's workplace.

Table 5.1 Workplace experiences of professional socialisation. Based on *Workplace realities and professional socialisation of recently graduated physiotherapists in New Zealand*, 2004, by M Roe-Shaw, Unpublished PhD thesis, Otago University

Context themes	Experience themes
1. Undergraduate preparation for workplace reality and professional role This refers to weaving together the impact of undergraduate preparation on recently graduated physiotherapists when placed in the reality role of being a physiotherapist in the workplace.	**1. Seeking a sense of professional direction and identity** Part of professional socialisation involves coming to understand what it means to be a member of a profession and gaining a unique professional identity in that profession, and includes a sense of where I might be going in the profession.
2. Mentoring and collegial support This refers to the mentors and senior staff who provide new members of the professional group with advice, support and encouragement as they develop a workplace ethic.	**2. Searching for professionalism in the workplace** Part of professional socialisation involves seeking to understand professionalism in the workplace by looking for role models who demonstrate qualities, standards and typical features of the profession, including skills, knowledge, attitudes, values and competence within the profession.
3. Professional recognition of person and role This refers to the recognition of physiotherapy as a profession that has a useful and defined role in the hospital or private practice context. It includes recognition of the skills and knowledge base of a recently graduated physiotherapist as well as the patients' perceptions of the role of physiotherapists.	**3. Coping with role dissonance** Part of professional socialisation involves coming to terms with and juggling differences in expectations and realities in the competing demands of roles and goals encountered in the workplace.
4. System support and resources This refers to the health care system, the supports, constraints and resources that are available for recently graduated physiotherapists in the workplace. It includes available resources and supports and their impact on physiotherapists' ability to provide best practice service to their patients.	**4. Developing the capability to address the different roles and functions in physiotherapy practice** Part of professional socialisation involves developing the capability, skills and attitudes to be able to perform the various roles that comprise professional responsibilities.
5. System rules, restrictions, norms and expectations This refers to the different health care systems in public hospitals and in private practices, which have a clearly defined role for physiotherapists, and the impact of these systems on each individual's practice.	**5. Coping with different practice models within and beyond physiotherapy** Part of professional socialisation involves recognising, choosing and dealing with different practice models, the espoused best practice model taught within the academic institution, and the different workplace practice models such as patient-centred care and evidence-based practice.

Table 5.1 Workplace experiences of professional socialisation. Based on *Workplace realities and professional socialisation of recently graduated physiotherapists in New Zealand*, 2004, by M Roe-Shaw, Unpublished PhD thesis, Otago University   *continued*

6. Professional development opportunities This refers to the professional development opportunities and restrictions within the workplace. It includes the expectations of recent graduates of professional development and supervision, and the reality of professional development opportunities.	**6. Seeking career and job satisfaction** Part of professional socialisation involves recent graduates seeking to find their feet, to consolidate their professional knowledge and see a future in the physiotherapy profession. It includes seeking and gaining a sense of satisfaction in the choice and the realities of job and career.

7. Career options
This refers to the career structures and opportunities that exist in physiotherapy in both the public and private sectors.

8. Financial issues
This refers to the loans that physiotherapy students take out to pay their course fees and the remuneration that recent graduates receive in the public and private sector.

When Table 5.1 and Figure 5.1 are compared, a number of common influences on recent graduates' workplace experiences can be identified. These include the level of workplace support, the effectiveness of mentors/supervisors, the availability of learning opportunities, the attributes of graduates and the quality of professional entry programs. Roe-Shaw's (2004) research findings emphasised socialisation, whereas Hummell's (2007) research findings placed a greater emphasis on graduates' work roles, yet both identified the significant impact of the workplace setting and culture on graduates' experiences. Most of Hummell's participants had positive experiences, but the majority of Roe-Shaw's did not. In both studies, graduates were active agents in their workplace integration and professional socialisation. They experienced marked challenges in their initial employment and many demonstrated resilience (Hummell 2007) or *saving grace* (Roe-Shaw 2004) when faced with high levels of work stress and limited workplace support.

GRADUATE NARRATIVES: FLOURISHING, COPING AND STRUGGLING

In Hummell's (2007) research, narratives constructed from the stories of allied health graduates' first year of employment reflected three experience modes: flourishing, coping and struggling. These modes are illustrated by the following quotes. The quality of graduates' educational preparation and workplace environment and their abilities and attributes influenced these experience modes. Graduates who were flourishing tended to have consistently positive experiences, transitions and outcomes throughout their first year of employment. Those who were coping or struggling tended to have experiences that varied from positive to highly negative. Some graduates moved from struggling to coping or vice versa during their initial employment.

Flourishing

I got set up really well from the start because I had an experienced therapist as my supervisor. She was just the best for making a new grad feel relaxed and confident and was very clear about her expectations. We met each week to start with and then each fortnight for about an hour. I got lots of informal supervision too.

The autonomy is fantastic. I've had to be pretty independent, that was just expected of us. But I knew that if I had any problems I could have called my supervisor or someone more senior and they would have been happy to help.

I think the biggest highlight has been treating someone and seeing a difference, seeing something work that I've done – it's huge. Also I'm lucky to get heaps of thank-yous every day from clients and families. The other therapists are also really fantastic at letting me know that I'm doing a top job.

I'm in a really supportive workplace, and I've learnt so much from watching what other therapists do, and listening to them and how they've dealt with certain situations or clients. You learn from experience, but also from listening and watching other people, talking about things with other people. I'm really glad I've had that. My manager and colleagues have been really receptive to any ideas I've had or new ways of doing things that I had learned at uni.

Coping

When I started I had total information overload. Part of me still felt like a student in the first few months of work too, and fair enough it was my first year out, but I got used to it all and it improved.

It took me about 6 months to feel confident with everything I do. One of the things that helped me gain confidence was having a good honest chat with my supervisor following a particularly difficult period. Realising that she was there to help me and didn't expect me to know everything without guidance was a relief.

Mostly work's pretty good. It's just the issues, like some of the staff who treat me like I don't know anything, the clients who don't improve and some of the bureaucracy, that's the hard part to deal with.

The last year has been a big achievement, pretty stressful too, especially in the early months. It's been a pretty big learning experience, that's for sure. I think I'd like to stay working here for a bit longer, increase my skills and then move on to a different workplace or client group.

Struggling

The lack of supervision has been hard, especially in my first couple of months. I came out of uni where I did highly supervised treatments to nothing – no supervision. Sometimes it's nice when I have patients and I know what to do, but I also get the patients who I don't have a clue about, and I have no-one to ask. Unless I seek out help, I've been more or less by myself.

I'm not learning a lot because I'm just treating the same small client group. There's a bit of learning in there, when I do something and it doesn't work and I think what else can I try and I talk to the other grade ones and they give me ideas. It took me about 6 months to feel confident with my clients. Some aren't making progress so that's hard.

The other grade ones in my section are lovely, without them I would have been ready to quit. Most have the same length of experience as me, others are 3 or 4 years out and they're really supportive, 'I know it's hard but you'll get through'.

With some staff there's a lack of respect for allied health professionals and some are such negative people. It's very stressful. Plus for the past 6 months we've been understaffed with senior staff so that's been hard. I've decided that if things don't improve soon, I'm going to look for another job. I love the client work that I do, but I realise that I don't get the support or the opportunities to learn that I want.

GRADUATES' ABILITIES AND ATTRIBUTES AND THEIR ROLE IN SOCIALISATION

Allied health graduates in their first year of employment can be and desirably should be active agents in their own workplace transitions and professional socialisation. Hummel's (2007) participants demonstrated the following key abilities and attributes: action-orientation, an ability to deal resiliently with work stress, and a capacity for intense learning. They used their initiative to enhance the quality of their client service provision, learning and skill development (see also Solomon & Miller 2005), to manage work stressors (see also Tryssenaar & Perkins 2001) and to obtain professional supervision and support (see also Steenbergen & Mackenzie, 2004). A number of the participants in Roe-Shaw's study (2004) were able to overcome the deficiencies and difficulties encountered in their workplaces due to an inherent strength of character that she called 'saving grace' and defined as graduates' valuing of their role, potential and rewards in patient care in the midst of angst and concern about difficulties faced in their work roles and settings.

SHARED RESPONSIBILITIES IN SHAPING THE PROFESSIONAL SOCIALISATION JOURNEY

Professional socialisation occurs in communities of practice. It is a responsibility shared by the individual professional, peers, mentors, supervisors, managers and organisations.

The professional's (own) responsibility

Responsibility for one's professional development comes with the title of professional. This responsibility involves making choices, including about career plans, commitment to the profession and clients, involvement in continuing professional education (CPE), and managing work challenges. For Hummell's (2007) participants, intense learning and a strong motivation to learn their work role as quickly and effectively as possible were key to enabling them to provide quality services to their clients. For Roe-Shaw's (2004) participants it was the value they placed on their role in helping their patients that helped them survive the angst of difficult workplaces. Physiotherapists use reflection, talking with supportive managers, supervisors and colleagues, and being action-oriented to cope with workplace demands and stress. These strategies are successful when stressors are short-term and when they achieve positive outcomes (Hummell 2007). When stressors are longer term and unresolved, graduates' coping strategies are undermined (Hummell 2007, Roe-Shaw 2004).

The potential contributions of mentors, supervisors and peers

The workplace contributes to professional socialisation by providing system support and people support. People support may include mentoring, supervision, collegial including peer support, and networking. Effective mentoring, supervision and collegial support have been identified as important in assisting recent graduates to learn their work roles and integrate into the workplace and workforce (Hummell 2007, Solomon & Miller 2005). Mentoring and supervision from senior physiotherapists in particular are perceived as playing key roles in facilitating the professional development and socialisation of these new graduates through providing support and feedback, monitoring clinical and professional behaviour standards and acting as role models (Miller et al 2005, Roe-Shaw 2004). Mentoring has been described as having chemistry, serendipity and reciprocity (Hawkey 1997) that is symbiotic by nature and mutually beneficial. Networking extends beyond the boundaries of the workplace to link up with colleagues via email, telephone or in person (e.g. at physiotherapy association branch meetings).

In some settings, such as regional and remote areas of Australia, support from senior colleagues is limited (Struber 2004). Roe-Shaw (2004) found that the shortage of senior physiotherapists in New Zealand hospitals resulted in a constant reliance on younger staff to take over supervisory duties for new graduates and professional entrants. In such circumstances new graduates, facing a steep learning curve, may lack feedback, collegial support, supervision, peer group learning and career role models.

The potential contribution of mentors, supervisors and colleagues, including peers, to the professional socialisation journey is significant. In both Hummell's (2007) and Roe-Shaw's (2004) studies, recent graduates who experienced positive mentoring/supervision and collegial support described themselves as *motivated* and *enthusiastic* about their physiotherapy practice. In contrast, those who were *thrown in the deep end* and received limited feedback about their workplace practice from supervisors or senior colleagues experienced fears that they were not effective practitioners.

The roles and responsibilities of managers and the organisations

Organisation and physiotherapy managers have a clear human and financial responsibility to provide supportive workplace environments that, according to recent research (Hummell 2007, Roe-Shaw 2004, Solomon & Miller 2005), promote the development of positive outcomes of good management frameworks for graduates, workplaces and clients. Supportive workplaces implement sound management practices, namely the provision of comprehensive workplace orientations, quality supervision, support, stress management and communication systems, multiple CPE opportunities and appropriate resources (Hummell 2007).

Organisation managers have a critical role in establishing supportive workplace cultures primarily through developing effective management systems. These aim to ensure adequate staffing levels that enable graduates in their first year of employment to receive appropriate levels of professional supervision and support, adequate physical resources that allow these graduates and other staff to work effectively, and the employment of skilled professional managers. Physiotherapy managers need to implement sound management practices and employ appropriately skilled supervisors or senior staff members who have a positive attitude towards helping others learn. Hummell (2007) recommended the following organisational features for professional managers relevant to each dimension of sound management practices:

- well-organised and welcoming workplace orientation
- effective supervision/mentoring systems that commence on the first day of employment
- well thought-out formal and informal support systems
- transparent communication systems
- structured and flexible stress management processes and systems
- broad-based continuing professional education opportunities
- appropriate human and physical resources.

SUMMARY

Several core themes inform this discussion of professional socialisation. The first is that acculturation occurs inevitably and novices or newcomers entering the workplace, profession or team are drawn into the culture, learning from existing members/staff what it means to be a member of the group. This places responsibility for the success and quality of work teams and client outcomes on the shoulders of incomers, insiders and system managers. Professional socialisation should not be left to chance. Newcomers should not be left to swim, sink or drop out of the system. Rather, given the investment in time, money and hope that all parties are committing to and the consequences to the health and wellbeing of therapists and their patients that could result, professional socialisation should be a collaboration in good practice evolution.

Reflective questions

- Consider your own journey of professional socialisation. What factors have influenced this journey?
- How are you influencing and enhancing the professional socialisation of students and colleagues you are working with?

References

Adamson B, Harris L, Heard R et al 1996 University education and workplace requirements. The University of Sydney Printing Services, Sydney

Boud D 1998 A new focus on workplace learning research. In: Boud D (ed) Current issues and new agendas. National Centre for Vocational Education Research, Leabrook, SA, pp 1–8

Cant R, Higgs J 1999 Professional socialisation. In: Higgs J, Edwards, H (eds) Educating beginning practitioners: challenges for health professional education. Butterworth-Heinemann, Oxford, pp 46–51

Ewan C 1988 Becoming a doctor. In: Cox K, Ewan, C E (eds) The medical teacher, 2nd edn. Churchill Livingstone, Edinburgh, pp 85–89

Hawkey K 1997 Roles, responsibilities and relationships in mentoring: a literature review and agenda for research. Journal of Teacher Education 48(1):325–335

Hummell J 2007 Allied health graduates' first year of employment. Unpublished PhD thesis, The University of Sydney, Australia

Hunt A, Adamson B, Harris L 1998 Physiotherapists' perceptions of the gap between education and practice. Physiotherapy Theory and Practice 14(4):125–138

Hunt A, Adamson B, Harris L 1999 Community and workplace expectations of health science graduates. In: Higgs J, Edwards H (eds) Educating beginning practitioners: challenges for health professional education. Butterworth-Heinemann, Oxford, pp 38–45

Miller P A, Solomon P, Giacomini M et al 2005 Experiences of novice physiotherapists adapting to their role in acute care hospitals. Physiotherapy Canada 57(2):145–153

Roe-Shaw M 2004 Workplace realities and professional socialisation of recently graduated physiotherapists in New Zealand. Unpublished PhD thesis, Otago University, New Zealand

Solomon P, Miller P A 2005 Qualitative study of novice physical therapists' experiences in private practice. Physiotherapy Canada 57(3):190–198

Southon G 1994 Professional autonomy and accountability. World Hospitals 30(4):4–9

Steenbergen K, Mackenzie L 2004 Professional support in rural New South Wales: perceptions of new graduate occupational therapists. Australian Journal of Rural Health 12(4):160–165

Struber J 2004 Recruiting and retaining allied health professionals in rural Australia: why is it so difficult? The Internet Journal of Allied Health Sciences and Practice 2(2):1–13. Available: http://ijahsp.nova. edu.articles 5 Aug 2006

Tryssenaar J, Perkins J 2001 From student to graduate: exploring the first year of practice. American Journal of Occupational Therapy 55(1):19–27

Wright S 1997 Examine what residents look for in their role models. Academic Medicine 71(3): 290–292

PHYSIOTHERAPY PRACTICE

CAREER PATHWAYS AND PROFESSIONAL DEVELOPMENT

six

Margot Skinner, Christine Bithell, Damian Mitsch and Matt Walsh

Key content

- Pathways leading to autonomous physiotherapy practice
- Factors that influence career pathways
- Professional development requirements for a variety of career pathways
- Constraints on career pathways

INTRODUCTION

Physiotherapy has been recognised as a career distinct from other health professions since the late 19th century. In this chapter we explore career pathways and the key factors that shape careers and continuing professional development pathways, including legal requirements, limitations around practice, professional socialisation and opportunities for specialisation.

THE PATHWAY TO BECOMING A PHYSIOTHERAPIST

Pre-registration professional degrees in physiotherapy range from undergraduate baccalaureate degrees of three to four years' duration with or without honours to graduate entry masters and professional doctoral degrees. There is an internationally accepted guideline for the preregistration curriculum, which should be the equivalent of 4 years' duration at university level (WCPT 2007). Prior to registration a person has no legal standing in terms of scope of practice and, therefore, by law is not entitled to practise before completing a prescribed course of physiotherapy education. However, the relevant legislation provides for students as long as they are practising within the academic confines of a school of physiotherapy recognised by the authority to provide the physiotherapy education, and they are under the supervision of physiotherapists licensed to practise.

Registration processes

In some countries including Singapore and India no legislation for registration is yet in place. However, in Western countries such as Australia, New Zealand, the USA and the UK, physiotherapy programs are accredited by the registering authority or its agent. Graduates are able to register under the relevant legislation and commence independent unsupervised practice within their scope immediately upon obtaining their qualification. Applicants applying for registration must make a statutory declaration that they are fit and able to meet the competencies set down by the registration authority for practice and that they will accept and adhere to codes of practice, professional behaviour and ethics.

The overriding purpose of registration is to protect the public from harm. A registration authority (Table 6.1) sets down the process of registration and prescribes the scope of practice under which a physiotherapist from an accredited school can practice. New Zealand and the UK have a system of national registration in place. As a result of agreement by the Council of Australian Governments (COAG) (2007), Australian state and territory governments are also implementing a system of national registration for health practitioners. National registration allows a physiotherapist to practise under a common legislative framework in all provinces, states and territories without requiring registration in multiple jurisdictions. Such legislation may also have provision for limited scope registration of visiting physiotherapists, such as visiting lecturers and postgraduate students.

Physiotherapists with qualifications obtained outside countries such as Australia, New Zealand and the UK who are seeking full registration need to undergo individual English language assessment, portfolio assessment and/or examination, unless there is a reciprocity agreement such as the *Trans Tasman Mutual Recognition Act*, 1997, an overarching statute between the Australian States and New Zealand. Similarly for the UK those with European Community citizenship have the right to be considered for registration.

The pathway to autonomous practice

Under general scope registration in most Western countries physiotherapists are autonomous and are entitled to practise in any field in which they are competent, being at the same time bound by the ethics set by the registering authority. The scope of practice is a statement that describes those qualified to use the title 'physiotherapist':

> Physiotherapists are registered healthcare practitioners educated to apply scientific knowledge and clinical reasoning to assess, diagnose and manage human function. They promote mobility, health and independence; rehabilitate; and maximize potential for activity. (Physiotherapy Board of New Zealand 2004)

The general scope of practice that applies to physiotherapists continuing in practice may be further described as in this example from New Zealand:

> Assessing, diagnosing, treating, reporting or giving advice in the capacity of a physiotherapist, using the knowledge, skills, attitudes and competence initially attained for registration as a physiotherapist in New Zealand and built upon in postgraduate and continuing physiotherapy education and wherever there could be an issue of public safety; advertising, holding out to the public, or representing in any manner that one is authorised to practise physiotherapy in New Zealand. (Physiotherapy Board of New Zealand 2004)

Physiotherapists' actual scope of practice, their ability to practise independently and the level of practice autonomy vary from country to country and sometimes also from state to state within a country. Independent practice, in countries such as Australia, New Zealand and the UK, which has been described in detail in Chapters 1 and 2,

Table 6.1 Examples of registration processes required in order to practise physiotherapy					
	National/ state legislation	Registration authority	Type of registration	APC* required	Ongoing requirements	Number of APC holders
Australia		State-based registration boards	Full, with limited registration available for overseas qualified physiotherapists and students in some states	Annually	Continuing professional development required in some states	14,000
ACT	*The Health Professionals Act* 2004					
NT	*Health Practitioners Act* 2007					
NSW	*Physiotherapists Act* 2001					
Qld	*Physiotherapists Registration Act* 2001					
SA	*Physiotherapy Practice Act* 2005					
Tas	*Physiotherapists Registration Act* 1999					
Vic	*Health Professions Registration Act* 2005					
WA	*Physiotherapists Act* 2005					
New Zealand	National – *Health Practitioners Competence Assurance Act* (2003)	Physiotherapy Board of New Zealand	Full Special scope (limited to a time and place) Vocational (not yet active)	Annually	Formal system of ongoing professional development based on a triennial cycle – random audits undertaken	3,300
USA	State – individual state practice acts	State departments of health	Full	Annually	Yearly continuing education hours requirement	65,000+
United Kingdom	National – *Health Professions Order* 2001	Health Professions Council	Full	Biennially	Formal requirement for ongoing continuing professional development. Random audits undertaken	40,000

*APC: Annual Practising Certificate

means that patients may see a physiotherapist as a primary contact practitioner without referral or supervision by a medical practitioner. It is similar to autonomous practice. The American Physical Therapy Association (APTA) defines autonomous practice as:

> Independent, self-determined professional judgment (as well as) an ability to refer to and collaborate with health care providers and others to enhance PT patient/client management. (APTA 2007)

However, the nature of autonomous practice is dependent upon its setting. Autonomous practice has been permitted for all physiotherapists in the UK since 1977 (Department for Health and Social Security (DHSS) 1997) and in Australia since 1976, as discussed in Chapter 2. Levels of education, the ability to diagnose and primary contact (with no doctor referral required) are probably the most tangible ways to differentiate physiotherapists from others who may work in a similar field, such as physiotherapy assistants.

Autonomy may also be limited by outside authorities. For example, certain health insurance companies in the USA or publicly funded services, such as the National Health Service (NHS) in the UK or Medicare in Australia, may set their own criteria regarding payment of fees to physiotherapists or referral for physiotherapy. Increasingly, however, in line with the clinical autonomy enjoyed by private practitioners, open access schemes, led by experienced physiotherapists (Chartered Society of Physiotherapy (CSP) 2004), have been introduced to provide a more efficient service to patients and reduce waiting lists. In addition, services are increasingly moving away from the hospital environment into the community, so practice opportunities will become more diverse and the need for autonomy greater (Bithell 2007). Thus factors such as practice knowledge, contextual experience and opportunities for professional development will substantially influence career pathways. These are explored further in the next section.

FACTORS THAT INFLUENCE CAREER PATHWAYS

Many experienced physiotherapists have developed their practice knowledge during very different times and have experienced a vastly different practice ontology or body of knowledge that supports their practice. Contextual experiences influence what is valued and/or discarded as practice knowledge, and knowledge construction, organisation and management are strongly influenced by the context of learning (Eraut 1994). The process of ongoing professional development is an expectation for all practising physiotherapists. It is a key part of what shapes a career pathway and occurs through a continual blending of learning new knowledge and moulding by the various influences on and contexts of practice. The use of the term *pathway* implies a journey or movement forward and a sense of advancement and new knowledge. This metaphor poses a number of questions regarding the professional development journey. These questions are now explored.

1. What contributes to the career pathway and who/what shapes its direction?

The rapidly changing global health environment has impacted upon practice and thus career pathways through changes in such factors as the body of knowledge, economics and accountability.

- **Knowledge** – Practice knowledge is dynamic and is constructed through social and historical factors. How we define practice knowledge influences what is valued and how clinical experiences are interpreted. The organisation and development of knowledge that occur through practice are key components of professional advancement. Advances in technology that have made vast amounts of knowledge easily accessible to both the general public and professionals also challenge the organisation and management of that knowledge. Knowledge and clinical reasoning have been shown to have an interdependent relationship in practice (Higgs et al 2004).
- **Economics** – Global economies have become more finance- and consumer-driven rather than socialised. This has led to shrinking health care dollars and more market competition within the health care sector (Neubauer 1998).
- **Accountability** – Demands for research-based treatment and fiscal accountability, more knowledgeable patients and the competitive nature of many other allied health professions vying for the same market of patients have led to the rise of evidence-based practice and quantitative research.

It appears that changes in our practice are driven by both internal as well as external factors. In education, reflection and transformative learning have been recognised as valuable aspects of advanced practice (Schön 1983, Mezirow 1991, Jensen et al 1999), and they have also been emphasised in pre-registration curricula.

2. What are the typical professional landscapes that I should expect to see around me and what might there be beyond?

Following registration physiotherapists often start their careers with a broad general interest in practice. They may be employed in work environments that offer excellent educational opportunities including mentoring programs. Many larger organisations have a series of in-service education programs, which may be accredited with a state or national continuing education body such as the New Zealand College of Physiotherapy Inc (NZCP). Over time, physiotherapists begin to take continuing education courses in their evolving areas of interest. This may involve the commencement of various levels of advanced certification and specialisation (see Fig 6.1).

Professional socialisation is an expected part of a typical career pathway. Therapists learn not only how to identify themselves within a profession but also how to interact and learn the politics, hierarchies and language of the various communities (Vygotsky 1978, Wenger 1998). However, the potential for professional socialisation and identity formation in a working environment may be limited when situations of professional isolation occur (e.g. in more remote working environments) or if practice limitations are imposed by external bodies such as medical insurers. It is vital, therefore, that professional organisations and their special interest groups take on the role of provider/facilitator of professional development opportunities as well as being major vehicles for professional socialisation.

As clinical experience accumulates the next stage of professional development begins. Physiotherapists start to focus on specialist areas of interest and the pathway of learning becomes more clearly defined. Work contexts, changes in jobs and travel to other parts of the country, or even internationally, all add to the depth of experience. For example, in sports physiotherapy practitioners often work with team sports, possibly travelling with a professional team or acting as a consultant to a dance company or

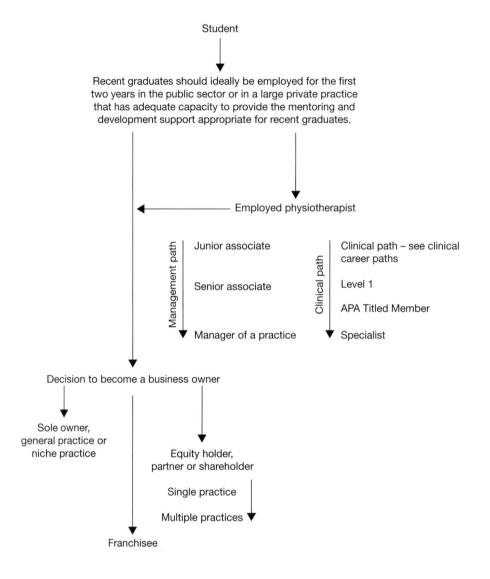

Fig. 6.1 Model for a possible career path in private practice, including the route to specialisation, as determined by the Australian College of Physiotherapy. Based on *Private Practice Career Pathway*, 2007, Australian Physiotherapy Association

an industrial manufacturer. Others may choose to take the pathway of more formal study that may comprise an advanced degree in a clinical specialty, research or even online programs such as professional doctoral study, which are now becoming readily accessible, particularly in the USA. Such stages of professional development have been examined more fully in the medical model (Schmidt et al 1992, Dreyfus & Dreyfus 1996), nursing (Benner 1992) and more recently in physical therapy (Jensen et al 2000, Higgs & Titchen 2001).

3. Where are the horizons of my profession and the boundaries of my pathway? How are choices made as to the directions that I can take?

Professional development is constantly being shaped by the various social influences and the contexts of practice experienced. Contextual experiences influence what is valued and/or discarded as practice knowledge. Likewise, knowledge construction, organisation and management are strongly influenced by the context of learning (Eraut 1994). As well, the culture in which one is embedded has an influence on the pathway that is taken. Practitioners are faced with the ever-expanding globalisation of information and portability of professionals, and are also challenged by cultural differences including language, gender biases and hierarchies that influence practice.

4. Who else is travelling on the path and what is their role?

Physiotherapists are often members of many different communities simultaneously. In older industrial models of work a person's identity was defined by work only. However, in the newer business models, creativity and personal identity are also recognised and valued, and social learning in all its forms contributes to what constitutes a professional identity (Wenger 1998).

Professional identity includes codes of practice, standards of conduct, skills, tools and methods that are deemed appropriate within the boundaries of physiotherapy. This is, like practice knowledge, a dynamic and evolving culture. As physiotherapists advance professionally, their personal pathways change but so, too, do the local and international identities and cultures of which they are a part. It is a constant challenge for practitioners to reason and interpret their way through this evolving professional culture, and collaboration with others travelling on the same path is an important part of this professional socialisation.

Specialisation (such as sports, Pilates or paediatric physiotherapy) creates a form of community that shares a commonality in language, methods and habits. Transfer of professional craft knowledge, a term used to describe a form of wisdom and connoisseurship that is learned through practical experience, mentorship and reflection (Eisner 1985, Higgs et al 2004), occurs within these specialisations, both formally and informally. Special interest groups formally recognised by professional bodies have certain standards of practice, share journal and research bases or have certain rites of passage such as levels of accreditation and forms of recognition of expertise. As well as these tangible forms of inclusion, communities share other tacit forms of knowledge that are learned through practice: acceptable behaviours, skills, tools and methods that are deemed appropriate for that group. Special interest groups may be seen as a microculture of the larger profession.

Just as language, role and identity form a part of any community, so too internationally we have the challenge of these boundaries of professionalism. Questions that beg further examination are 'Who are the gatekeepers that define what these boundaries are?' and 'How do novices recognise, negotiate and shape these boundaries as they move on the pathway to being advanced clinicians?'

5. Where are the various roadmaps and checkpoints that I should expect to see?

Health care practitioners have ways of recognising the pathway from novice to advanced practitioner. These may include national exams and credentialling, or less tangible rites such as learning the shared language of a specialty group or the use of its methods, tools and hierarchies.

At a specialisation level, physiotherapists educated elsewhere in the world must undergo the same national examination as local graduates unless there is a reciprocity agreement for qualifications. Physiotherapists must recognise, when moving from one place to another, that state or national laws may differ in their requirements for regulation of documentation, and in the use of modalities and techniques such as acupuncture or manipulation.

Whether practitioners choose to accept or reject the notion that professional development is both an uncertain pathway and influenced by their practice epistemology (frames of reference) has an influence on the career pathways taken. In a complex dynamic health care environment health care providers need to be adaptable and critical in order to build on the historical strengths of the profession and discard those now outmoded.

EMPLOYMENT OPPORTUNITIES AND CAREER PATHWAYS

The job market has some bearing on where the entry-level practitioner works initially. Some entry-level practitioners prefer to take a rotational position in a large publicly funded hospital or health authority, where they have the opportunity to spend a few months in a variety of inpatient, outpatient and community settings. Others move into a setting with a specific focus such as women's health; still others select an academic route and enrol in research-based higher degrees. The career paths for physiotherapists are diverse and may be dependent on: their physical environment and context, e.g. a remote rural setting; an opportunity to take ownership of a practice; successful application for a management opportunity arising from a vacancy or creation of a new tier in a department structure; or a research grant that sets the path for a research career. Whatever the path, continuing professional development is a professional responsibility, and may also be mandatory by law. A typical career pathway for a graduate may include a mixture of management and formal postgraduate education, and one or more memberships of professional special interest groups. For another physiotherapist the route may be more direct and follow a path leading to specialisation and consultancy status without the broad experience base.

Newly qualified physiotherapists are encouraged to choose employment in environments where there are mentors and peer support, and where they can experience a variety of placements. A rotational position can include placements in a musculoskeletal outpatient clinic, intensive care, neurology, elderly rehabilitation, or other areas such as mental health, women's health, or paediatrics. This allows for consolidation of knowledge and skills learned as a student moves through six to eight different short-term placements. Ideally some of these placements will cross the boundary between acute and primary care and involve working in the community. Although some may choose to continue to consider themselves generalists, after around two years' experience staff normally begin the route to specialisation by progressing into a more senior post in one area. Continuing professional development may then be more focused on the acquisition of further knowledge and skills leading towards expertise in the chosen specialty.

Employment conditions for physiotherapists include two high level structures, contractor and employee. Some employment arrangements are clearly one or the other. A practitioner who is offered a permanent position to work five days a week at a hospital is generally considered an employee. A person who contracts to provide occasional occupational health services to a local business is generally classed a contractor.

Determining a person's status as an employee or contractor is based on what legal systems refer to as the balance of probabilities, that is, what is more likely to be the case. The types of factors considered include whether the person

- is presented to the outside world as an emanation of the business
- uses the equipment and assets of the employer
- is subject to the policies and procedures of the business
- decides starting and finishing times
- is paid a salary or by invoice
- must personally undertake the work or may delegate it to subcontractors.

Two examples of employment situations are described in Table 6.2. A number of key court cases have helped to define criteria for assessing a person's status. For example, Stevens v Brodribb Sawmilling Co Pty Ltd (1986) is an important case in Australian law as it established a set of indicia that may be used to assist the process of assessment.

Table 6.2 Examples of employment situations for a physiotherapist		
	Scenario	**Commentary**
Example 1	A practitioner leases a space in a medical centre. The practitioner pays an administration fee to cover reception, bookkeeping, telephone and general marketing. The practitioner chooses to be available during the open hours of the centre but is bound to follow certain rules as part of the lease and management agreement. The centre collects fees on behalf of the practitioner and deducts the management fee before paying the balance to the practitioner. The practitioner is a sole trader and may employ additional staff to meet peak demand.	*The practitioner is not likely to be deemed an employee as she is effectively running her own small business within the centre. Although there are some rules that apply, they are part of a commercial lease or part of the practitioner's obligations to assist in managing her business affairs. The practitioner has a high degree of control over business decisions like fees and staffing.*
Example 2	A practitioner is offered a contract to work at a physiotherapy practice. The practitioner will be paid a percentage of the income he generates and is required to work a minimum 30 hours a week. The practitioner must attend all staff meetings and must comply with practice policies. Equipment is provided but part of the proportion kept by the practice is listed as rent, management, equipment fees. The practitioner is paid in the same cycle as other employees and is not required to furnish an invoice.	*This is likely to be deemed an employment arrangement on the balance of probabilities. The practice has made the arrangement look like a contract on the surface but the circumstances that define the relationship suggest it is a standard employment relationship. Where the arrangement is deemed an employment relationship by a court, all the usual employment conditions apply. These may include minimum provisions for annual leave, sick leave, long service leave, minimum pay rates during quiet or non-income-producing times, coverage for workers compensation and the payment of compulsory superannuation (which may also apply under Example 1).*

There is a wide range of employment models within physiotherapy. The more common ones include:

- common law contracts – an agreement between two parties outside of industrial relations legislation
- enterprise wide agreements – a registered agreement between the collective employees and the employer
- individual agreements – a registered agreement between an individual employee and an employer
- award-based employees – employees who are paid in accordance with a mandated minimum set of conditions established in law.

Finding out which structure may be used in individual states or countries is outside the scope of this text. However, most governments provide access to basic employee advice about minimum employment conditions. Health unions also offer support for members on industrial relations matters.

Management of physiotherapy services as a career pathway

There are increasing opportunities for physiotherapists to be involved in management in a part-time or full-time capacity, e.g. as a professional advisor, or in a broader sense. Management pathways for clinicians include managing the clinical leadership of health care delivery in a role such as a clinical director, mainstream management such as a director role in a large hospital, or management or ownership in the private sector.

There are few barriers to physiotherapists moving into a management career in the health sector. To be successful in a management role physiotherapists usually need to learn additional skills to those acquired in their undergraduate education. Undertaking formal education in a relevant area like human resource management, business law or finance will often assist. For example, the challenges in the public sector relate more to public demand, budgets, resourcing and government policy, whereas the private sector tends to face business pressures such as access to loans and other forms of funding, pressures from private heath insurers and funding bodies, and market competition.

Clinical specialisation as a career pathway

Credentialling for practice-specific specialisation within physiotherapy follows a similar model in countries in which this term is recognised. Credentialling is administered in Australia by the Australian College of Physiotherapists (ACP) and in New Zealand by the NZCP. Practitioners may specialise in a number of areas that offer specialisation through the professional body. Figure 6.1 shows a model for the pathway to specialisation. The model requires postgraduate study, a commitment to research and teaching, an ongoing commitment to professional development, and examination. Passing the specialisation examination confers the right to become a member of the ACP and to the title of 'specialist physiotherapist', which is included on the register under national registration (see Ch 2).

Eminent specialists may also be inducted as fellows of the College. Fellowship is an honour bestowed on physiotherapists to recognise their contribution at the highest level of research, learning and professional practice.

The opportunities for clinical specialist and extended scope practice (ESP) posts are evolving in Australia (see Ch 2). In the UK the NHS formally recognised the need to establish higher clinical grades in the allied health professions in 2000 (Department of Health 2000, 2001), to facilitate the recruitment and retention of those with high level clinical skills and to improve patient care and outcomes. ESP and clinical specialist posts were already developing without formal recognition, and these were consolidated into a career progression towards newly created consultant physiotherapist posts. Clinical specialists are senior physiotherapists who are regarded by their peers and managers as expert practitioners within a specific area of practice, such as continence care or sports injuries. Their roles include teaching others, taking referrals of complex patients from other therapists and advising on complex problems. Alternatively, and at an equivalent point within the grading structure, ESPs are those who for part of their time work outside the scope of practice normally carried out by a physiotherapist. ESPs work alongside consultant medical staff, receiving in-service training and supervision within the medical team until they are able to practise with less supervision but still with access to the consultant for guidance. These posts were designed to improve the efficiency of services to patients. Examples include an ESP physiotherapist in an emergency department as first contact for all apparent musculoskeletal trauma without bony injury, ordering X-rays and other tests, providing immediate advice and treatment,

Table 6.3 Special interest groups and sections within national professional bodies				
Physiotherapy special interest group/section	APA	NZSP	CSP	APTA
Acupuncture		✓	✓	
Animal	✓		✓	✓
Aquatic	✓			✓
Cardiorespiratory /acute care	✓	✓	✓	✓
Educators/research	✓			✓
Gerontology	✓	✓	✓	✓
Hand		✓	✓	✓
Manipulative	✓	✓	✓	
Neurology	✓	✓	✓	✓
Occupational	✓	✓	✓	✓
Oncology				✓
Paediatrics	✓	✓	✓	✓
Private practice	✓	✓	✓	✓
Sports/orthopaedic	✓	✓	✓	✓
Women's health	✓	✓	✓	✓
Electrotherapy and wound management				✓
Health policy and administration	✓			✓

and referring for physiotherapy as appropriate. Consultant physiotherapy posts were approved in 2000 to work alongside doctor and nurse consultants to develop clinical protocols and improve services to patients (Department of Health 2000). The posts are service-specific and may be created only with specific service improvements in view, such as cutting waiting lists and times or improving services for older people. They are not primarily management posts, and although the consultant will work with a supportive team that may include a clinical specialist and other physiotherapists, they are not line managers. The configuration of the work of the consultant is determined by local need with maximum flexibility. Different models of practice are emerging and work is being undertaken currently to determine how these new posts are developing.

Academia as a career pathway

Physiotherapists who are aspiring to an academic career are normally expected to have gained several years of post-qualification clinical experience and a masters or research degree (CSP 2003). Universities have an expectation that all newly appointed staff who do not have previous university teaching experience will undertake an in-service postgraduate certificate in learning and teaching (or equivalent) in their first year, to acquire an understanding of teaching, learning and assessment and effective teaching skills.

Entry into an academic career pathway is by successful appointment to an academic post. The exact requirements for each academic post will differ in terms of particular clinical specialties and also in the emphasis that is placed on holding a research degree and/or a record of publications in peer-reviewed journals. Research active universities have a clear expectation of postgraduate qualifications and publication history. A visit to a university's website will provide insights into its mission and aspirations that will direct its staff appointments policy and indicate whether a PhD or other doctoral award is essential or desirable. As physiotherapy education requires that academics who teach aspects of the theory and practice of physiotherapy must have clinical backgrounds, clinicians who enter university lectureships without higher degrees are normally offered an opportunity to undertake (or complete) a professional doctorate or PhD in the early years of their career.

All universities require from their academic staff excellence in teaching quality, energetic involvement in research and scholarly activity with tangible research outputs, and community service both within the institute and outside. A number of schools offer post-qualifying education in the form of masters and shorter continuing professional development programs in addition to qualifying programs, and academic staff are required to teach across levels and programs. In addition there is now a strong policy-driven requirement to develop interprofessional learning and teaching opportunities for all health students; academic staff may be expected to teach interdisciplinary groups for topics such as communication skills, health policy and case-based learning seminars.

University structures differ and physiotherapy may be placed as a single department or school within a larger faculty, or it may be clustered into a larger multiprofessional school. Either case presents the opportunity for a head of department/school post with academic leadership and development responsibilities as well as the continuation of personal research, consultancy or teaching interests.

Research as a career pathway

The university career structure offers the opportunity for research posts graded as reader or professor, with an established or personal chair. These posts require a considerable track record such as specialisation, personal research and publications, grant monies obtained, and research supervision of PhD and postdoctoral research students.

In Australasia most of these research posts are within the universities, though they are often grant funded and therefore do not hold long-term job security. There are relatively few research posts for physiotherapists within state and national health funded authorities, though there is a growing trend. In contrast in the UK such posts have been held within the NHS where no career structure for clinical academic researchers exists in physiotherapy. Although a recent report under the aegis of the UK Clinical Research Collaboration has concluded that the situation of clinical academic careers for nurses and also allied health professions requires considerable investment in training and infrastructure as there is currently no formal career structure or support, it is not clear when physiotherapists could expect implementation of the recommendations as further work is needed (UK Clinical Research Collaboration 2007).

CONSTRAINTS ON CAREER PATHWAYS

Physiotherapists need to practise within the constraints of their knowledge and skill. As in all professions, it falls back on individual practitioners to determine the point at which they do not have the knowledge or skill to continue to progress treatment. Thus the treating practitioner must consult colleagues with specialist skills or refer to a different health professional or other consultant. Professionals are judged harshly by the legal system if they move outside their scope of practice.

Some constraints on professional practice are defined by external factors such as policy, tradition, statute or finance. For example, it could be argued that it is tradition that limits physiotherapists from having a role in an emergency department, as they have the skills and knowledge base to work with many acute orthopaedic or respiratory patients. In some countries legislative boundaries preclude physiotherapists from providing elements of health delivery such as acupuncture, injecting, prescribing medication, and the use of certain imaging equipment. However, financial and access barriers have by far the greatest impact on the scope of practice for physiotherapists. An example of a financial and access barrier in Australia is the lack of direct referral access to medical specialists for real-time ultrasound, as there is no statute that limits physiotherapists from requesting ultrasound to assist in diagnosis.

Limitations on practice are a complex combination of what is deemed acceptable behaviour and moral and ethical factors. The decisions that shape professional boundaries are influenced by personal, professional and global factors. Therapists' world views, for example, have been shown to influence their clinical reasoning (Unsworth 2004). The boundaries that exist are not linear or constant; they shape, change and shift according to the historical context, local health care environment, and interactions with the patient and other professionals.

SUMMARY

Career pathways in physiotherapy are many and varied. They may lead to specialisation in clinical practice, management or research for some, while others may choose a combination. The career pathway is influenced by choices in continuing professional development as well as by factors such as professional socialisation and the landscape surrounding the practice location.

Reflective questions

- What are the requirements of a graduating physiotherapist who wishes to practise in my country?
- What are the factors that determine the scope of physiotherapy practice and how do these change during a career?
- What factors should I consider when taking up employment as a physiotherapist?
- What is meant by the route to specialisation? Interview an experienced physiotherapist and track their career pathway.

References

APTA 2007 Autonomous Physical Therapy Practice, HOD P06-06-18-12, Program 32, American Physical Therapy Association. Available: http://www.apta.org/AM 01 Sep 2007

Australian Physiotherapy Association 2007 Private practice career pathway. APA, Melbourne

Benner, P T C 1992 From beginner to expert: gaining a differentiated clinical world in critical care nursing. Advances in Nursing Science 14(3):13–28

Bithell C 2007 Entry-level physiotherapy education in the United Kingdom: governance and curriculum. Physical Therapy Reviews 12:145–155

CSP 2003 Entering physiotherapy teaching. CSP, London

CSP 2004 Making physiotherapy count: a range of quality assured services. CSP, London

Council of Australian Governments 2007 COAG Meeting 13th April 2007. Available: http://www.coag.gov.au/meetings/130407/index.htm#health 19 Oct 2007

Department of Health 2000 Meeting the challenge: a strategy for the allied health professions. DH, London

Department of Health 2001 Investment and reform for NHS staff: taking forward the NHS plan. DH, London

DHSS 1977 Health service development – relationship between the medical and remedial professions. Health circular HC (77)33. DHSS, London

Dreyfus H L, Dreyfus S E 1996 The relationship of theory and practice in the acquisition of skill. In: Tanner C, Chesla C (eds) Expertise in nursing practice. Springer, New York, pp 29–47

Eisner E 1985 The art of educational evaluation: a personal view. Falmer, London

Eraut, M 1994 Developing professional knowledge and competence. Falmer, London

Health Practitioners Competence Assurance Act 2003 New Zealand Government, Wellington

Higgs J, Jones M, Edwards I et al 2004 Clinical reasoning and practice knowledge. In: Higgs J, Richardson B, Abrandt Dahlgren M (eds) Developing practice knowledge for the health professions. Butterworth-Heinemann, Oxford, pp 181–198

Higgs J, Titchen A (eds) 2001 Practice knowledge and expertise in the health professions. Butterworth-Heinemann, Oxford

Jensen G, Shepard K, Gwyer J et al 1999 Expertise in physical therapy practice. Butterworth Heinemann, Boston

Jensen G, Gwyer J, Shepard K 2000 Expert practice in physical therapy. Physical Therapy 80(5):44–52

Mezirow J 1991 Transformative dimensions of adult learning. Jossey-Bass, San Francisco

Neubauer D 1998 Impacts of globalization on health and health care policy. CPEA, University of Sydney, occasional paper no. 1

Physiotherapy Board of New Zealand 2004 Recertification guidelines. Wellington

Schmidt H, Boshuizen H, Norman G 1992 Reflections on the nature of expertise in medicine. In: Keravnou E. (ed) Deep models for medical knowledge engineering. Elsevier, Amsterdam, pp 231–248

Schön D 1983 The reflective practitioner: how professionals think in action. Basic Books, New York

UK Clinical Research Collaboration 2007 Developing the best research professionals: qualified graduate nurses: preparing and supporting clinical academic nurses of the future. Available: http://www. ukcrc.org 27 Aug 2007

Unsworth C 2004 Clinical reasoning; how do pragmatic reasoning, worldview and client-centredness fit? British Journal of Occupational Therapy 67(1):10–18

Vygotsky L 1978 Mind in society: the development of higher psychological process. Harvard University Press, Cambridge, MA

WCPT 2007 Guidelines for Physical Therapist Professional Entry-level Educational Programmes (Accepted June 2007). WCPT, London

Wenger E 1998 Communities of practice: learning, meaning and identity. Cambridge University Press, Cambridge

MODELS AND PHILOSOPHY OF PRACTICE

Franziska Trede and Joy Higgs

seven

Key content

- Values
- Assumptions
- Different ways of knowing and practising

INTRODUCTION

Physiotherapy is practised in many different ways and physiotherapists work in many different contexts ranging from acute care settings, private practice and professional sports clubs to chronic care in community settings including nursing homes. Physiotherapy clients come from a diverse range of backgrounds and include older people, professional athletes, prematurely born babies, rehabilitation groups and their families and carers. These different practice situations and this diversity of clientele have an impact on how physiotherapy is practised in each of these contexts.

One way of understanding the choices and approaches of different physiotherapists in their practice is through *practice models*. Physiotherapists develop their own practice models as they accumulate and learn from their professional and life experiences. In some cases this involves conscious choices based on personal values and philosophy, deliberate learning and reflections on practice, whereas in other cases practitioners may unquestioningly follow dominant practice approaches engendered through their education and practice settings.

In this chapter we explore practice models and the philosophy underpinning them. We discuss the ways that different models of practice are framed by values, interests and world views. We argue that it is important to appreciate these different perspectives and become aware of personal professional practice values and interests in order to make conscious choices, provide clients with options, and clearly articulate practice among colleagues and in multidisciplinary teams. Three key sources inform this discussion. The first is Franziska Trede's doctoral research in which she investigated the philosophical perspectives underpinning physiotherapy practice. All data quoted in this paper are from this research (Trede 2006). The second is a book (Higgs, Richardson & Abrant Dahlgren 2004) that examined the epistemology of practice (or the way practice knowledge is developed and used in practice). The third is Habermas' (1972) theory of knowledge and human interest.

WHAT IS PROFESSIONAL PRACTICE?

Professional practice does not occur in isolation. It is shaped by internal and external forces. Internal forces include professional ideology and what a physiotherapist identifies with and aspires to become. Physiotherapists may identify themselves predominantly as scientists, therapists, educators, advocates or trainers. External forces include social, economical, political and cultural aspects that change with time. A profession such as physiotherapy is a community of people who share practice knowledge, practice interventions and practice goals. Professional practice reflects a structured body of knowledge, expertise, regulations, autonomy and accountability. Members of a profession are accountable to themselves, their profession, the system within which they work, their service receivers and society at large (Eraut 1994). A key question is: what criteria determine the nature of accountable professional practice? Should physiotherapy practice be informed predominantly by empirico-analytical frameworks of the natural sciences or by hermeneutic frameworks of the social sciences as well? In discussing these issues we need to reflect on how practice knowledge is defined, what counts as evidence (Abrandt Dahlgren 2002), and what role patients' experiences play in health care practice. Dimensions of professional practice have been described as context relevance, people-centredness, authenticity and wisdom (Higgs & Titchen 2001). However accountability, credibility and standards of professional practice are defined, practice is underpinned firstly by values and interests, and these are located in philosophical perspectives.

A key notion of clinical professional practice is that it is concerned with, relates to, and is practised with people (Ewing & Smith 2001). Physiotherapy in particular is frequently concerned with helping people in pain or with physical limitations, and with promoting their self-management of health conditions. A professional practitioner needs technical knowledge and technical skills, but it is equally important to apply these technical aspects in ethical and appropriate ways that are carefully tailored to each client. The relational nature of professional practice is especially relevant for physiotherapists because practitioners rely on patients' active participation during treatments and adherence to exercise prescriptions between treatments. Physiotherapists liaise with other health care professionals and work as part of a health care team. Building and maintaining professional relationships is part of good practice. The way professionals relate to their clients and each other has an impact on the way they practise.

There are many aspects of physiotherapy where there are no set rules and where decisions are based on moral and ethical grounds. Physiotherapists who are aware of their ethical practice and the values that underpin their practice are better able to articulate, argue or justify their professional decisions, clinical interventions and evaluation. They appreciate the importance of communicating clearly with others and working collaboratively. A people-centred, relational approach to practice clarifies expectations, helping practitioners to consider a diversity of health beliefs and to avoid misunderstandings and inappropriate care.

WHAT HAS PHILOSOPHY TO DO WITH PHYSIOTHERAPY?

Physiotherapy is not a straightforward mechanical technical profession that applies scientific truths to practice. Practice is shaped by the models or frameworks that physiotherapists choose, consciously or unconsciously, to adopt. These frameworks are reflected in questions like: How do we practise physiotherapy? How do we know what model or philosophy underpins our way of practising? Models are mind maps and abstract representations of practice. They can be articulated and conscious, or implicit in practice. Most practitioners have probably never drawn up a model of their practice and would find it hard to articulate their practice approach at a philosophical level. In her doctoral research, Franziska (Trede 2006) found that most of the physiotherapists in her study did not think in terms of models. To explore what philosophical underpinnings shaped their model of practice she asked them:

- What kind of physiotherapist are you?
- What kind of physiotherapist do you identify with?
- How do you know what your patients need?
- What are your main practice challenges?

Many of the participants said that these questions were difficult for them to answer, indicating that they had not thought in great depth about their practice. For example:

> These are things I haven't given a great deal of thought to. You do things automatically without thinking why you do them.

> I don't really … I haven't really thought about that, actually, it's a hard question. You're making me really think about what I'm doing, aren't you? It's great.

The diverse responses from the participants were evidence of the complexity of physiotherapy and professional practice. Although physiotherapy is informed by science and evidence-based practice, the pure application of technical textbook knowledge is problematic. Clients bring multiple variables (including preferences and concerns) to physiotherapy consultations that are often not considered as evidence worthy of informing practice alongside knowledge derived from rigorously designed randomised trials where most variables are controlled (Jones et al 2006). For example, prescribing physical exercises can mean different things with different clients, such as professional athletes recovering from an injury, sleep-deprived young mothers, older men with Parkinson's disease and women from cultural backgrounds that do not value women exercising. Each of these clients brings different perceptions, past experiences, expectations, barriers and supportive environments to exercising. Physiotherapists deal with diversity and complexity on a daily basis. The workplace environment also shapes professional practice. Colleagues, managers and other health care professionals influence the way we practise. Awareness and acceptance of different world views as well as flexibility are required to provide ethical, culturally appropriate professional practice.

Practice models are shaped by philosophical perspectives, their key values and ways of seeing the world. Philosophy can be understood as the pursuit of knowledge and wisdom. It deals with fundamental questions about the nature of reality, justification of beliefs and the conduct of life. Philosophy meets physiotherapy at the crossroads of the following questions:

- What type of knowledge is regarded as valuable professional knowledge?
- Which beliefs about health, illness and fitness are adopted?
- Which ethical positions and values guide clinical professional practice?

- What influences the way we reason about a case, assess certain functions and not others, come to a diagnosis, make professional judgements, set goals and decide on evaluation strategies?

All of these questions are philosophical questions that cannot be answered with simple short responses. They are best addressed by understanding the different views and philosophical stances that people adopt with regard to their practice and by discussing ethics, values and humanity.

Philosophical stances

To create knowledge we need to understand what it is that we can know and what 'really' exists. This falls under the heading of ontology, the branch of philosophy that deals with the nature of reality and what can be known. To effectively use knowledge in practice we need to understand what we mean by knowledge. Epistemology is the branch of philosophy that deals with how something can be known.

Do practitioners need to know about these challenging topics? The answer is 'yes', for two reasons: first, because as professionals they are required to demonstrate a duty of care, to provide high quality care informed by critically appraised practice knowledge of all relevant forms; and second, because they have a professional responsibility to contribute to the body of knowledge of their discipline. Higgs, Andresen & Fish (2004) and colleagues have deeply and critically examined the nature of knowledge and its development and provide strategies for understanding this challenging field.

Here are two examples of ontological and epistemological stances (Higgs et al 2007) and their influence on practice approaches:

1. In the positivist/empiricist research tradition the world is objective, since it is said to exist independently of the knowers, and consists of phenomena or events that are orderly and lawful. To positivists or empiricists, knowledge arises from the rigorous application of the scientific method and is measured against the criteria of objectivity, reliability and validity. This philosophical stance underpins (largely invisibly) the medical model, with its focus on biomedical knowledge as evidence for practice decisions.
2. In the social constructivist view reality and knowledge are socially constructed (Berger & Luckmann 1966). That is, reality exists because we give meaning to it in our different lives and cultures. The social constructionist approach (McCarthy 1996) construes knowledge as a changing and relative phenomenon that is socially defined and produced. Wellness practice models that reflect cultural diversity in clinical decision making fit in this category.

Ethics

Ethical practice honours rights, obligations and fairness. Clients have a right to privacy, confidentiality, freedom of choice and refusal of treatment. It is good practice to be familiar with the patient charter in your workplace. As a physiotherapist you have ethical obligations to your clients, your profession and society at large to show respect for people and their autonomy (Beach et al 2005). Ethics in health is underpinned by values of compassion, empathy and caring (Halpern 2003). Ethics describe what humans ought to do in a reasonable, moral, well-supported framework. They are fundamental moral principles that are translated into codes of ethics by professional organisations. Ethics apply to conducting research, to professional practice with clients and to teaching students. Ethics underpin professional conduct and professionalism, and ethical standards should impact on the way physiotherapists practise and justify their choice of treatment.

Humanity

For the purpose of this chapter, humanity means being mindful of the quality of being human. To be human means to have values, to be driven by interests, willpower and motivations. Although we would like to think that we make rational decisions based on commonsense reasoning, we know that this is not always the case. For example, most chain smokers know that it is unhealthy to smoke but they do not all act on this knowledge and medical advice. Humans are complex beings. Often much more is needed than scientific knowledge, well written brochures and statistical facts to help clients learn to make changes, be more responsible for their wellbeing and take greater control over their health. Although largely concerned with the biophysical aspects of health, physiotherapists are wise to consider clients as whole beings and remember that clients also have their own will, self-understanding and concepts about health.

Values

Values and professional identity are not directly visible but become apparent in the way physiotherapists practise. Physiotherapists bring their personal professional values to professional practice, just as clients bring their personal values to the clinical encounter. Clients' values may become apparent when they express their priorities and concerns. Some physiotherapists may place more value on technical skill than on human engagement, others may emphasise pragmatic aspects to get their work done and cope with a heavy workload in a busy hospital, yet others may focus on honouring patient dignity and facilitating patient self-determination over any other competing interest. Each of these values informs the way physiotherapy is practised. Values influence what is seen as valuable knowledge in practice, and shape the attitudes that underpin professional identities.

FOUNDATIONS OF PRACTICE MODELS – INTERESTS

Physiotherapy can be seen as a science that combines applied science and social science. Each of these perspectives is located in a different practice paradigm or model, which in turn is underpinned by different philosophical values. Habermas, a prominent philosopher of critical social sciences, argued that all knowledge is influenced by interests. In his theory of knowledge and human interest Habermas (1972) contended that there would be no knowledge if there was no interest in asking questions. The types of questions we ask and the types of questions we do not ask indicate what we want to know about the world (ontological interest) and how it can be known (epistemological interest). The way we learn and practise is influenced by what we are interested in, what we listen to, what we want to engage with. What we do not want to hear or learn we tend to exclude and forget.

Habermas contended that asking certain questions and not other questions exposes our interests and biases. What we understand as knowledge and what we consider valuable knowledge are informed by our interests, values and motivations. These interests, values and motivations guide our behaviour. Habermas differentiated between three types of interest: technical, practical and critical interests. Each interest develops different types of knowledge and defines reality differently. Practice models can be located in one of these three interests.

Technical interest

Technical interest entails a bias towards predicting outcomes, controlling environments and asserting certainty and expert authority. Technical interest guides a one-way, cause-and-effect type of reasoning by controlling or excluding other variables. Technical interests generate context-free, universal, generalisable knowledge that has widespread applicability. Practice can be seen as routine. This predictive knowledge can be used confidently to prescribe rational purposive actions. From the technical perspective, facts and value-free knowledge are differentiated from personal, cultural knowledge and emotions, and objective rationality is considered superior. Physiotherapists who predominantly follow technical interests assume an expert role, tell patients what is best for them and measure outcomes with quantitative tools. The following two quotes (Trede 2006) are from physiotherapists whose practices were located in technical interest:

You look at their [clients'] past history, you look at their deficiencies and just plan to correct those deficiencies, if it's possible. I find that a bit straightforward. You see what you see and see what is needed and just react to that.

I don't like to give them [clients] a choice between stretching and strengthening exercises because I don't think they can decide which one is more appropriate. I think it is a decision that is made with my assessment. I am clinically trained. I don't think that they could do that. I guess I always decide what exercises to do. Then I let them work out how they are going to do that throughout the day. I wouldn't think of giving them total control. I think it lies in their best interest to do what I say. I explain why the exercises need to be done, what they are trying to achieve. That makes a big difference.

These quotes illustrate how these physiotherapists placed importance on technical knowledge, which meant that treatment plans were relatively rigid and the emphasis was on expertise and professional authority.

Practical interest

Practical interest pursues pragmatic goals and seeks common ground. Professional practice guided by practical interest aims for consensus and is conducted in the spirit of collaboration. Physiotherapists with these interests assume that understanding is based on prior experiences that need to be considered and incorporated into treatments. The focus for these physiotherapists is on understanding their observations within clients' contexts and working with them to achieve shared goals. The following quotes (Trede 2006) are from physiotherapists who could be said to embody perspectives driven by practical interest:

I use anatomical models and pictures and also make analogies, I'll ask the patient to repeat back to me what their understanding of it is. Particularly with some sort of postoperative guidelines that are quite complex and there's a lot required of the patients. And I'll give them written exercises with pictures and some other guidelines as well, to try and – well, from my point of view, to try and improve their compliance, but also from their point of view, to increase their understanding of the reason that they're doing this physiotherapy program.

You really need that skill [of negotiation] because conflict and didactics doesn't get you anywhere. It sets up two polar opposites, which is a great way to fuel conflict (laughter). But if you try to acknowledge someone else's point of view whether you agree or not, at least I mean to give them a little bit might make them give you a little bit and get that concept going. Like there is this threatening kind of a guy. I have spent hours and hours with this person on a few occasions. He came up to me the day he left and said he really appreciated all that interaction. And it was like 'Oh, OK'. Whereas to stand back and say 'No you are on the wrong track. That's wrong; let's do it my way' – that is not realistic.

These physiotherapists make the point that there is no one best way of treating clients. Instead their focus is on providing appropriate treatments and offering learning tools that suit clients. This people-centred approach to practice involves listening, negotiating and collaborating with clients, activities that are underpinned by practical interests.

Critical interest

Critical interest pursues critique and change. Critique does not mean criticism but implies skepticism and curiosity. A critical interest encourages physiotherapists to question their practice, their clients' beliefs and the policies that frame their practice. This type of critique separates reason from authority and draws out the ideology and hidden agenda behind truth claims and facts, and may result in behaviour and process changes. Such changes are initiated through critique; they liberate people from unnecessary constraints. These changes mean a shift in attitudes and perspectives, and they empower self and others. Physiotherapists with critical interests engage in open transparent dialogues with clients. Clients are encouraged to be involved participants and to collaborate in decision making with their therapist. The aim is to preserve self-identity and self-determination. The following quotes (Trede 2006) illustrate such critical practice:

The penny dropped for me only after 10 years of clinical experience. I had [a patient with] an above-knee amputation and he had a prosthesis. He walked perfectly in the gym. I had him walk without a limp. I was really pleased with all this. Then I met him downtown in the shopping centre: he had his knee locked, he was walking on the inner quarter of his foot, foot stuck out at right angle and he was perfectly happy. I stood and looked at him and thought, 'I can make you walk perfectly without a limp but you don't want to do that'. And you know when he came to treatment he would do it but obviously he wasn't feeling safe and he didn't want to do it that way and that is that. I think I wanted him to do what I wanted. I was trying to be a perfectionist. And it has also to do with all the other physiotherapists. They are checking on you that you are doing it all properly.

I can really only learn by trying to be as honest as possible with my clients about outcomes of treatments. Every time a patient walks into the room I ask them, 'How do you feel today compared to last time I saw you?' If they are looking vague I ask them, 'Do you feel better or worse or about the same?' I try to ask open questions and secondly to give them options and free them to say, 'Well, I actually feel worse. I know you do not want to hear that but I feel worse or I feel the same'.

Therapists who adopt a critical perspective question further and deeper to find out the assumptions and motivations that influence what people think, say and do. These quotes describe a democratic and emancipatory quality in therapist–client professional relationships where clients' contributions to treatment are valued and incorporated. Emancipatory interests drive critical reflection, sincerity and honesty in interpersonal communication between therapists and clients. Goals and outcomes of treatments are defined not only by biomedical parameters but by personal and social considerations that foster integrity and self-identity as well as liberate people from unreflected, unnecessary constraints.

The way physiotherapists practise is influenced by their philosophical underpinnings, which in turn shape practice interests and professional identity. Table 7.1 highlights how technical, practical and critical interests influence practice.

Table 7.1 Influences of interests on aspects of practice			
Practice aspects	**Critical interests**	**Practical interests**	**Technical interests**
Professional identity	Self-awareness	Awareness of others	Scientific awareness
Critique and clinical reasoning	Starts with self, with the aim to transform	Starts with patients, with the aim to empower	Starts with technique, with the aim to master
Clinician power	Equalising power sharing	Clinician may share some power	Clinician has power
Patient power	Empowered in a way that can be sustained	Empowered	Disempowered
Focus of disease	Political	Practical	Technical
Practice knowledge	Propositional–technical, experiential and critical	Propositional–technical and experiential	Propositional–technical
Questioning technique	Open, strategic questions	Open questions	Closed, explanatory questions
Context of decision making	Historical–political context	Psychocultural context (definitely not political)	Out of context
Clinicians helping patients	To empower and liberate	To cope	To survive and comply
Identifying treatment options	Based on self-determination and liberation	Based on clinical complexity and diversity	Based on randomised controlled trials

PRACTICE MODELS – SCENARIOS

Using the three types of interest described by Habermas we can identify three different practice models: the medical model, the psychosocial model and the emancipatory, critical social sciences model. Table 7.2 illustrates how these practice models are shaped by different interests, knowledge and definitions of reality.

This table makes clear the distinctions between the three practice models with the aim of demonstrating their differences. Although physiotherapists have a tendency to favour one of these models, in the reality of practice the models are blurred. It is useful to remember that clinicians do not think about practice models in their work, but rather justify their way of practising as a response to practice contexts. We argue that *professional* practice should be informed and 'knowingly practised'. This requires a higher level of informed decision making in determining and enacting practice models.

Table 7.2 Practice models and their ways of knowing, interests, knowledge and definitions of reality. Informed by *Knowledge and human interest*, by J Habermas

Practice models	Ways of knowing (epistemology)	Interests	Knowledge	Definitions of reality
Empirico-analytical and medical model (natural science)	Controlled observation	Technical cognitive: ■ prediction ■ objective evidence	■ Facts ■ Truths	Technical control
Historical-hermeneutic and psychosocial model (social science)	■ Understanding meaning ■ Interpretations of texts	Practical cognitive: ■ mediation ■ finding consensus	Intersubjectively negotiated meaning	Mutual understanding in the conduct of life
Emancipatory and wellness model (critical social science)	Self-reflection	Emancipatory cognitive: ■ transformation ■ emancipation	Critical of natural and social influences and negotiated understandings	Toward emancipation from seemingly natural constraints

Consider the following scenario from a biomedical perspective that demonstrates a technical interest.

Scenario 1a

In his role as a physiotherapist in an outpatient amputee unit Lee teaches clients to walk with prostheses. His new client, Dora, has an above-knee amputation. As a diligent physiotherapist Lee places emphasis on equal weight-bearing phases to teach Dora to avoid circumduction of the hip. Lee provides a lot of feedback to help Dora learn how to walk properly again. He gives Dora a handout with anatomical diagrams and explanations to help her memorise and understand the biomechanical functioning of gait. Dora is doing quite well and is compliant, but Lee notices that after three sessions she does not turn up to appointments regularly. When Dora keeps her next appointment Lee asks her why she didn't come, and explains how inconvenient it is for him. He has a long waiting list and it is her responsibility to communicate. Dora seems shy, smiles apologetically but does not provide a good reason. Lee stresses the importance of walking well to avoid low back pain and to be safe, but has a feeling that Dora is not really taking it in and is not listening. Dora does not turn up for further treatment sessions and Lee is left wondering why. He is also a bit angry that this client is not grateful for all his efforts, and he feels tired.

In this scenario the physiotherapist teaches gait from a medical–functional perspective. Gait training is gait training, and all amputees have to learn the same things. He uses a therapist-centred perspective, providing the client with information, giving her a brochure, explaining to her how she has to fit into the booking system and why exercising is important from a biomedical perspective.

The same scenario from a bio-psychosocial perspective demonstrates a practical interest.

Scenario 1b

Lee explains the importance of gait training and makes his perspective known to Dora. He also listens to Dora's account to gain a more holistic picture of her life situation, learning that she is not interested in sport, nor is she fussed about people noticing that she walks with a prosthesis; she simply wants to be able to get around. Dora had physiotherapy previously when she had pneumonia and did not like the rough percussions on her chest. She says she only wants a few treatments. Lee uses this information to ensure that he remains sensitive to Dora's wishes and perception of touch. As soon as Dora is reasonably able to walk safely she is discharged, even though her gait is not perfect.

In this situation the physiotherapist also teaches gait but integrates his biomedical knowledge with the personal experiences and beliefs of his client. Patient and therapist learn from each other and work together towards shared goals. The physiotherapist is proud to have adopted a patient-centred approach.

The same scenario from a wellness perspective demonstrates a critical interest.

Scenario 1c

Lee starts by asking Dora why she is here, what she expects to get out of treatment and what her major concerns are. He quickly notices that communication is difficult and prompts her to discuss her ethnic background. He finds out that Dora is from Greece, left school early to help the family on the farm, is illiterate even in Greek, and has limited proficiency in English despite living in Australia for 20 years. When offered a health care interpreter Dora refuses. After asking why she refuses, Lee finds out that she believes interpreters are only for signing consent forms before operations or in more important cases than hers. She is only an old Greek woman. Lee explains that interpreters provide a free, confidential, professional service and she agrees to have an interpreter. Now there can be a three-way dialogue where Lee can explain the fine details of gait training to Dora, who in turn can provide feedback and ask questions that are answered to her satisfaction.

Open dialogue is placed at the centre of practice in this scenario. The physiotherapist is not satisfied with initial responses such as 'I don't want an interpreter' and tries to find the reasons behind this statement. He aims to liberate clients and himself from taken-for-granted assumptions by reducing unnecessary (sometimes even self-imposed) constraints. For example, he demystifies this client's perception that interpreters are only used for signing consent forms. Learning from this critique results in change: the client agrees to use an interpreter. Lee critically uses biomedical knowledge in each clinical situation. This physiotherapist does not routinely hand out brochures to clients who cannot read them, and avoids assumptions by engaging clients in critical dialogues. Both therapist and client explore assumptions and work together towards best outcomes for the client.

These scenarios are stereotypes of the three practice models that are discussed in the health literature: the biomedical, psychosocial and wellness models, respectively. In clinical reality these models are blurred and various situations could demand different aspects of each approach. We have deliberately contrasted the different perspectives in a simplistic way to demonstrate the difference in their philosophical underpinnings, different emphases on what is valuable practice knowledge and different interests and values that shape how physiotherapists practise.

SUMMARY

In this chapter we have discussed how philosophy interfaces with physiotherapy practice. Three different practice models were identified based on the theory of knowledge and human interest (Habermas 1972). Physiotherapy practice today operates in increasingly more complex, diverse and uncertain environments. Patients are better informed, technology is advancing and health care practice is constantly changing. Many different human interests collide in physiotherapy practice. We have argued that awareness of different philosophical viewpoints and interests illuminates practice models and assists physiotherapists to develop their professional practice.

Becoming aware of their own interests and philosophical viewpoints enables practitioners to practise in a more conscious and intentional way. Professional practice biases influence many professional activities such as clinical reasoning, decision making, history taking, goal setting and evaluation. Practice interests shape professional identity, professional authority, professional practice knowledge and professional roles. The clinical reality of physiotherapy is influenced by many, often competing interests and forces. Being aware of these influences and forces helps practitioners to make conscious decisions that are based on critical thought and to choose the kind of physiotherapist they want to become. Awareness of philosophical influences on physiotherapy practice enables practitioners to engage in informed, articulate and mature debate with colleagues and the wider health care community. By knowing what they are doing practitioners feel more in control of what they are doing. Reflecting on the values and biases they bring to practice enables them to determine their future direction and enhances them as valuable team members and mature citizens.

Reflective questions

- How would you respond to the answers posed at the beginning of this chapter, e.g. what kind of physiotherapist would you like to become?
- Observe how other professionals practise and critique their way of practising. What do you like about their way of practising and what would you not adopt into your way of practising and why?
- What difference do you want to make in your professional practice?
- How do you decide what is valuable knowledge?
- How would you describe and critically appraise your practice model?
- What questions do you need to ask to understand your clients' perspective? Try formulating some questions.

REFERENCES

Abrandt Dahlgren M 2002 What is the evidence – and where does it take us? Advances in Physiotherapy 4(1):1

Beach M C, Sydarman J, Johnson R L et al 2005 Do patients treated with dignity report higher satisfaction, adherence, and receipt of preventive care? Annals of Family Medicine 3(4):331–338

Berger P, Luckmann T 1966 The social construction of reality. Anchor Books, Garden City

Eraut M 1994 Developing professional knowledge and competence. Falmer, London

Ewing R, Smith D 2001 Doing, knowing, being and becoming: the nature of professional practice. In: Higgs J, Titchen A (eds) Professional practice in health, education and the creative arts. Blackwell Science, Oxford, pp 16–28

Habermas J 1972 Knowledge and human interest (trans Shapiro J J). Heinemann, London

Halpern J 2003 What is clinical empathy? Journal of General Internal Medicine 18:670–674

Higgs J, Titchen A 2001 Framing professional practice: knowing and doing in context. In: Higgs J, Titchen A (eds) Professional practice in health, education and the creative arts. Blackwell Science, Oxford, pp 3–15

Higgs J, Andresen L, Fish D 2004 Practice knowledge – its nature, sources and contexts. In: Higgs J, Richardson B, Abrandt Dahlgren M (eds) Developing practice knowledge for health professionals. Butterworth-Heinemann, Oxford, pp 51–69

Higgs J, Richardson B, Abrandt Dahlgren M, 2004 Developing practice knowledge for health professionals. Butterworth-Heinemann, Oxford

Higgs J, Trede F, Rothwell R 2007 Qualitative research interests and paradigms In: Higgs J, Titchen A, Horsfall D et al (eds) Being critical and creative in qualitative research. Hampden Press, Sydney, pp 32–42

Jones M, Grimmer K, Edwards I et al 2006 Challenges in applying best evidence in physiotherapy. The International Journal of Allied Health Sciences and Practice 4(3):1–8

McCarthy E D 1996 Knowledge as culture: the new sociology of knowledge. Routledge & Kegan Paul, London

Trede F 2006 A critical practice model for physiotherapy, PhD thesis, The University of Sydney, Australia. Available: http://ses.library.usyd.edu.au/handle/2123/1430 15 Nov 2007

CLINICAL REASONING IN PHYSIOTHERAPY

Megan Smith, Rola Ajjawi and Mark Jones

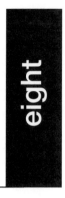

Key content

- Physiotherapy clinical reasoning strategies
- Physiotherapy clinical reasoning capabilities
- Factors that influence physiotherapy clinical reasoning
- Activities that facilitate learning to clinically reason

INTRODUCTION

Clinical reasoning is an inherent component of physiotherapy clinical practice. The term *clinical reasoning* refers to the thinking and decision making processes used by practitioners. It encompasses related terms such as clinical decision making, problem solving and professional judgement. Learning to do clinical reasoning requires novice practitioners to engage in ongoing critical examination of their reasoning processes and the factors that influence their reasoning.

APPROACHES TO REASONING IN PHYSIOTHERAPY PRACTICE

Clinical reasoning is a complex, multi-dimensional phenomenon consisting of a number of overlapping approaches or ways of thinking about clients and their problems within the clinical context (Higgs 2006, Norman 2005). It is both an independent cognitive process undertaken by practitioners and a collaborative and narrative process involving clients and others (Edwards, Jones & Carr 2004, Higgs et al 2006). Clinical reasoning has been portrayed visually as circular (or spiralling) and interactive in nature rather than linear, demonstrating the evolution of the reasoning process via repeated interactions with the client (Higgs & Jones 2000).

Physiotherapy reasoning incorporates the cognitive strategies of hypothetico-deductive reasoning and pattern recognition (Edwards 2001, Smart & Doody 2007). Hypothetico-deductive reasoning has components of data acquisition, hypothesis generation, data interpretation and hypothesis evaluation (Jones & Edwards 2008, Rivett & Higgs 1997). If we consider the case study overleaf, physiotherapists might use hypothetico-deductive reasoning to identify, propose and narrow possible reasons for Anna's ongoing high levels of pain and limited progress in mobility. Pattern recognition involves practitioners rapidly identifying clients' problems as they draw upon their existing practice-based knowledge of the illness or disorder and typical clinical presentations. Pattern recognition contrasts with the more deliberative testing of possible explanations for the client's presentation associated with hypothetic-deductive reasoning. Pattern recognition has been linked primarily to the reasoning of experts. However, Eva (2004) has suggested that pattern recognition or less deliberative methods of reasoning can also be demonstrated by novice practitioners. The less established knowledge base of novice practitioners, however, may result in a more limited consideration of diagnostic options and potentially less accuracy in forming diagnoses.

Case study 1

Anna is in the orthopaedic ward having undergone a total knee replacement (TKR) five days ago. Her progress has been slow and she continues to experience high levels of pain and knee swelling. She is walking with a pick-up frame. The physiotherapist has been visiting her twice daily and has been asking Anna to perform a range of motion exercises and strengthening exercises, and encouraging her to walk more on the ward. At times Anna becomes teary during physiotherapy sessions and is reluctant to perform her exercises or try to increase her walking distance. Anna lives alone in a house with three outside steps but no internal steps.

Recent research has extended our understanding of the reasoning approaches adopted by physiotherapists. Edwards (2001) identified a range of reasoning strategies used by expert physiotherapists in neurological, orthopaedic and domiciliary settings (Table 8.1). These strategies include the more familiar approaches to reasoning about clients and their physical problems and planning interventions (diagnostic and procedural reasoning). (These terms overlap with hypothetico-deductive reasoning and pattern

Table 8.1 Clinical reasoning strategies used by physiotherapists. Based on Edwards, Jones & Carr (2004).

Strategies of clinical reasoning	Explanation
Diagnostic reasoning	The thinking processes used to form a physiotherapy diagnosis or identification of the client's physical problems
Narrative reasoning	The processes used to appreciate and understand clients' interpretations of their illness experiences
Procedural reasoning	Reasoning used to make decisions about physiotherapy intervention strategies
Interactive reasoning	Reasoning used to develop, establish and maintain effective interaction with the client and others
Collaborative reasoning	The processes involved in engaging with clients in a shared and consensual approach to interpreting their problems, planning interventions and making decisions
Reasoning about teaching	Reasoning about the use of teaching in therapy
Predictive reasoning	The processes of identifying the likely progression of a condition and responses of the client to physiotherapy
Ethical reasoning	The processes of identifying and resolving the ethical and pragmatic or contextual issues in a clinical situation

recognition strategies.) In addition, Edwards found that physiotherapists use narrative, interactive, collaborative, teaching, prognostic and ethical reasoning. The physiotherapists in his study combined these approaches or strategies of reasoning in varying ways according to the characteristics of the clinical situation and problem.

Understanding the interrelationship between clients' biophysical problems and any predisposing or co-existing psychosocial factors involves understanding (and discussing) clients' experiences with their health problems (i.e. narrative reasoning), combined with reasoning about the more biophysical aspects of clients' problems. Applying the notion of narrative reasoning to our case study, the physiotherapist might engage in narrative reasoning by asking Anna about her experience of surgery and post-operative management and how she felt those experiences impacted on her recovery. This could include exploring Anna's understanding of her current physical impairments and the management recommended, her expectations and goals, and any concerns or fears she might have with respect to her management or what the future holds. This narrative reasoning would then enable the practitioner to understand more deeply how Anna is interpreting the experience of her condition and her recovery. This information, when combined with reasoning about her medical diagnosis, could be used to develop a broader understanding of the client and her problems and to guide appropriate management.

Collaborative reasoning and shared decision making are important aspects of physiotherapy practice. The goals of adopting a shared approach to decision making are to respect the self-knowledge of clients and their capacity to share in decision making about their health and to facilitate their collaboration in genuinely client-centred (person and situation-specific) care. Shared decision making involves both parties (and, as relevant, carers, families and friends) collaborating in the process of treatment decision making, and being satisfied with their level of involvement (Charles et al 1999). The shared decision making model utilises scientific information (or evidence) to better inform clients and enhance both their capacity and permission to make choices about their health. Collaborative reasoning highlights the interactive or social nature of reasoning that is embedded in the client–health professional relationship (Siminoff & Step 2005).

CAPABILITIES REQUIRED FOR PHYSIOTHERAPY CLINICAL REASONING

Clinical reasoning has key dimensions of knowledge, cognition, metacognition, the clinical problem, the environment and the client's input (Higgs & Jones 2000). Smith's research in acute care settings (2006) identified that physiotherapists use a range of capabilities in their clinical decision making that incorporate and expand these key dimensions. These capabilities include:

- the ability to develop, organise and access their own unique multidimensional knowledge base for practice
- cognitive abilities to identify and process multiple data inputs to understand clients and their problems and the contexts of practice, and to make decisions for action
- metacognitive and reflexive capabilities to monitor, critique and refine clinical knowledge and reasoning
- social capabilities to interact effectively with clients, carers and other health care professionals

- emotional capabilities to make ethical decisions in the face of challenging personal and emotional circumstances, to respond appropriately to the emotional circumstances of others and to form effective relationships.

Clinical reasoning requires an organised, multidimensional knowledge base

Effective clinical reasoning requires the ability to develop, organise and access a unique multidimensional knowledge base for practice (Norman 2005). More experienced and expert practitioners have a broader, deeper and more organised knowledge base (Phillips et al 2004, Schmidt & Boshuizen 1993) that is client-centred and has evolved through reflection (Jensen et al 2000). Studies of clinical reasoning in medicine indicate that the experience of solving clinical problems contributes to the organised nature of knowledge (Norman 2005). In the case study introduced earlier, practitioners would have knowledge of the surgical procedures used in a TKR, typical presentations of patients following such a procedure, interventions that are effective in restoring mobility and function, and the usual rates of progress. This knowledge is organised in a way that makes it accessible when clients present similarly.

Different types of knowledge, drawn from different sources, are used in clinical reasoning related to a particular problem. Physiotherapists' knowledge can be categorised as propositional knowledge, professional craft knowledge and personal (life-based) knowledge (using the categories of Higgs & Titchen 1995). Propositional knowledge refers to knowledge acquired from theory and research. Novice practitioners acquire this knowledge through formal university studies, continuing education and reading. Professional craft knowledge is knowledge derived from clinical practice experience. It develops from critical reflection on the practitioner's knowledge and practice experience as well as that of clients, work colleagues and mentors (Ajjawi 2006, Beeston & Simons 1996, Jensen et al 2000, Resnik & Jensen 2003). Smith

Table 8.2 The nature of knowledge in acute care physiotherapy. Based on Clinical decision making in acute care cardiopulmonary physiotherapy, 2006, by M C L Smith, Unpublished PhD thesis, The University of Sydney, p 274	
Type of knowledge	Explanation
Propositional knowledge	Knowledge of published scientific principles, theory and research
Procedural knowledge	Knowledge that underlies action, including knowing what to do, when to do it and how to perform the skills of practice
Predictive/comparative knowledge	Experiential knowledge of previous instances, which provides the framework for interpreting the current situation; used to predict likely outcomes and consequences
Situational/contextual knowledge	Knowledge of the physical, social and organisational features of the context
Interpersonal knowledge	Knowledge of people (e.g. this client, the illness, and the response of other workers in the workplace)
Personal/self-knowledge	Knowledge of oneself and one's life experiences

(2006) found that practitioners developed and used a body of knowledge specific to their unique experience and practice settings (see Table 8.2), reflecting these different categories and sources of knowledge.

Clinical reasoning requires a range of cognitive strategies

Clinical reasoning requires the ability to think and process complex concepts and information in order to formulate decisions and plan actions. Physiotherapists' reasoning occurs in the midst of practice; this requires them to *think on their feet*, sometimes rapidly, as the client's condition changes in response to their action. Smith (2006) found that physiotherapists used a range of cognitive capabilities that included the ability to: identify and collect client information relevant to the clinical problem; make mental representations of clients and their problems as a basis for understanding them; process a multitude of client and contextual inputs to make ethical and justified decisions; predict the consequences of decisions and actions; make pragmatic decisions in the face of uncertainty and contextual demands; and adapt practice decisions to new and changing circumstances. Readers will recognise that these cognitive capabilities are consistent with being able to integrate the multiple strategies of reasoning we have previously described.

Physiotherapy cognition during practice is multi-layered, with practitioners being required to make highly skilled judgements on three levels: micro-, macro- and meta-judgements or decisions (Paterson et al 2005). Micro-judgements involve making process decisions; for example, if we consider our case study, how to respond immediately to Anna's tears during therapy. Second, macro-judgements involve making output decisions, such as determining the reason for Anna's high levels of pain and working out a plan of management for her. Third, meta-judgements involve reflective evaluative decisions regarding practice. In our case study this could be asking, 'Did my strategies to motivate and encourage Anna have a positive effect?' These layers of complexity associated with making decisions further demonstrate the extent of cognition required for clinical reasoning during practice.

Clinical reasoning requires skills in metacognition and reflection

Although much initial clinical reasoning research has focused on trying to identify the cognitive processes used in clinical reasoning and the knowledge used in reasoning, increasing recognition has been given to the role of metacognition and reflection as key dimensions of clinical reasoning. Metacognition refers to higher level thinking processes used by practitioners to monitor and critique their cognitive and decision making processes when reasoning. Practitioners undertake these metacognitive or monitoring processes concurrently with making decisions (Higgs & Jones 2000, Smith 2006). They continue to identify and incorporate new data into their reasoning throughout client interactions. This capacity to monitor and adapt reasoning in response to changing circumstances and to growing understanding of the client and his/her condition is necessary for safe and effective clinical practice.

Clinical reasoning also makes use of reflective strategies to critically evaluate practice and as the means to add to knowledge and refine reasoning skills ready for subsequent action (Jensen et al 2000, Resnik & Jensen 2003, Smith 2006). Effective reflection to enhance practice involves critiquing one's decision making and using this critique in the development of knowledge structures to inform subsequent decision making. In relation to our case study, reflection could lead the physiotherapist to realise that he/she had focused too much on diagnostic reasoning and associated procedural management for Anna's physical impairments and insufficiently on the narrative reasoning of Anna's experiences. Anna's pain and lack of desire to progress could relate to anxiety about returning home to live on her own, and this anxiety might be compounding her physical impairments, creating a barrier to progress.

Clinical reasoning requires social and emotional capabilities

Clinical reasoning is not an isolated process; it requires interaction and collaboration with clients, carers and other health professionals (Edwards, Jones & Higgs 2004). Strategies such as narrative and collaborative reasoning, where the emphasis is on understanding the illness experience of others and nurturing of consensus, require more than just cognitive and metacognitive capabilities. These strategies require social and emotional capabilities (Smith 2006).

Social capabilities are needed to engage effectively with others. They include the ability to interact effectively with others in the decision making context, to involve others (both clients and other health professionals) meaningfully and appropriately in collaborative decision making, to critically learn from others for knowledge and guidance, and to manage relationships where differentials in power exist to achieve effective decision-making autonomy.

The clinical problems faced by physiotherapists frequently have an emotional and ethical dimension. Physiotherapists require emotional capabilities to form effective relationships and to engage in ethical reasoning (as described by Edwards, Jones & Carr 2004). A physiotherapist working with Anna would need to acknowledge, understand and address her distress during therapy. Emotional capability involves the ability to identify and manage clients' and caregivers' emotions as they impact on physiotherapy management. It also includes the ability to establish and maintain effective relationships in the workplace with clients, caregivers and work colleagues, through consideration of and appropriate responses to the emotions of others. Emotional capability also enables practitioners to be aware of and deal with problematic emotions in order to make difficult decisions for client management. Clinical reasoning is 'shaped by the professional's underlying humanity and self-knowledge, and underpinned by moral and ethical sensitivity to the individual client and particular context' (de Cossart & Fish 2005, p 132).

FACTORS INFLUENCING CLINICAL REASONING

Clinical reasoning in physiotherapy is a dynamic process that is dependent upon the nature of the problem and cannot be isolated from the context in which it occurs. It is also influenced by factors related to practitioners themselves. Competent clinical practice requires the ability to identify and understand factors that positively or negatively influence decision making. Clinical reasoning in physiotherapy is more appropriately viewed as a process of making decisions that are optimal given the situation and circumstances rather than as a single 'right' process to be enacted regardless of context.

The influence of clients and their problems on clinical reasoning

Clients have beliefs about their illness and its relationship to their management. These beliefs can function as either facilitators or barriers to recovery, and must be understood and either supported or challenged within the different management strategies employed.

The nature of the problem, such as its chronicity (ranging from acute to chronic), also impacts on clinical reasoning (Ajjawi 2006). Ajjawi found that reasoning about acute problems often represented a short-term analysis of the problem, with intervention directed to short-term goals such as stabilising the client's respiration or reducing acute pain and swelling. Reasoning about a chronic problem involves a long-term view of the client's life story, including the client's functional limitations and quality of life. Psychosocial factors, including the clients' thoughts, feelings, self-efficacy and coping strategies have been demonstrated (Craig 2006, Flor & Turk 2006) to contribute significantly (positively and negatively) to clients' disability experiences. Therapists must develop narrative reasoning capabilities and teaching skills to effectively address the psychosocial dimensions of a client's presentation, with referral to other health professionals if required (Jones & Edwards 2008).

Smith (2006) found that the difficulty of the reasoning task influenced decision making. Where decisions were considered simple, practitioners adopted reasoning strategies that required less cognitive effort, often choosing preferred interventions. Indeed, reasoning associated with these less complex problems may appear automatic and subconscious to practitioners as they engage in their everyday activities. Smith found that as decisions were perceived to be increasingly difficult, uncertain and complex, reasoning was raised to greater consciousness, with increased instances of deliberate focused reasoning, seeking the assistance of others and using controlled experimentation in intervention.

The influence of context on clinical reasoning

There has been increasing recognition that clinical reasoning is contextually dependent (Higgs & Jones 2000, Jette et al 2003, Thornquist 2001). Physiotherapists practise in a range of diverse contexts that include intensive care units, community-based private practices, rehabilitation facilities, nursing homes and clients' homes. The contexts that surround physiotherapists' clinical reasoning incorporate multiple physical factors, organisational factors and social factors that physiotherapists engage with daily.

Physical factors that can influence reasoning include location (e.g. distance that the client has to travel to receive services), venue (e.g. room layout, ambience, security) and resources (e.g. the location, supply and availability of equipment).These factors can facilitate or impose constraints in physiotherapy practice and client services/options. Social factors in the context may include the opinions, attitudes and actions of other physiotherapists, medical and nursing staff. Organisational factors include such aspects as workloads, interruptions and organisational systems that guide decision making such as clinical pathways, policies and protocols, but also system definitions of acceptable practice that are represented in the norms, criteria and standards (or assumed knowledge) that individuals working in a particular practice setting adhere to.

Awareness and analysis of contextual factors are important for optimal decision making. Smith (2006) found that cardiorespiratory physiotherapists modified their decisions in response to contextual factors, but also developed strategies to manage and control the context of their practice to achieve desired outcomes. In this study contextual factors assumed different levels of importance according to the unique circumstances that occurred at a given time.

Factors related to practitioners

It has long been established that the reasoning of novice practitioners differs from that of expert practitioners in a number of ways (Benner 1984). Recent research in physiotherapy has identified that expert practitioners have a more organised knowledge base specific to their area of work, a broader and deeper understanding of clients and their problems, faster reasoning processes and more effective outcomes of decisions (Edwards, Jones & Carr 2004, Jensen et al 2000, Resnik & Jensen 2003). A key difference between novice and expert practitioners is their confidence in their reasoning (Ajjawi 2006, Smith 2006). Smith (2006) found that in clinical decision making by acute care physiotherapists, self-efficacy and confidence in decision making were important determinants of the decisions that were made. Where self-efficacy was higher there was a greater willingness for participants to appropriately balance the risks and benefits of intervention rather than to avoid performing interventions due to fear and anxiety. Feelings of higher self-efficacy resulted from the physiotherapists evaluating their levels of knowledge (particularly in comparison to the knowledge levels of other health professionals with whom they were working), having experienced success and failure, and knowing the likely responses to interventions compared with the likelihood of adverse events occurring. All of these factors involve metacognitive ability, essential for ongoing learning, self-appraisal and confidence.

Other practitioner factors that impact on reasoning include practitioners' personal and professional frames of reference (Trede 2006). These include practitioners' beliefs and attitudes that are related to cultural and philosophical views and life experiences (Jones et al 2002), both personal and professional. Trede's (2006) research highlights the importance of collaboration, i.e. clinicians' models of practice and patterns of dialogue in shaping practice process and outcomes. Clinical reasoning is informed by the professional's ideology (i.e. values, interests and prejudgements that guide thinking and are shaped by social, economic and political forces). Understanding existing personal and professional philosophies of practice is essential for the continual critical appraisal required to promote change and revise habits of practice as warranted.

LEARNING TO DO CLINICAL REASONING

Clinical reasoning is a skill to be learned that should continue to evolve and develop throughout a physiotherapist's career path. Learning to do clinical reasoning should focus on the capabilities we have described above. Here we suggest possible strategies that practitioners can use to learn and refine their clinical reasoning.

- **Develop an extensive, accessible knowledge base.** Strategies such as literature searches, reading of journal articles and attending continuing education lectures and courses are key ways of increasing practitioner knowledge. However, the answers to many clinical problems as experienced by clinicians are not always found in these sources. Learning through experience of professional practice and critical reflection on clinical reasoning is an essential aspect of developing a sound, relevant and organised knowledge base to support professional clinical reasoning.

- **Develop skills in the range of physiotherapy reasoning strategies and their integration in practice.** It is relatively easy when learning to reason to limit the reasoning focus to identifying diagnoses and choosing interventions. Specific attention also needs to be given to developing capabilities in narrative reasoning, collaboration, interaction and teaching, ethical practice and integrating contextual factors. As we have noted, clinical reasoning requires practitioners to process information rapidly and to make decisions within the context of practice. Learning to reason requires practising reasoning skills under a range of conditions such as time pressure, changing circumstances and uncertainty. It is useful to practise reasoning with peers and to gain feedback on your reasoning from mentors.

- **Experience authentic clinical cases either in actual clinical settings or in simulation.** Practising reasoning with many real client cases and associated contextual cues is essential for developing flexibility and responsiveness in reasoning strategies in response to authentic context cues (Eva 2004). Practice of authentic clinical cases is essential to promote meaningful knowledge acquisition and use in clinical reasoning. Authenticity refers to the clinical features of the case as well as the narrative and contextual aspects of clients' presentations. Case studies from journals and books (e.g. Jones & Rivett 2004) are an excellent resource for acquiring knowledge and practising clinical reasoning. To lay the foundation for effective hypothetico-deductive reasoning and pattern recognition we would encourage practice of multiple instances of particular conditions where the emphasis is on learning the commonalities in clinical presentation but also the possible diversity. Cases should range in complexity, requiring accessing various degrees of deliberation in reasoning.

- **Learn from (and about) communicating reasoning.** Communication of clinical reasoning is an important aspect of learning to reason. Articulating clinical reasoning contributes to the development of reasoning ability by focusing learners' attention and facilitating conscious self-monitoring and self-critique. Learning is enhanced by receiving feedback from others about reasoning processes and outcomes (Ajjawi & Higgs 2007). In addition, the practice of explaining clinical reasoning promotes reflection and feedback, and the development of processes necessary for communicating reasoning, such as the ability to break down and 'unbundle' thought processes and then to frame and present the message to match the communication abilities and needs of co-communicators (Ajjawi 2006). Creating formal (and informal) opportunities for discussion of client cases is an achievable strategy to promote the development of clinical reasoning abilities. Clinical reasoning can be formally communicated with clinical educators or lecturers and informally communicated with peers, other staff and clients. Probing questions used by those listening to reasoning during these client case discussions can help to elaborate thinking processes. For example, we can ask, 'Why did you apply that treatment?', and encourage learners to consider both supporting and opposing evidence behind clinical hypotheses or decisions.

- **Engage in storytelling or narratives.** Narratives where client stories are preserved and where listeners are personally and professionally engaged are an alternative way of presenting and viewing case studies (Bleakley 2005, Rosenbaum et al 2005) that may be useful for developing social and emotional capabilities in clinical reasoning. Storytelling offers a way of communicating information that promotes coherent recall and explanation of complex information because stories are an ideal way of relating what is learned to what is already known (Fairbairn 2002). Hence stories help students to construct new knowledge and to integrate it with their existing body of knowledge (Titchen & Higgs 2000). Active listening and thinking about the story being told allows students to visualise the situation, setting and characters. This facilitates linkage between that story and other similar situations (Koening & Zorn 2002), which may lead to knowledge transfer between situations. Interacting with stories about professional practice, where physiotherapy students and practitioners may discuss decisions, reasons and justification and identify moral and ethical dilemmas, is a useful strategy outside of the clinical environment for learning to empathise (Fairbairn 2002) and to reason ethically. Storytelling is also likely to promote reflection in individuals telling or creating stories and in the audience engaging with the story being told (Cortazzi et al 2001). It may be for this reason that informal discussions and telling of and listening to client 'stories' in the staffroom continue to be important activities for personal and professional development. In such discussions it is important to maintain respect for clients and ensure ethical issues such as confidentiality are addressed.

- **Develop and enhance metacognitive skills.** Metacognition is a skill that develops with practice; it is described by experienced physiotherapists as a deliberate attitude/action of self-reflection, monitoring and critique (Ajjawi 2006). These activities require learners to become aware of their cognitive strategies and potential sources for error. To identify specific errors in their thinking and to develop strategies to overcome them, learners need to consider alternatives, by 'stepping back' and reflecting on their decision making, by practising mentally, using simulation and seeking feedback (Croskerry 2003).
- **Establish skills in reflection and make this a critical aspect of your practice.** The clinical environment provides rich opportunities for the application, critique and development of practice-based (experiential) knowledge and refinement of existing knowledge networks. Learning in the clinical setting requires processing of and reflection upon the experiences gained and the available learning opportunities (de Cossart & Fish 2005).
- **Identify factors about yourself that influence your clinical reasoning.** Critical self-reflection on your beliefs, attitudes, confidence and self-efficacy is an important aspect of learning to reason. Because aspects of self evolve, this process should be ongoing, particularly as habits of practice start to form.
- **Learn critically from others.** Mentoring and support from colleagues and other health professionals enhance clinical reasoning at all stages of development (Ajjawi & Higgs 2007), particularly during the phase of being a novice physiotherapist, when the steep learning curve and responsibilities of practice may be overwhelming. Experiences gained during physiotherapy practice that are shared with others help in understanding clients' conditions and needs, as well as giving practitioners an understanding of their role within the health care system. Established norms, values and circumstances in which practice takes place influence learning to reason (Ajjawi & Higgs 2007). Physiotherapists should be critically aware of the impact of workplace and professional cultures on their learning. The behaviour of others and knowledge and guidance from our colleagues are sources of knowledge that we draw upon. Novice practitioners need to be mindful of the knowledge they acquire from others (as well as their own practice-based knowledge), and they should critically evaluate such knowledge and its source before incorporating it into their practice. In this way

they can challenge unsubstantiated or routine practices and, thereby, pursue quality assurance and reflective personal development.

SUMMARY

In this chapter we have described clinical reasoning in physiotherapy. In summary, clinical reasoning involves multiple ways of thinking about clients and their problems, the context of clinical practice, and ourselves as practitioners. The process of clinical reasoning requires a range of capabilities that practitioners should regard as elements of being a physiotherapist. Although clinical reasoning is less visible than other aspects of physiotherapy practice, such as applying manual techniques, it should not be viewed as an invisible process that develops opportunistically; rather, it requires focused learning, critical appraisal and refinement with clinical experience.

Reflective questions

- For each of the capabilities described in this chapter, how would you rate your current ability?
- How would you judge the quality of your clinical reasoning?
- What are your learning needs in relation to clinical reasoning?

Further reading

Edwards I, Jones M, Carr J et al 2004 Clinical reasoning strategies in physical therapy. Physical Therapy 84(4):312–335

Edwards I, Jones M, Higgs J et al 2004 What is collaborative reasoning? Advances in Physiotherapy 6:70–83

Higgs J, Jones M, Loftus S et al 2008 Clinical reasoning in the health professions, 3rd edn. Butterworth Heinemann, Oxford

Smart K, Doody C 2007 The clinical reasoning of pain by experienced musculoskeletal physiotherapists. Manual Therapy 12(1):40–49

References

Ajjawi R 2006 Learning to communicate clinical reasoning in physiotherapy practice. Doctoral thesis, University of Sydney. Available: http://hdl.handle.net/2123/1556 12 Sept 2007

Ajjawi R, Higgs J 2007 Learning clinical reasoning: a journey of professional socialisation. Advances in Health Sciences Education p 1-18 DOI 10.1007/s10459-006-9032-4 12 Sept 2007

Beeston S, Simons H 1996 Physiotherapy practice: practitioners' perspectives. Physiotherapy Theory and Practice 12:231–242

Benner P 1984 From novice to expert: excellence and power in clinical nursing practice. Addison-Wesley, Menlo Park, CA

Bleakley A 2005 Stories as data, data as stories: making sense of narrative inquiry in clinical education. Medical Education 39(5):534–540

Charles C, Gafni A, Whelan G 1999 Decision-making in the physician-patient encounter: revisiting the shared treatment decision-making model. Social Science and Medicine 49(5):651–661

Cortazzi M, Jin L, Wall D et al 2001 Sharing learning through narrative communication. International Journal of Language and Communication Disorders 36(Suppl):252–257

Craig K D 2006 Emotions and psychobiology. In: McMahon S, Koltzenburg M (eds) Wall and Melzack's textbook of pain, 5th edn. Elsevier, Philadelphia, pp 231–240

Croskerry P 2003 The importance of cognitive errors in diagnosis and strategies to minimize them. Academic Medicine 78(8):775–780

de Cossart L, Fish D 2005 Cultivating a thinking surgeon: new perspectives on clinical teaching, learning and assessment. tfm, London

Edwards I 2001 Clinical reasoning in three different fields of physiotherapy: a qualitative study. The Australian Digitized Theses Program. Available: www.library.unisa.edu.au/adt-root/ 24 Nov 2005

Edwards I, Jones M, Carr J et al 2004 Clinical reasoning strategies in physical therapy. Physical Therapy 84(4):312–335

Edwards I, Jones M, Higgs J et al 2004 What is collaborative reasoning? Advances in Physiotherapy 6:70–83

Eva K W 2004 What every teacher needs to know about clinical reasoning. Medical Education 39(1): 98–106

Fairbairn G J 2002 Ethics, empathy and storytelling in professional development. Learning in Health and Social Care 1(1):22–32

Flor H, Turk D C 2006 Cognitive and learning aspects. In: McMahon S, Koltzenburg M (eds) Wall and Melzack's textbook of pain, 5th edn. Elsevier, Philadelphia, pp 241–258

Higgs J, Jones M. 2000 Clinical reasoning in the health professions. In: Higgs J, Jones M (eds) Clinical reasoning in the health professions, 2nd edn, Butterworth-Heinemann, Oxford, pp 3–14

Higgs J, Titchen A 1995 The nature, generation and verification of knowledge. Physiotherapy 91(9): 521–530

Higgs J, Trede F, Loftus S et al 2006 Advancing clinical reasoning: interpretive research perspectives grounded in professional practice. CPEA Occasional paper 4. Collaborations in Practice and Education Advancement, The University of Sydney

Jensen G M, Gwyer J, Shepard K F et al 2000 Expert practice in physical therapy. Physical Therapy 80(1):28–43

Jette D U, Grover L, Keck C P 2003 A qualitative study of clinical decision making in recommending discharge placement from the acute care setting. Physical Therapy 83(3):224–236

Jones M, Edwards I 2008 Clinical reasoning to facilitate cognitive-experiential change. In: Higgs J, Jones M, Loftus S et al (eds) Clinical reasoning in the health professions, 3rd edn, Elsevier, Edinburgh, pp 319–328

Jones M, Edwards I, Gifford L 2002 Conceptual models for implementing biopsychosocial theory in clinical practice. Manual Therapy 7(1):2–9

Jones M A, Rivett D A 2004 Introduction to clinical reasoning. In: Jones M A, Rivett D A (eds) Clinical reasoning for manual therapists. Butterworth-Heinemann, London, pp 3–24

Koening J M, Zorn C R 2002 Using storytelling as an approach to teaching and learning with diverse students. Journal of Nursing Education 41(9):393–399

Norman G 2005 Research in clinical reasoning: past history and current trends. Medical Education 39:418–427

Paterson M, Higgs J, Wilcox S 2005 The artistry of judgement: a model for occupational therapy practice. British Journal of Occupational Therapy 68(9):409–417

Phillips J K, Klein G, Sieck W R 2004 Expertise in judgment and decision making: a case for training intuitive decision skills. In: Koehler D J, Harvey N (eds) Blackwell handbook of judgment and decision making. Blackwell, Malden, MA, pp 297–315

Resnik L, Jensen G M 2003 Using clinical outcomes to explore the theory of expert practice in physical therapy. Physical Therapy 83(12):1090–1106

Rivett D, Higgs J 1997 Hypothesis generation in the clinical reasoning behavior of manual therapists. Journal of Physical Therapy Education 11(1):40–45

Rosenbaum M E, Ferguson K J, Herwaldt L A 2005 In their own words: presenting the patient's perspective using research-based theatre. Medical Education 39(6):622–631

Schmidt H G, Boshuizen H P A 1993 On acquiring expertise in medicine. Educational Psychology Review 5:205–221

Siminoff L A, Step M M 2005 A communication model of shared decision making: accounting for cancer treatment decisions. Health Psychology 24(4 supplement):S99–S105

Smart K, Doody C 2007 The clinical reasoning of pain by experienced musculoskeletal physiotherapists. Manual Therapy 12(1):40–49

Smith M C L 2006 Clinical decision making in acute care cardiopulmonary physiotherapy. Unpublished doctoral thesis, University of Sydney

Thornquist E 2001 Diagnostics in physiotherapy – processes, patterns and perspectives, Part II. Advances in Physiotherapy 3:151–162

Titchen A, Higgs J 2000 Facilitating the acquisition of knowledge for reasoning. In: Higgs J, Jones M (eds) Clinical reasoning in the health professions, 2nd edn. Butterworth Heinemann, Oxford, pp 222–229

Trede F 2006 A critical practice model for physiotherapy. Doctoral thesis, The University of Sydney. Available: http://hdl.handle.net/2123/1430 12 Sept 2007

CONTEXTS OF PRACTICE

WORKING AND LEARNING IN COMMUNITIES OF PRACTICE

nine

Joy Higgs, Rola Ajjawi and Megan Smith

Key concepts

- Communities of practice
- Participating in practice communities
- Working in multiple practice communities
- Using communities of practice as a mentoring framework

INTRODUCTION

Health professional students, teachers, practitioners and researchers work and learn in communities of practice (CoP). In using this term we are referring to the idea of communities or groups in a particular field having a considerable influence over and support for the way individuals entering those communities learn to meet the expectations and develop the capabilities for working in their practice communities. A core feature of these communities is that learning is embedded in practice rather than being a separate and even optional activity.

Vickie's story – day 1

There were six of us allocated to this hospital for our first year out. When Simon and I heard about our allocation we were thrilled – a hospital with lots of opportunities for rotation to good units and wards – and other new grads had reported having a great year there. Then – lots to do getting ready, a holiday, packing up uni books and papers. But now – it's DAY ONE. So much different from being a student – I'm here for a year – and employed – not just visiting for 6 weeks. I'm responsible. I'M responsible. Can I do it all on my own? Arrived early – but still a lot of busy people already there in the staff room – what are the rules? Where do I go? Pleased that some of the other first years are there too – we chat together in a corner – waiting …. Next a meeting – rather formal – with the Head of Department – orientation. Quite a bit about rosters, contact people, support systems, regulations – the system rules. And so – to work …

Vickie – 3 months later

Looking back – well – I thought I knew a lot when I left uni. And that orientation on Day 1 seemed organised but overwhelming. But neither prepared me for the steep – very steep – learning curve I would be on for the next month especially – and then every time I went to a new work area – or worked weekends for the first time – or gave my first ward meeting report – or had my first disagreement with the ward manager or – well the list goes on. It wasn't just one group of people – the physio department – and their expectations I had to meet – but each work area, each professional group – the nurses, doctors, OTs and so on … and the bureaucracy, the system – and beyond the workplace the physio profession – and health care. It was a bit like being owned by lots of groups. And it took a lot of getting to know each of these groups and their expectations of me. But it was worth it – the more I learned and the better I coped with all the work demands, the more I belonged. Here's what it looked like to me (see Fig 9.1.).

COMMUNITIES OF PRACTICE – THEORETICAL PERSPECTIVES

The concept of CoP is relatively new, and has become popular in academic fields such as education, organisational learning and management. Since the introduction of this term its meaning has undergone change, from its original presentation as a theory of situated learning that occurs during socialisation into a practice (Lave & Wenger 1991), to a guide for managing informal groups, to a framework for enhancing organisational performance (Wenger et al 2002). In the field of education, for example, the term CoP has been used to describe learning in online and virtual communities, in schools and in tertiary institutions, as well as continuing professional development and higher degree research studies.

There are two key features in CoP that transcend all these applications and continue to underpin the concept (Cox 2005): *situated negotiation of meaning* (which refers to locally and socially constructed knowledge) and *identity being central to learning*. In a critical review of the literature, Cox (2005) argued that the ambiguity of the terms *community* and *practice* is a source of the concept's reusability (and strength), allowing it to be reappropriated for different purposes. In contrast, Eraut (2002) argued that certain aspects of CoP may be useful for theory building and new conceptualisations of workplace learning but that the concept itself is too limiting considering the wide range of workplace contexts. In this chapter we take a broad view of practice, meaning the performance of the role of the profession or occupational group in serving or contributing to the community. We therefore see wide application for CoP across multiple workplaces and occupational and professional work contexts.

A CoP was initially defined as a 'set of relations among persons, activity and world, over time and in relation with other tangential and overlapping communities of practice' (Lave & Wenger 1991, p 98). This notion of CoP allows for participation at multiple levels in these tangential and overlapping communities (e.g. you can take a peripheral role in some communities and a more central role in others). Taking this definition we see a clear parallel with the experiences of 'Vickie' upon entering the workforce and her multiple CoP (see Fig. 9.1).

Individuals are both part of and distinct from workplace communities, and may belong to several communities simultaneously (Wenger 1998). Such communities are not necessarily well-defined identifiable groups with socially visible boundaries (Lave & Wenger 1991). Classrooms or work teams become communities in which learning can be collaboratively sought, knowledge can be collaboratively constructed, and practice can be collaboratively pursued as all participants engage together in activities to which they are committed and to which they contribute based on the demands of the situation.

Originally CoP was presented as a theory whereby learning is seen as a historical and

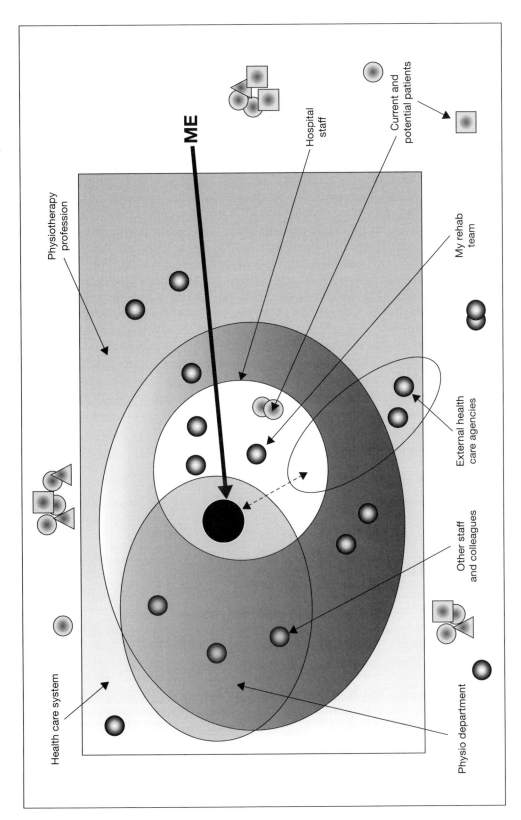

Fig. 9.1 Vickie's mind map of belonging to communities of practice

situated dimension of social practice (Lave & Wenger 1991). Lave and Wenger proposed that learning is a process of participation in a CoP. Part of the process of becoming a full member of that community is *legitimate peripheral participation*. This is the process of transition from newcomer to expert or 'old timer' and involves movement from the periphery of a sociocultural CoP to its centre as the individual becomes progressively more engaged and active in community activities and more imbued with that sociocultural perspective. This perspective of practice and development emphasises the social rather than (simply) cognitive dimensions of learning, highlighting the subconscious and informal nature of learning that occurs through normal working practice.

Legitimate peripheral participation is a construct that helps us to understand learning. It takes place regardless of any intentional educational objective. The strength of this view of learning is to move beyond a mechanistic view of learning as cognitive transmission towards an active social participation (cultural) view of learning. Hay (1993) argued that, for legitimate peripheral participation to work constructively, newcomers must not be left powerless at the periphery until they become 'masters', by which point they may be socialised into following routines of practice. Instead, learners need to be placed at the centre of the interaction in a dialogic relationship with a CoP, where they have the freedom to emulate (and change) what they choose of the practices of the community. In this way learners may follow the path of legitimate peripheral participation, and they can shape and be part of a new community, become part of several communities or find new ways into the centre of the community from the periphery.

Vickie and Simon at 6 months

S: I was watching you today in the team meeting. It was good to hear you question the rehab protocol – I haven't liked it for some time – but today you came up with a good argument for changing it.

V: Thanks – yes, I've been trying to figure out what was bugging me about it – and partly it was the actual protocol and partly it was having a protocol that no one questioned. I was glad that the team supported me in speaking up – and changing the 'rules' was good too – seeing the protocol as a starting point or a guide, not a requirement.

PARTICIPATION IN PRACTICE COMMUNITIES

Wenger (1998) extended CoP theory to include three dimensions of participation: mutual engagement, joint enterprise and shared repertoire. He referred to people 'being active participants in the *practices* of social communities and constructing *identities* in relation to these communities' (p 4). He defined CoP as groups that form through sustained mutual engagement in a shared purpose or 'joint enterprise', developing a shared repertoire of discourse and action. They learn to 'talk the talk' and 'walk the walk' of their group. This revised concept of CoP recognised that relationships can be harmonious or conflicting. Communities do not necessarily always display the positive or warm connotation associated with the term; they may also be diffuse, fragmented and contentious (Brown & Duguid 1996); in these cases participation and learning may be hindered (if not inhibited completely). Individuals working within a CoP need to recognise the power forces that exist within a community and learn to function within them; relationships may involve challenge, criticism, conflict and disagreement

(Cox 2005).

Wenger (1998) focused on how individuals construct identities based on different levels of participation as members in multiple communities, and he considered the dilemmas this may present. Cox (2005) argued that the nature of work in the 21st century involves frequent restructuring and part-time or temporary contracts, and that this work is at times competitive and individualised, time-poor, spatially fragmented and heavily mediated (by computers, for example). Such conditions inhibit sustained collective engagement (a condition needed for the formation of CoP according to Wenger). The value of using CoP to understand and shape practice is in the types of knowledge and skills that emanate from the patterns and actions built up historically in a community into which health professionals are socialised through social interaction and active participation. A critical knowing stance among health professionals (based on an understanding of the processes through which professional knowledge develops) can ensure that professional knowledge and activities are not limited by practitioners simply reproducing past practices (Abrandt Dahlgren et al 2004).

WORKING IN MULTIPLE COMMUNITIES OF PRACTICE

Vickie's mind map of her working situations in Figure 9.1 demonstrates how she saw herself belonging to multiple CoP, which included:

- *The work team in the rehabilitation department.* Here Vickie was the sole physiotherapist with her own caseload as well as a participant in team activities such as case conferences. This community was directly involved in Vickie's day-to-day work and professional behaviour and role.
- *The physiotherapy department.* Vickie was one of 15 staff members in her department, where she was a member of the whole group and part of the 'first years' subgroup. Both groups influenced Vickie's professional identity and development, her sense of self as a professional and her confidence and self-appraisal as a competent practitioner.
- *The hospital.* This was a larger community group where system rules and regulations, working conditions and the physical environment created the setting for Vickie's employment.
- *The physiotherapy profession.* This community set the standards of practice, established the ethical code of conduct, contributed to professional education (formal and informal) and regulated the conduct of members of the profession that set expectations of Vickie and other members of the profession.
- *External agencies.* Vickie worked from time to time with people employed in other health care agencies such as nursing homes. She had to learn how to deal with each new community's procedures and cultures.
- *The health care system.* Indirectly Vickie was a member of a large, complex, multi-layered CoP called the health care system.

Vickie and Simon at 12 months

V: It's amazing really. I thought I understood all these multiple levels of interaction involved in physio. But only now near the end of first year out do I feel I've got a handle on it.

S: I know what you mean. But I think it's going to take me years to really get it.

USING COMMUNITIES OF PRACTICE AS A MENTORING FRAMEWORK

CoP can serve as a framework for mentoring. To explore this potential we return to the story of 'Simon' in his first year of clinical practice.

Simon's story

In the large metropolitan hospital Simon rotates through a number of different clinical areas. He has recently rotated to the intensive care unit, where he will spend the next three months. During this rotation he will be mentored by 'Marnie', who works permanently in the unit as the senior physiotherapist.

In this example we assume that a CoP has developed through the shared work experiences and goals of the individuals who work together in the intensive care unit. Through their shared work they also engage in shared learning opportunities to solve common problems. Intensive care units are typically complex work environments where patients are critically ill, complex technology is used and patient situations may change rapidly. For beginning practitioners, or any practitioner for that matter, entering these settings can be daunting. Intensive care units also typically have expected protocols of practice (explicit and codified as well as implicit and informally communicated) and established modes of communication that those who work in the unit are aware of and adhere to. Practitioners in Simon's situation need to learn these ways of practice. By using a framework that recognises the characteristics of a CoP Marnie can play an important role in facilitating Simon's integration into the CoP and facilitating Simon's learning experience.

An initial role that Marnie could play in this case is to facilitate Simon's admission to the CoP. Hay (1993) noted that novices are not automatically included in a CoP. Likewise Bleakley (2002) observed that in medical practice junior doctors needed to gain legitimate entry into the working group. Marnie could facilitate Simon's access by introducing him to the other members of the community, explaining to him the community's ways of communicating and acting, and also by providing him with practice opportunities that are seen as legitimate by the community. Cope et al (2000, p 851) explained that 'a critical part of the socialization into practice is the opportunity to make an authentic contribution to the communal enterprise'.

A second role of a mentor is to facilitate learning. Effective clinical practice requires knowledge of the context, knowledge and skills of discipline practice, and the integration of these (Eraut 2004). Within CoP knowledge of context is held collectively by the community. As a new member of the community, Simon needs to learn how to access this knowledge, as well as how to critique it in the development of his own practice within the community. In this case Marnie could model how learning occurs in relation to other members of the community by asking questions and engaging Simon in dialogue and shared decision making about patient care as well as articulating her own learning. Marnie could also engage in a number of strategies that enable Simon to access and learn the contextual aspects of practice, including discussing common episodes, working together on tasks, articulating more difficult aspects of tasks, explaining cultural and situational norms, discussing cases and describing stories, articulating her own knowledge of the context and how it influences her decision making and practice, and discussing how she prioritises her practice activities by sharing and negotiating with other members of the community and how she balances this with her own professional role (see Eraut 2004). An additional role for Marnie would be to ensure that Simon incorporates the contributions of other members of the practice community in his learning, thereby moving away from the notion that learning is focused only within the newcomer–mentor dyadic relationship.

Marnie may also guide Simon's learning by enabling him to participate in tasks at a level commensurate with his experience. As Simon becomes increasingly capable of independent practice Marnie can progressively withdraw her support and provide him with increasingly complex activities to perform. This process builds on the concept of legitimate peripheral participation. The move from peripheral to full participation is one that entails a shift in power and responsibility. The roles of student physiotherapists are clearly viewed in terms of peripheral participation. However, a new graduate of physiotherapy may (prematurely) be given full participation status within an overstretched system with limited resources and support. 'Credible learning is not limited to the acquisition of structured knowledge, but involves the provision of increased access to participating roles in expert performances' (Bleakley 2002, p 13). As Simon performs activities that are typical of the community and appropriates its language, his contribution is considered legitimate. Legitimacy is also enhanced when Simon's actions are considered trustworthy by other members of the community.

Bleakley (2002) observed that novices entering a CoP may seek to emulate the behaviour of more senior staff to further their practice development without understanding the tacit/implicit knowledge and professional judgements that guide such behaviours or critically evaluating them. That is, apparent acculturation into the community may occur, but without the establishment of individual meaning and identity this outcome is undesirable. As a mentor Marnie could provide a safe environment in which novices can share their experiences and enhance their awareness of their practice. She could also support efforts by the novice to question and critique the practice of the community and offer new perspectives. In this way novices become critical (thoughtful) members of the community, contributing to its advancement rather than unquestioningly joining in community activities and perhaps sustaining existing sub-optimal practices.

Organisational system factors such as heavy workloads, time pressures and staff shortages have been found to interfere with physiotherapists' ability to supervise or mentor novice practitioners (Ajjawi 2006, Sellars 2004). Sellars called for a change in culture, starting with managers providing vital resources and quality training, and contended that clinical supervision and mentoring should become embedded in policy. She also urged health professionals to value their capabilities and the time taken to reflect on the complexities of clinical practice. Developing learning communities within health care teams distributes the responsibility for mentoring and support across several health professionals. In such communities, learning would be a primary goal embedded in daily practice, rather than an additional responsibility or chore. Opportunistic learning can thus be enhanced through collaboration in CoP, effective role modelling and informal focused discussions about practice.

Vickie and Simon at 18 months

S: Hi Vickie, I'm having a fabulous time in ICU.

V: That's great – you were nervous about going there, weren't you?

S: Sure – but it's made a big difference working with Marnie. She's showing me the ropes – not just doing physio but also how to work with the team. Instead of panicking about what I have to do, I'm learning more about working with others in the team.

SITUATED LEARNING

Situated learning is closely related to learning within CoP. The construct is based on the notion that knowledge is contextually situated and is fundamentally influenced by the activity, context and culture in which it is used (Billett 1996, Brown et al 1989). That is, knowledge is co-produced through activity in context. This can be seen in the example of Marnie and Simon. Full participation in the real context of practice allowed Simon to select elements that he perceived as meaningful to his learning, guided by Marnie. Brown et al (1996, p 24) compared knowledge to a set of tools, arguing that tools can be understood only through use, and that using them appropriately requires understanding and adopting the belief system of the community and culture in which they are used. 'The culture and the use of a tool act together to determine the way practitioners see the world; and the way the world appears to them determines the culture's understanding of the world and of the tools'. For students and novices to be able to use tools as practitioners, they must enter the practitioners' community and its culture.

In this way learning can be seen as a process of acculturation that occurs by joining and participating in CoP rather than merely by the application of skills or principles that operate independently of social context. This is a much richer process and outcome than learning knowledge and skills in isolation; it extends to understanding one's profession and its role in health care and internalising what is expected of that profession both from within and outside. Understanding the relationship between the CoP and the individual's dispositions toward working, learning and participating in the community is crucial to understanding the learning that takes place. For example, an important capability of health professional practice that has been found to develop through acculturation in CoP is communication of clinical reasoning (see Ajjawi 2006, Ajjawi & Higgs 2007). Both of the concepts that Cox (2005) argued underpin CoP (situated negotiation of meaning and identity being central to learning) were valuable in conceptualising how physiotherapists learned to communicate their reasoning.

Ajjawi (2006) found that learning to communicate reasoning was enhanced through participation in everyday work practices where the contexts of learning and practice are identical, that is, situated learning. Formation of a professional identity with professional responsibilities including accountability and duty of care for patients encouraged such learning in her participants. They were further motivated to improve their reasoning and communication abilities when facing challenging work situations that extended or stretched them beyond what they could accomplish independently. The notion of developing beyond one's individual ability through interaction and cooperation with others encapsulates the concept of learning within the zone of proximal development (ZPD) (Vygotsky 1978). Vygotsky (p 85–86) defined the ZPD as 'the distance between the actual developmental level as determined by individual problem solving and the level of potential development as determined through problem solving under the guidance or in collaboration with more capable peers'. This collaboration occurs when members of CoP, including clients, caregivers, peers, colleagues and mentors, extend or

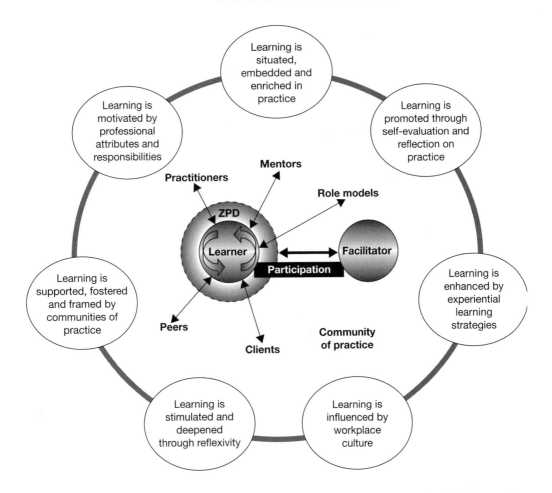

Fig. 9.2 A model of learning for practice. Derived from *Learning to communicate clinical reasoning in physiotherapy practice*, 2006, by R Ajjawi, PhD thesis, The University of Sydney

scaffold the novice's learning through guidance, modelling, discussion and feedback in the context of the challenging situation. Multiple ZPDs can occur in multidisciplinary settings, where every health professional provides scaffolding for all the others, and where the problems are so complex that no individuals are expected to perform at the expert level on their own (Loftus 2006).

The model developed in Ajjawi's (2006) research is adapted here to illustrate how physiotherapists can utilise CoP for their professional practice development (see Fig 9.2). This model represents a cross-sectional image of interaction and development within one CoP. The learner occupies the central circle and learns within his or her ZPD (represented by the dashed circle surrounding the learner) in participation with various members of the CoP. Professional attributes and responsibilities for each learner drive their learning, e.g. motivation, passion, excitement, and level of challenge or responsibility. The facilitator in the adjacent circle is in direct interaction with the learner. Any member of the community, including clients, caregivers, colleagues and mentors, may act as a facilitator in participation with the learner; these people are also learners, depending on the context or situation in their respective journeys. The curved arrows within the learner's circle represent reflexivity as the learner develops and enhances professional capabilities through raised awareness, focusing of attention, and lifelong and self-directed learning. Reflexivity is evident in heightened awareness and self-critique of practice, with a genuine desire to continue to improve. Learning occurs largely within the boundaries of the CoP, represented in the model by the outer bold circle. Although not demonstrated in the figure, we recognise that CoP influence and are influenced by wider social, cultural and political contexts. Dotted along the boundary of a CoP are themes that help us to conceptualise how learning in practice is facilitated. A longitudinal image would reflect how these themes interact and overlap throughout health professionals' career journeys as professional capabilities such as reasoning and its communication develop and improve.

SUMMARY

We have used the example of two new graduate physiotherapists to illustrate how the concepts of CoP and situated learning can be employed to understand and facilitate physiotherapists' learning to practise. Beginning practitioners can use these concepts to identify CoP within their workplace and consider the role of these communities in their learning. Practitioners might also consider how learning to practise physiotherapy is a social and cultural activity as much as it is an individual pursuit, and reflect on the implications for their approach to learning and the facilitation of learning in others.

Reflective questions

- How have you learned to adjust your interactions when working in different practice communities?
- How could you use the ideas on CoP in this chapter to shape your professional development?

References

Abrandt Dahlgren M, Richardson B, Sjostrom B 2004 Professions as communities of practice. In: Higgs J, Richardson B, Abrandt Dahlgren M (eds) Developing practice knowledge for health professionals. Butterworth-Heinemann, Edinburgh, pp 71–88

Ajjawi R 2006 Learning to communicate clinical reasoning in physiotherapy practice. PhD thesis, University of Sydney, Australia. Available: http://hdl.handle.net/2123/1556 21 Oct 2007

Ajjawi R, Higgs J 2007 Learning clinical reasoning: a journey of professional socialisation. Advances in Health Sciences Education pp 1–18 DOI 10.1007/s10459-006-9032-4. Available: http://www.springerlink.com/content/g5211k5824q1p630/?p=285e0532d77a4cc1a191672fbcd9e914&pi=1 14 Dec 2007

Billett S 1996 Situated learning: bridging sociocultural and cognitive theorising. Learning and Instruction 6(3):263–280

Bleakley A 2002 Pre-registration house officers and ward-based learning: a new 'apprenticeship' model. Medical Education 36:9–15

Brown J S, Collins A, Duguid P 1989 Situated cognition and the culture of learning. Educational Researcher 18(1):32–42

Brown, J S, Collins A, Duguid P 1996 Situated cognition and the culture of learning. In: McLellan H (ed) Situated learning perspectives. Educational Technology Publications, Englewood Cliffs, NJ pp 19–44

Brown J S, Duguid P 1996 Stolen knowledge. In: McLellan H (ed) Situated learning perspectives. Educational Technology Publications, Englewood Cliffs, NJ pp 47–56

Cope P, Cuthbertson P, Stoddart B 2000 Situated learning in the practice placement. Journal of Advanced Nursing 31(4):850–856

Cox A 2005 What are communities of practice? A comparative review of four seminal works. Journal of Information Science 31(6):527–540

Eraut M 2002 Conceptual analysis and research questions: do the concepts of 'learning community' and 'community of practice' provide added value? Paper presented at the annual meeting of the American Educational Research Association, New Orleans, LA, April 1–5. Eric Database 466030

Eraut M 2004 Informal learning in the workplace. Studies in Continuing Education 26(2):247–273

Hay K E 1993 Legitimate peripheral participation, instructionism, and constructionism: whose situation is it anyway? Educational Technology 33(2):33–38

Lave J, Wenger E 1991 Situated learning: legitimate peripheral participation. Cambridge University Press, Cambridge

Loftus S 2006 Language in clinical reasoning: Learning and using the language of collective decision making. PhD thesis, University of Sydney, Australia. Available: http://hdl.handle.net/2123/1165 3 Oct 2007

Sellars J 2004 Learning from contemporary practice: an exploration of clinical supervision in physiotherapy. Learning in Health and Social Care 3(2):64–82

Vygotsky L S 1978 Mind in society: the development of higher psychological processes (trans M Cole). Harvard University Press, Cambridge

Wenger E 1998 Communities of practice: learning, meaning, and identity. Cambridge University Press, Cambridge

Wenger E, McDermott R and Snyder WM, 2002. A guide to managing knowledge: cultivating communities of practice, Harvard Business School Press, Boston, MA

CULTURE AND PHYSIOTHERAPY PRACTICE

Louisa Remedios, Heather Dawson and Ian Edwards

ten

Key content

- Culture as the lens we use to interpret the world and as an influence on how we think, feel and act
- Cultural literacy and cultural competence as two frameworks for understanding cross-cultural encounters
- Integrating concepts of culture with clinical reasoning and an evidence-based practice model of physiotherapy delivery

MEET THE AUTHORS

By introducing ourselves with some stories about cultural experiences, we highlight our diverse backgrounds and our personal experiences of working in cross-cultural contexts in clinics and classrooms, both in Australia and overseas. We also highlight that everyone carries cultural stories and that we see value in listening to individuals' stories as important in building 'cultural wisdom', an attribute we see as fundamental to physiotherapy practice.

> **Heather**: Living and working as a physiotherapist in Afghanistan, Australia, India, Indonesia, UK and Zimbabwe has taught me that we need to be aware of our different belief systems and values and that it can be easy to misunderstand each other. As an Australian physiotherapist from an Anglo white middle class background, I am still teaching myself to question my assumptions whenever I interact with other people. This was illustrated on a recent visit to a country I have visited many times previously. The waiter asked me if I wanted more coffee, I smiled and said 'thanks' in the local language, meaning 'yes, thanks'. He walked away. My colleague laughed and told me that by saying thanks I was saying 'no, thanks' in that context. Even the same behaviour can be interpreted differently by persons from different cultures. For example, some overseas students avoid eye contact. In my culture, avoiding eye contact means you may be hiding something or are shy. I learned that in their culture it was considered rude to look an elder or authority figure in the eye. So the students were showing me respect, while I may have made them feel uncomfortable by trying to make eye contact. We live and learn!

Heather is an experienced physiotherapist who has worked extensively in the public health arena both locally and overseas.

Ian: Some years ago I was working in the physiotherapy department of a hospital in the Punjab in India. I had not long been in India, having arrived fresh from living in the working class area of Port Adelaide, South Australia. I was invited to have 'chai' at morning tea by one of my male colleagues, who offered his hand. Not wishing to offend and considering myself a friendly guy, I took the offered hand. However, to my growing unease, my colleague held my hand as we walked through the department, and continued his firm grip as we walked outside and through the hospital grounds before continuing to a stall down the street. My thought processes, translated into words, went something along the lines of 'If only the boys back in Port Adelaide could see me now!' With further experience of life in India and Afghanistan, I came to see that holding hands was just 'how it was' between male friends in public, whereas male and female friends would hardly dare to hold hands in public. This situation was the reverse to that at home. It certainly contrasted with what I think in retrospect was a fair representation of the views of Port Adelaide males (at least those I knew) that such a practice would constitute an occupational health and safety hazard. This experience occurred many years ago but its lesson has remained with me: much of what we know is socially constructed and there can be more than one 'valid' reality or perspective for a particular phenomenon.

Ian lived and worked in Afghanistan as a physiotherapist for several years in the 1980s and has also spent time in rural Mexico learning about community-based rehabilitation in poor communities.

Louisa: Born and bred till 14 years of age in India, I moved with my family to Melbourne in the 1970s. I have vivid memories of contrasts and confusion and quite a bit of embarrassment in those early years. Moving from the noises, smells and chaos of the streets of Calcutta to the empty, quiet, clean streets of suburban Melbourne, where all life seemed to occur indoors, I felt like I was living in a science fiction movie. The classroom was a change from a Catholic convent run by nuns to a public co-educational school in Melbourne, where miniskirts were tolerated by teachers, cooking (home economics) was to be learned at school, and debating and disagreeing with older people was acceptable (a behaviour I still have trouble with). I also had to learn Auslish (Australian English) fast. For example, 'Would you like to wash the dishes?' meant the same as 'Please wash the dishes' in Indian English; and when you were invited out to a meal, bringing a plate (with something on it) was a way of life and not a failure in hospitality. Needless to say, it took a while to develop my cultural literacy (see below) of Australian life and Australian classrooms and I have lived through several misunderstandings on the way to acculturating (to some extent) to the Australian way of life. However, the experiences of living in a new culture have been fun more than frustrating, more pleasure than pain. It has only been difficult when I have not been respected for my values, and have been made to feel that my way is not the right way, rather than simply a different way.

Louisa is an academic at the School of Physiotherapy, The University of Melbourne. Her PhD was on the experiences and responses of overseas educated students to classroom cultures in Australia.

INTRODUCTION

Our objective in this chapter is to introduce the notion of culture and its important role in our practice as physiotherapists, at both local and global levels. We highlight two frameworks that can be used to sensitise ourselves to cross-cultural encounters (cultural literacy and cultural competence), and we draw attention to the influence of culture on our clinical decision making and therefore on the quality of our health care service.

There is a clear rationale for understanding culture and its influences on the health care systems in Australia. Government statistics indicate that individuals living in Australia come from 185 different countries. Nearly one in four Australian residents was either born overseas or has at least one parent from overseas (Australian Bureau of Statistics 2007). The main message here is that we, as physiotherapists, are likely to come from one of the diverse cultures that are represented in Australia. Further, we will all work with patients/clients from different cultural backgrounds, as well as colleagues who have different cultural beliefs. Since many of us are likely to choose to work overseas, understanding our own cultures and being sensitive to the cultures of others will be essential skills. We believe that increasing our knowledge of how cultures operate and how we operate within our own cultural frames and developing our skills at recognising and respecting the cultural preferences of others are central to the development of 'cultural wisdom', an important attribute for physiotherapists.

CONCEPTUALISING CULTURE

Culture is a complex concept and there are many different definitions and descriptions of the term. It has been described as one of the most 'complex and differently interpreted word(s) in the human language' (Wadham et al 2007, p 4). Table 10.1 gives examples of some approaches to describing culture.

Common to most definitions is the emphasis on *learned knowledge* related to *values, beliefs and norms* that are *shared by a group* of people. It is essentially the lens through which we view, interpret and respond to the world around us. A definition that captures the pervasive and fundamental aspect of culture in our lives describes it as:

> whatever it is one has to know in order to operate successfully, and in a manner acceptable to the members of a given society. It is the form of things that people have in mind, their models for perceiving, relating, and interpreting. Culture consists of guides or standards for deciding what is, for deciding what one feels about it, for deciding what to do about it, and for deciding how to go about doing it ... Culture informs, influences and shapes fundamental beliefs and values and thereby shapes expectations, attitudes, behaviours and practices. (Goodenough, cited in Minas & Klimidis 1994, p 4)

If we take this definition into the health care domain, we can see culture as profoundly influencing how we think, feel and act, both as therapists and as patients. Culture influences how we view our own health status, when we judge ourselves to be sick or healthy and who we see as responsible for our state of wellness. Every judgement we make is influenced by our cultural education. Culture even dictates whether we prefer to say *patient* or *client* when referring to health service users (we use the terms interchangeably in this chapter).

Author(s) (date)	Definition*
Table 10.1 Definitions of culture	
Mead (1837)	Culture means the whole complex of traditional behaviour which has been developed by the human race and is successively learned by each generation. A culture is less precise. It can mean the forms of traditional behaviour which are characteristics of a given society, or of a group of societies, or of a certain race, or of a certain area, or of a certain period of time
Dewey (1916)	The capacity for constantly expanding the range and accuracy of one's perception of meaning
Kroeber, Kluckhohn (1952)	Culture consists of patterns, explicit and implicit, of and for behavior acquired and transmitted by symbols, constituting the distinctive achievements of human groups, including their embodiments in artefacts; the essential core of culture consists of traditional (i.e. historically derived and selected) ideas and especially their attached values; culture systems may, on the one hand, be considered as products of action, and on the other as conditioning elements of future action
Geertz (1966)	Culture … denotes an historical pattern of meanings embodied in symbols, a system of inherited conceptions expressed in symbolic forms by means of which men communicate, perpetuate, and develop their knowledge about and attitudes to life
White, Epston (1990)	An extrasomatic (nongenetic, nonbodily), temporal continuum of things and events dependent upon symbolling
Hofstede (1994)	The collective programming of the mind which distinguishes the members of one group or category of people from another
Eisenhart (2002)	A set of symbolic and material forms, affected but not determined by history and structure, actively appropriated or 'produced' in groups to bring order and satisfaction to experiences. In consequence, culture includes both enabling and disabling dimensions, both reproductive and transformative possibilities for those who produce and live by it
Wadham et al (2007)	Culture is the 'toolbox' by which we interpret and attempt to fix the problems we face as humans

*Definitions sourced from: Varenne H (n.d.) The culture of CULTURE. Available: http://varenne.tc.columbia.edu/hv/clt/and/culture_def.html 10 Dec 2007.

Because different societies have evolved different beliefs over time, persons from different cultural backgrounds can have vastly different views about health and the appropriate way to manage it. We may view someone as sick when in fact they see themselves as perfectly healthy and vice versa (Jorgensen 2000). Different cultural beliefs and values can lead to a rich variation in how individuals experience their health and the degree to which they wish to manage their own health. It can also be a potential source of misunderstanding and conflict (overt or hidden) between patients and health professionals.

CHALLENGING THE NOTION OF CULTURE AS A CATEGORY OF CONSTRAINT

One approach to the study of culture has been to focus on people as belonging to categories, with the emphasis on their differences (for examples see Hall & Hall 1990, Hofstede 1980). In this approach, people labelled as belonging to one culture are seen as very similar to each other, with the tendency to stereotype individuals, assuming that an individual from a culture represents the behaviour of all persons from that culture. For example, if one student from a cultural group prefers not to make eye contact, it is inferred that all students from that group will avoid eye contact. Culture appears as an inflexible system that is so powerful, deep-seated, collective and binding as to limit our freedom to act outside our cultural comfort zone!

Current understandings of culture see individuals as internalising the learned rules and nuances of their culture to different extents, and as acting out varying attachments to cultural values (Gudykunst 1997). The individual's response to any social context, whether familiar or unfamiliar, is seen as a creative process, although with some constraints imposed by our understanding of 'what is possible, appropriate, legitimate, properly radical and so forth' (Eisenhart 2001, p 215). As there is always ongoing and continual reassessment of meanings and understandings, we are capable of adapting our cultural understanding through interactions with others in different cultural settings.

Another take-home message is that culture itself is always hybrid and heterogeneous (Wadham et al 2007), with individuals carrying multiple cultural influences. To some extent we choose the cultures we expose ourselves to and the value systems we engage with. We construct identity as we interact with other individuals, developing our history to make stories about who we are and how we wish others to see us. We are always actively, if not always consciously, shaping our value systems and evolving our cultural identity.

PHYSIOTHERAPY AS A CULTURE

It is important to recognise that we have been socialised to be physiotherapists, learning and internalising rules and values we share within the physiotherapy community. Dahlgren and Dahlgren (2002) point out that academic disciplines are 'powerful forces in the articulation, maintenance and reproduction of the perspectives, values and beliefs embedded in their cultures' (p 125), essentially becoming 'carriers of ways of thinking that rule their communities of practice' (p 115). Our socialisation into physiotherapy is a vivid example of how individuals develop new cultural understandings, buying into a culture and slowly constructing an identity that incorporates values of what matters in practice and in our *reality* of what constitutes good practice. Our notion of how a *good* patient should behave tells us a lot about our own value system. The degree to which we share these notions with our peers and, more especially, the sharing of why we judge them to be ideal are evidence of our socialisation into the physiotherapy community. However, our views may vary substantially from those of physiotherapists operating in different health settings, especially in different countries. More importantly, our training may be at odds with the cultural preferences of the patients we work with. Two frameworks for considering how we can respond in cross-cultural contexts are outlined in the following sections on cultural literacy and cultural competence.

CULTURAL LITERACY

Cultural literacy has been defined as knowledge and understanding of meaning systems and a way to negotiate these meaning systems appropriately in different cultural contexts (Schirato & Yell 2000). To any health care setting individuals bring varying levels of cultural literacy, depending on their previous exposure and knowledge of what is valued within the setting. Cultural literacy allows us to predict how an interaction will play out, the major values that are operating within the system, and how we can shape the outcome of an interaction to align with our own agenda. Literacy in this sense reflects reading the legitimate choices available to us, and it allows us to act intentionally. When we are culturally literate, we can be confident that when we give offence it is because we want to.

This notion is helpful for understanding the difficulty we would experience when working as a physiotherapist in an unfamiliar health context as well as the difficulties patients from different cultural backgrounds experience in the various Australian health settings. The individual entering a new domain needs to become familiar with the value systems operating, develop the capacity to sum up the priorities of the time, and act in a manner that produces desired outcomes. It is a common expectation that patients are culturally literate with regard to the health system. Knowledge of the subtleties of how the health system works allows the clients some control over the quality and quantity of care received. The risk is that a patient who is not fluent in the operating culture may inadvertently fail to perform as a 'good' patient, become labelled a 'bad' patient and then suffer the consequences of such labelling. We see it as part of the physiotherapist's role to be aware of the patient's cultural literacy and their ability to manage the health system as they would wish. Further, physiotherapists should make an effort to make key institutional values explicit to the patient.

CULTURAL COMPETENCE

Although it is considered an essential skill for health service providers (O'Shaughnessy & Tilki 2007, Stewart 2002), there is currently no generally accepted definition of cultural competence (Bhui et al 2007). Our preferred definition is: 'the ability of individuals to establish effective interpersonal and working relationships that supersede cultural difference' (Cooper & Roter 2003, p 552). Typically, definitions of cultural competence focus on the knowledge and skills required to work effectively in cross-cultural encounters. Culturally competent physiotherapists are required to have an awareness of cultural diversity, an understanding of and sensitivity to the health beliefs and values of health care users, awareness of their own cultural beliefs and biases, and the ability to respond appropriately to the cultural preferences of patients. (For further reading on cultural competence see Beach et al 2005, Kumas-Tan et al 2007, Niemeier et al 2003.)

The importance of cultural competence as a skill for health workers has grown out of a concern that some groups within the health system are being systematically privileged, while other groups (typically minority groups) are systematically marginalised at both an institutional level (Beach et al 2005) and at a therapist interaction level (Hunt 2007). Misdiagnosis and ineffective assessment and treatment outcomes, as well as poor patient adherence to management strategies, have been highlighted as risks in culturally incompetent practice (Bhui et al 2007). In contrast to cultural literacy, where agency and obligation for negotiating the context lie with the individual *unfamiliar* with the dominant cultural context, cultural competence places the obligation on the individual *who has knowledge of and is part of* the dominant culture. That is, the physiotherapist is responsible for the success of the health interaction. Cultural competence is directed to the physiotherapist's behaviour and ability to both listen to and respond appropriately to patients' values and beliefs. The focus is typically on the physiotherapist's understanding, acknowledging and accepting the culture the patient brings to the therapeutic encounter. In addition, some authors argue that *valuing difference* and *cultural humility* (Juarez et al 2006, Tervalon & Murray-Garcia 1998) are essential components of cultural competence. Recognising cultures as different but equal is the key.

A useful model for developing cultural competence presented by O'Shaughnessy and Tilki (2007) focuses on four stages of development: 1) awareness of personal culture, 2) knowledge of other cultures, 3) cultural sensitivity and 4) cultural competence. Stage one focuses on self-reflection and attending to our own cultural roots, beliefs, value systems, assumptions, interpretations, etc. (i.e. factors that influence our own cultural lens). At this stage our personal biases and ethnocentricity need to be acknowledged. Ethnocentricity has been defined as the unconscious belief that one's own way is proper and morally correct (O'Shaughnessy & Tilki 2007). A deeply held belief that our way of interpreting and judging the world is the right and proper way is often difficult to shake.

Stage two calls for knowledge of other cultures. There are obvious difficulties here in the amount of knowledge that we can effectively gather about the multiplicity of cultures our patients bring with them. However, some knowledge of general patterns of health beliefs in different communities is of value (Bonder et al 2002, Lee et al 2006) although, as noted previously, care must be taken to avoid stereotyping individuals. Pilotto et al (2007) remind us that patients may be stressed when seeking care and might not be 'typical' representatives of their cultural group. Further, if we accept that we have all taken different cultural paths, we are likely to interpret our own health status differently from those with identical conditions (Jorgensen 2000), even if they share our primary culture.

Stage three is cultural sensitivity, which calls for performance of respect, trust, acceptance, empathy and respectful attentiveness to the patients' values. Jensen and Paschal (2000, p 42) advised that physiotherapists should recognise 'a plurality of moral perspectives and for health workers to *tolerate* [italics added] moral differences and uncertainties while respecting and understanding various cultural traditions'. Notions of cultural humility (Tervalon & Murray-Garcia 1998) and a valuing of other cultural preferences, rather than a pragmatic acceptance (and tolerance) of differences, should also be considered. The need for patients to tolerate the moral choices of the physiotherapist should also be given some thought if we are to practice in a culturally sensitive manner.

Stage four, the final stage, is cultural competence. This stage calls for responding to the patient's explanatory model of health. Our understanding of how well we are and how much control we like in managing our own health is important in relation to how we should be treated by health care providers. According to O'Shaughnessy and Tilki, cultural competence is only achieved 'when power lies with the person being served' (2007, p 9).

CULTURE AND DECISION MAKING IN CLINICAL PRACTICE

Evidence-based practice, defined as the integration of best research evidence with clinical expertise and patient values (Sackett et al 2000), emphasises the imperative for practitioners to actually explore and understand patient values. Adopting the broader view of culture expressed in this chapter, practitioners will commonly find themselves with the challenge of exploring patients' values and beliefs in a cross-cultural enterprise where patients' lived experiences and interpretations of what is happening to them are not familiar or immediately identifiable. The cultural knowledge and skills described in the sections on cultural literacy and cultural competence must be expressed at some stage in the decision-making process in clinical practice.

The dominant method of clinical reasoning (defined as the thinking that is the precursor to decision making) in physiotherapy has been the hypothetico-deductive process. In this process, hypotheses regarding diagnosis and management are generated by the clinician and then, through questioning and testing, either confirmed or negated (Edwards et al 2004, Elstein et al 1978). Firmly situated within the biomedical model, this method is based on assumptions that truth or knowledge is fundamentally objective, measurable, predictive and generalisable. Allopathic medicine, with its diagnostic methods of measuring phenomena such as patient blood counts, blood pressure and body temperature, illustrates the idea that such important clinical knowledge is not only objective and measurable but is predictive of what such values should be for an individual, based on population norms. Physiotherapy, with its mandate of assessing and managing physical impairment and the pain associated with it, has traditionally harnessed these methods of reasoning and decision making (Daykin & Richardson 2004, Jorgensen 2000). However, contemporary understandings of the complexity and interrelatedness of factors influencing health, expressed in the WHO International Classification of Functioning, Disability and Health (2001) and in emerging findings from the pain science literature, point to the need for a broader framework of clinical reasoning, one which promotes understanding of the patient's illness or disability experience and the interpretation of that experience in terms of its role in subsequent decision making and actions (or inaction) on the part of the patient (Edwards et al 2006). As Geertz (1973) explained, culture is one of the webs in which we are all enmeshed and by which we interpret experience and make meaning of our existence.

Narrative reasoning (see Ch 8) in the context of health care reflects people's innate need to create a coherent and meaningful sense of their life experiences (Brody 2003). In their narratives, patients interpret their experiences and edit them in order to fit the meaning and direction they perceive in their life paths. The theory of narrative reasoning also contends that the meaning(s) that people attribute to their situations, expressed in their narrative or story, may also be constitutive of subsequent actions and decision making (White & Epston 1990). Indeed, Lindemann Nelson (2002) has argued that it is the retelling of the story that brings a sense of who the person before us really is.

Ascertaining and understanding a person's narrative requires acceptance of a set of assumptions regarding truth and knowledge that is different from those in the biomedical model. These alternative assumptions include that truth and knowledge are context dependent and socially constructed, and allow for the notion of multiple realities rather than a single objective reality (Edwards et al 2006). Ian's anecdote introducing himself to the reader illustrates that truth and knowledge can be socially constructed and lead to multiple realities (in this case the reality that it is usual practice for male friends to hold hands in many parts of Asia and not so in other settings, particularly in conservative working class areas such as Port Adelaide as it has been up till now). In clinical practice this insight finds application in understanding why patients with similar pathologies and impairments may have vastly different experiences and levels of disability.

So where does culture come into this? Given that the main enterprise of narrative reasoning is to ascertain and understand a person's story or narrative from that person's rather than our own perspective, the notion of what facilitates or extinguishes voices becomes highly relevant. Narrative reasoning has an aim of hearing and understanding the story, as a particular interpretation of the realities experienced and told by the person with whom we engage in clinical practice. It is not hard, therefore, to see how the use and practice of narrative reasoning in conjunction with other forms of problem solving in clinical practice enables practitioners to both develop and translate skills of cultural literacy and competence into the decision making of clinical practice.

SUMMARY

The main message of this chapter is that it is the responsibility of all physiotherapists to be sensitive to (a) the cultural influences in/on their practice, (b) how their own personal and professional culture develops and (c) health service users' cultural preferences. In effect, physiotherapists should be active in developing their cultural wisdom, incorporating their knowledge of culture into their clinical practice.

Reflective questions

- Consider your cultural beliefs about health and wellness. Explore your assumptions about 'good' and 'bad' patients. Reflect on the beliefs and values that you bring to your answer.
- Consider working in a country you have not worked in previously and where you think the culture may be very different from yours. What research would you conduct before going to work in this new cultural setting? What skills will you need to take with you?
- Do you view yourself as culturally competent? What would you need to do to 'give power to the person being served'?

References

Australian Bureau of Statistics 2007 Migration: permanent additions to Australia's population. Australian Social Trends article 4012.0. Available: http://www.abs.gov.au/websitedbs/D3310114.nsf/home/home 10 Dec 2007

Beach M, Price E, Gary T, et al 2005 Cultural competence: a systematic review of health care provider educational interventions. Medical Care 43(4):356–373

Bhui K, Warfa N, Edonya P et al 2007 Cultural competence in mental health care: a review of model evaluations. BMC Health Services Research 7:15

Bonder B, Martin L, Miracle A 2002 Culture in clinical care. Slack, Thorofare, NJ

Brody H 2003 Stories of sickness, 2nd edn. Oxford University Press, Oxford

Cooper L, Roter D 2003 Patient-provider communication: the effect of race and ethnicity on process and outcomes of healthcare. In: Smedley BD, Stith AY, Nelson AR (eds) Unequal treatment: confronting racial and ethnic disparities in health care. Institute of Medicine, National Academy Press, Washington, pp 552–592

Dahlgren M, Dahlgren L 2002 Portraits of PBL: students' experiences of the characteristics of problem-based learning in physiotherapy, computer engineering and psychology. Instructional Science 30:111–127

Daykin A, Richardson B 2004 Physiotherapists' pain beliefs and their influence on the management of patients with chronic low back pain. Spine 29:783–795

Edwards I, Jones M A, Carr J et al 2004 Clinical reasoning strategies in physical therapy. Physical Therapy 84:312–335

Edwards I, Jones M, Hillier S 2006 The interpretation of experience and its relationship to body movement: a clinical reasoning perspective. Manual Therapy 11:2–10

Eisenhart M 2001 Changing conceptions of culture and ethnographic methodologies: recent thematic shifts and their implications for research on teaching. In: Richardson V (ed) Handbook of research on teaching, 4th edn. AERA, Washington DC, pp 209–225

Elstein A, Shulman L, Sprafka S 1978 Medical problem solving: an analysis of clinical reasoning. Harvard University Press, Cambridge, MA

Geertz C 1973 The interpretation of cultures. Basic Books, New York

Gudykunst W 1997 Cultural variability in communication. Communication Research, 24(4):327–339

Hall E, Hall M 1990 Understanding cultural differences: Germans, French and Americans. Intercultural Press, Yarmouth, MA

Hofstede G 1980 Culture's consequences: international differences in work related value. Sage, London

Hunt M 2007 Taking culture seriously: considerations for physiotherapists. Physiotherapy 93(3): 229–232

Jensen G M, Paschal K A 2000 Habits of mind: facilitating student transition toward virtuous practice. Journal of Physical Therapy Education 14(3):42–47

Jorgensen P 2000 Concepts of body and health in physiotherapy: the meaning of the social/cultural aspects of life. Physiotherapy Theory and Practice 16:105–115

Juarez J, Marvel K, Brezinski K et al 2006 Bridging the gap: A curriculum to teach residents cultural humility. Family Medicine 38(2):97–102

Kumas-Tan Z, Beagan B, Loppie C et al 2007 Measures of cultural competence: examining hidden assumptions. Academic Medicine 82(6):548–557

Lee T, Sullivan G, Lansbury G 2006 Physiotherapists' perceptions of clients from culturally diverse backgrounds. Physiotherapy 92(3):166–170

Lindemann Nelson H 2002 Context: backward, sideways and forward. In: Charon R, Montello M (eds) Stories matter: the role of narrative in medical ethics. Routledge, New York

Minas H, Klimidis S 1994 Cultural issues in posttraumatic stress disorder. In: Watts R, de L Horne D J (eds) Coping with trauma: the victim and the helper. Australian Academic Press, Brisbane, pp 137–154

Niemeier J, Burnett D, Whitaker D 2003 Cultural competence in the multidisciplinary rehabilitation setting: are we falling short of meeting needs? Archives of Physical Medicine and Rehabilitation 84(8):1240–1245

O'Shaughnessy D, Tilki M 2007 Cultural competency in physiotherapy: a model for training. Physiotherapy 93(1):69–77

Pilotto L, Duncan G, Anderson-Wurf J 2007 Issues for clinicians training international medical graduates: a systematic review. Medical Journal of Australia 187(4):225–228

Sackett D, Strauss S, Richardson W et al 2000 Evidence-based medicine: how to practice and teach EBM, 2nd edn. Churchill Livingstone, Edinburgh

Schirato A, Yell S 2000 Communication and cultural literacy: an introduction. Allen and Unwin, St. Leonards, NSW

Stewart M 2002 Cultural competence in undergraduate healthcare education. Physiotherapy 88(10): 620–629

Tervalon M, Murray-Garcia J 1998 Cultural humility versus cultural competence: a critical distinction in defining physician training outcomes in multicultural education. Journal of Health Care for the Poor and Underserved 9(2):117–125

Wadham B, Pudsey J, Boyd R 2007 Culture and education. Pearson Education Australia, Frenchs Forest, NSW

White M, Epston D 1990 Narrative means to therapeutic ends. W W Norton, New York

WHO 2001 International classification of functioning, disability and health. World Health Organization, Geneva

THE EXPANSION OF COMMUNITY-BASED PHYSIOTHERAPY

eleven

Leigh Hale, Anne Croker and Di Tasker

Key content

- Core concepts in community-based physiotherapy – community, health, community-based physiotherapy, primary health care, health promotion, community-based rehabilitation
- The scope and expanding role of physiotherapy practice within the community
- The role of physiotherapy in the promotion of wellbeing and fitness in community-based groups
- Useful attributes and skills required to work as a community-based physiotherapist
- Factors influencing effective delivery of physiotherapy services in the community

INTRODUCTION

Community-based physiotherapy would appear to be a simple concept: physiotherapy provided in the community. However, this simplistic viewpoint conceals the multifaceted, stimulating and evolving nature of the role and work of community-based physiotherapists. Community-based physiotherapy is a rapidly developing area of future importance for the profession. This area provides opportunities to expand areas of practice in innovative ways and increase the role and profile of the profession in addressing future global health needs. This chapter explores the concept of community-based physiotherapy, the practice opportunities it provides and the requirements to work in this exciting field.

CONCEPTUALISING COMMUNITY-BASED PHYSIOTHERAPY

Physiotherapists work in metropolitan, regional, rural and remote communities in developed and underdeveloped countries in an array of interesting locations. These include health centres, sporting venues, clients' homes, schools, workplaces, organisations, recreational parks and facilities, government and council bodies (both local and national), retirement homes and hospices. Community-based work has been conceptualised broadly by Stricklin (1997, p 159): 'a community health care worker sees people where they live, work, play, worship, study and die'.

Physiotherapists working in the community have not only the possibility to practise in a wide range of locations and contexts, but also the scope to integrate broad conceptualisations of health, health promotion and rehabilitation into their practice. As autonomous professionals trained in client-centred practice and skilled in teamwork, communication and problem solving, physiotherapists are well positioned to work in the community and support the vision of the World Health Organization (WHO) for the 'integration of biomedical/technological and social approaches to health' (WHO 2005).

Principles underlying community-based physiotherapy

Community-based physiotherapy is embedded within the WHO's philosophy of primary health care (PHC), health promotion and community-based rehabilitation (CBR). The concepts of PHC, health promotion and CBR (as delineated in Table 11.1) are far richer in complexity than simply the concept of having first contact with a patient. Key concepts embedded in PHC are empowerment and inclusion (Kendall et al 2000). For example, in CBR the locus of control lies within the community, and it is (ideally) disabled people, their families and their community who decide what the priorities of the service should be (Stabbs 2004).

The global adoption of PHC has precipitated a greater community focus on health and health care (Stricklin 1997) and has the led to a reconceptualisation of health as being more than the absence of illness. Health is now viewed as a resource for living. Furthermore the responsibility for health is considered collective, to be shared among individuals, health professionals, health service institutions, government and other organisations (WHO 1986). Thus, the health of individuals is now seen to reflect a range of factors, including the performance of the health system, the environment, income and education levels, and health behaviours (AIHW 2004). Achievement of good health requires people to make appropriate choices, and health promotion enables people to make sound health choices more easily. Good health promotion strategies can permeate all aspects of daily life: the home, school, workplace and leisure activities.

In the area of rehabilitation, initiatives such as CBR (ILO et al 2002) and community-based physiotherapy have enabled physiotherapists to reach out into their communities rather than be confined to their practice cubicles. Physiotherapists working in the community address issues across the whole spectrum of the WHO's International Classification of Functioning (ICF) (WHO 2001), with particular emphasis on client participation and community involvement (see Table 11.1). Terms such as *client-centred approach, enablement, enhancing quality of life* and *empowerment* drive such physiotherapy practice.

The practice of physiotherapy is influenced by social trends, including the way society and health care leaders (e.g. WHO) conceptualise health. Further, health care practices, including physiotherapy, are shaped by economic, political and historical influences such as economic rationalisation and legislative changes relating to workplace efficiency and safety. In some ways these constraints on the health care system in general have expanded employment opportunities for physiotherapists working within the community. Economic rationalisation of health care services prompts early discharge from hospital, expanding the role of physiotherapists in the community. Changes to occupational health and safety laws requiring organisations in Australia and New Zealand to ensure safe working conditions and the ability to return to work after workplace accidents and injuries have increased the role played by physiotherapists in the workplace environment.

The scope of physiotherapy practice within the community

Community-based physiotherapy, based on a holistic philosophy of care, takes practitioners away from the more ordered confines of hospital wards, private practices

Table 11.1 WHO documents related to primary health care, community-based rehabilitation and health promotion	
WHO document	**Key concepts included**
Alma-Ata Declaration of Primary Health Care (WHO, 1978, 2005)	Primary health care is 'essential health care made universally accessible to individuals and families in the community by means acceptable to them, through their full participation and at a cost that the community and the country can afford. It forms an integral part both of the country's health system of which it is the nucleus and of the overall social and economic development of the community' (WHO 1978, p 2)
	Primary health care involves the concepts of:
	■ *level of care*, with primary health care being the first level of contact with the national health system by individuals, the family and community
	■ *philosophy of health work*, with primary health care being part of the community's overall social and economic development
	■ *governing principles*, being equity, community involvement, focus on prevention, use of appropriate technology, and a multi-sectorial approach
Community-based rehabilitation joint paper from the International Labour Organisation (ILO), the United Nations Educational, Scientific and Cultural Organisation (UNESCO) and the WHO (ILO et al 2002)	**Community-based rehabilitation** is 'a strategy within community development for the rehabilitation, equalization of opportunities and social integration of all people with disabilities. CBR is implemented through the combined efforts of disabled people themselves, their families and communities, and the appropriate health, education, vocation and social services' (ILO et al 2002, p 1)
Ottawa Charter of Health Promotion (WHO 1986)	**Health promotion** is the process of enabling people to improve and increase control over their health:
	■ Strategies involve *enabling, mediating and advocating*
	■ Priority action areas are to:
	■ build healthy public policy
	■ create supportive environments
	■ strengthen community action
	■ develop personal skills
	■ reorient health services
Jakarta Declaration on Leading Health Promotion into the 21st Century, 1997 (WHO 1997)	**Priorities for health promotion** are to:
	■ promote social responsibility for health
	■ increase investments for health development
	■ consolidate and expand partnerships for health
	■ increase community capacity and empower the individual
	■ secure an infrastructure for health promotion
	Health promotion should:
	■ be carried out *by and with people, not on or to people*
	■ improve:
	■ the ability of individuals to take action
	■ the capacity of groups, organisations or communities to influence the determinants of health
International Classification of Functioning (ICF) (WHO 2001)	The ICF was developed by the WHO as a framework and classification system for international use to describe and measure the function and disability relating to a health condition. To understand and classify the health of a person, the ICF takes into account the interrelationship of personal, social, environmental and medical factors that impact on the individual

and well equipped, staff-supported gyms. They enter an almost bewildering and infinite array of contextual variables and possibilities requiring an expanded range of practice skills, knowledge and competencies. Physiotherapists working in the community have scope to integrate health promotion approaches into their practice; and they may work with individuals or, more broadly, with a range of people, organisations and community groups.

Scope for the care of individuals

Providing care for individual patients who require ongoing physiotherapy management following discharge from hospitals or rehabilitation units is one of the roles of community-based physiotherapists. Client-centred and family-centred practice may be facilitated by engaging with patients, families and carers in their own surroundings. Care provided in this context enables the patient to take ownership of the situation while the therapist takes on the role of an invited guest (Hale & Piggot 2005). Home-based physiotherapy enables movement problems to be addressed in context, facilitating involvement of family and carers in health care, as illustrated in the following scenarios.

Scenario 1
Home visit for a baby with developmental delay

Marie (11 months old) sits in her highchair at the kitchen table with her mum, dad and her physiotherapist, Sue. Marie has poor head control and is not yet able to sit by herself. Sue's fortnightly visits provide a chance for Marie's mum and dad to check on her movement development, and to ensure that they are holding and handling Marie in a way that will help her learn to move well. On this visit Marie's dad says they would love to take her on a bushwalk, and wonders if she can be carried in a backpack carrier like other babies. Sue helps them devise a safe and supportive way to do this.

Scenario 2
Home-based stroke rehabilitation

Jenny, the community-based physiotherapist, is working with Ben, a 65-year-old recently discharged from hospital following a stroke. Jenny spends a great deal of time during the first visit discussing with Ben what he would like to achieve. Ben's greatest wish is to walk his daughter down the aisle at her wedding, without using any assistive device. Jenny then focuses her physiotherapy program on helping Ben to walk safely without assistance, and includes a plan for practising walking down the aisle at the church where the wedding will take place. This involves walking with Ben up and down the aisle, both on their own and with the family watching, demonstrating to Ben's daughter how she could assist her father.

In both scenarios the physiotherapist listens carefully to the desires of the patient and/or family and works collaboratively to arrive at a positive solution that takes into account the environmental context.

Scope for promoting health within the community

Physiotherapy roles within the community have expanded beyond traditional individual-based care. Community-based physiotherapists have opportunities to work with a range of individuals, community groups, organisations and policy-makers, and to be involved with the implementation of strategies promoting health within the community. Examples of different community-based physiotherapy engagements with clients are outlined in the following scenarios.

Scenario 3

Education for volunteers undertaking elderly support visits

A group of people meet at their local neighbourhood centre. They have all volunteered their time to visit people in their homes and in nursing homes. However, not many of them have had any experience with people with disabilities or health care problems. The local community physiotherapist leads a session to explore issues they might face in this situation and how to conduct themselves physically. How do you approach a person with dementia? Is it OK for a volunteer to help the person up from the chair? The volunteers are keen to help but uncertain how to do it well and with safety. After the education session, the physiotherapist stays to have a cup of tea with them and to answer some more questions, some of which are more confidential in nature and need specific advice and referral.

Scenario 4

School access and integration for a disabled child, with back care education for staff

Tom, the physiotherapist from a primary school's therapy team, makes his way through the school playground to the classroom where Erin is being helped into her walking frame so she can walk to the assembly hall. Erin has a developmental disability. Her teacher, the teacher's aide and other staff are getting aching backs from bending over to hold the frame. Tom notices that Erin's enthusiastic efforts to walk make the frame veer to one side. Tom discusses options with Erin and the staff, including using a different route, engaging a student to help on one side and stopping for rests to correct Erin's movement and help her concentrate better. During the discussion members of staff tell Tom that they enjoyed the back care workshop he ran at their previous staff meeting and appreciated his follow-up visit.

Scenario 5

Access to public areas for people with disability and their carers

The local hall is buzzing with people, wheelchairs and talk as the stroke club gets ready for its weekly meeting and education session. Individuals with stroke and their carers have arranged for the community physiotherapist and occupational therapist to come to this meeting to discuss the issue of access in public areas. Three people are unable to get their power wheelchairs up the slope to the post office and one carer has sore wrists as a result of helping her husband up the steps to the local dentist's rooms. After showing different ways of assisting with stairs, the physiotherapist and occupational therapist help arrange a meeting with the local council to address access issues.

Each scenario contains elements of constructive health promotion strategies. Each exemplifies working *by and with people* rather than *on or to people*; development of personal skills; enabling and empowering individuals; creating supportive environments; and strengthening community action. Scenario 5 also involves advocating.

Community-based physiotherapists may also have the opportunity to work with generic health workers or community-based disability workers. A generic health worker or community-based disability worker is an individual who is 'either a local community resident or who has close ties to a community, and who is trained and empowered by a liaising physiotherapist to take on a service delivery role in the provision of functional skill training programs for members of their community' (APA 2004, p 3). The concept of a community-based disability worker is closely linked to that of CBR.

Physiotherapists promoting wellbeing and fitness in the community

Chronic noncommunicable diseases, in particular metabolic and cardiovascular diseases, are a major public health issue for industrialised nations such as Australia and New Zealand (Vuori 2007). Most chronic noncommunicable diseases are caused by a small number of known and preventable risk factors, three of the most important being unhealthy diet, tobacco use and physical inactivity (WHO 2005). By virtue of their knowledge and skills, physiotherapists are well placed to play a leading role in health promotion and the prevention of chronic noncommunicable diseases (Heinonen & Sipilä 2007). In particular, physiotherapists can enable physical activity to be an easy choice for individuals and for community groups.

Participation in physical activity need not be burdensome, and physiotherapists can facilitate engagement of individuals in meaningful physical activities. They can conduct or supervise group community activities such as falls prevention programs for older adults and exercise classes for people with diabetes, obesity or hypertension. Barriers to participating in physical activities of the client's choice can be removed or negotiated by physiotherapists attending the activity with the individual, for example, by taking a woman who has had a stroke to the local swimming pool to set her up with an aquatic program or problem-solving to help a man with arthritis become engaged in lawn bowls. The possibilities are endless. It requires physiotherapists to reach out and collaboratively work with both individual clients and other health professionals to identify and develop strategies to overcome the barriers preventing clients' engagement with physical activity. Participation can be facilitated, whether the activity option is an organised exercise program or a physically related leisure pursuit. Furthermore, physiotherapists can become involved in policy making and can advocate for accessible and affordable physical activity opportunities, liaising with groups such as the local city council, government, or boards of retirement complexes or primary schools.

Engaging in physical activity is important to people both with and without disability (Rimmer 1999). For people with disability facing a large number of barriers, the ICF, discussed earlier in the chapter, provides a model for problem-solving in the community (Mulligan et al 2007). Using the ICF framework (WHO 2001), perceived personal and environmental barriers to inclusion in recreational activities can be identified and possible solutions suggested. For example, Mulligan et al (2007) described the use of the ICF framework to examine how environmental and contextual factors affected personal factors and acted as barriers to participation by an adolescent with autism in a community gym setting. Although their client's short attention span and cognitive impairments could not be modified, behaviours such as his need to explore a new environment and the signals he made under distress were identified as potential strategies to be managed. Thus he attended the gym at a quieter time of day, with a picture board used to cue him into the sequence of exercises; his use of the word 'finished' was respected, after which he moved to the next piece of equipment shown on the picture board. These strategies prevented the violent outbursts he had previously demonstrated (which caused him to be sent home) and meant that he could maintain an exercise program over a prolonged period of time.

PUTTING COMMUNITY PHYSIOTHERAPY INTO PRACTICE

After graduation, many physiotherapists work in hospitals or private practices to gain experience and further develop skills in communication and clinical decision making. Working in the community enhances these skills, as practitioners apply physiotherapy principles and strategies in complex situations where clients may have multiple medical and social problems that are seen in the context of their home and community environments (Heckman & Cott 2005). In such situations, physiotherapists may perceive themselves as a 'Jack/Jill of all trades' (Roberts 2006); however, the multi-skilled and multi-tasked nature of community physiotherapy is in itself highly skilled work. The focus of community physiotherapists on people's ability and participation can positively impact on their movement, comfort and function, and can add great depth and quality to the care provided by the inter-disciplinary team.

'Hands on' and 'hands off'

The physiotherapy profession has always prided itself on being a 'hands on' profession, but for the community-based physiotherapist the emphasis may also be on education, encouragement, counselling (Heckman & Cott 2005) and advocating. In such situations it is necessary to develop enhanced skills in ethical decision making, advocacy and mediation with clients and within the wider context of the health care team and the community. For example, within residential care facilities and schools, physiotherapists may need to advise and advocate, to ensure that restraints are not used inappropriately within the daily care routines of people with cognitive and physical disabilities such as dementia and developmental disability. This role may involve education, modelling and negotiation with carers and administrators to maximise clients' potential for independent mobility and comfort while ensuring safety.

Useful attributes and skills

As a result of their training, physiotherapists have a wide variety of attributes that prepare them well for the stimulating but uncertain world of community-based health care. These include:

- high levels of knowledge of anatomy, pathology and physiology
- advanced competencies in exercise prescription and rehabilitation knowledge
- the ability to think critically and solve problems
- organisational, communication and planning skills
- the ability to work independently and autonomously (Soever 2006).

These attributes are reinforced by life skills developed through experience and living. In a qualitative study in which community-based physiotherapists working with people with stroke described their practice, one participant highlighted the need in her job for experience in life: 'You need to have lived a little … I think life skills give you that little bit more realism …' (Hale & Piggot 2005, p 1937). The study highlighted skills considered necessary for physiotherapists to work in the community (see the box below). Although many of these skills are used in acute care settings, it is the combination of skills that is unique to practising in the community.

Life skills considered necessary in home-based stroke rehabilitation

Hale and Piggot (2005), p 1935

Tolerance

Acceptance

Patience

Honesty

Respect

Cultural competence

Being realistic

The ability to work around social circumstances

The ability to be flexible

The confidence to work in isolation

The ability to keep things simple

Good listening and communication skills

Counselling skills

The ability to build confidence in others

Knowledge of the roles of other rehabilitation team members

Knowledge of own limitations

Skills in educating and motivating people

Working in context

Working with clients within their community contexts facilitates demonstrable and relevant personal progress for individual clients and their families. The direction of the rehabilitation process, customised to suit clients in a timely and directed way, can enhance their sense of self and help them to re-establish control of their life process. For clients, this control can help to promote independence and participation in community and family life. Doolittle (1991, in Cott 2004) found that, although many health professionals may view stroke recovery in terms of movement return, people who had suffered a stroke viewed recovery as returning to previously valued activities. A participant in the Hale and Piggot study (2005, p 1934) was quoted as saying, 'In inpatient rehabilitation, we prepare a patient for discharge, whereas in home-based rehabilitation, we prepare a patient for life'.

Establishing trust is important when visiting and treating people in their homes. As a visitor, the therapist is the guest in the client's house, as opposed to the client being a visitor in the therapist's workplace. The therapist therefore needs to relinquish some of the control over goal setting and treatment choices that physiotherapists may assume within the more formal biomedical care arrangements (Heckman & Cott 2005).

Being part of the community health care team and the community

While they are addressing movement problems, visiting physiotherapists may also have opportunities to offer their clients assistance and referrals for other problems, such as social and psychiatric issues. The 'first contact' component of the community-based physiotherapists' role thus enhances health team coordination. Friendly, approachable and well-informed physiotherapy team members in community health teams can become valued by their team colleagues, local medical practitioners and hospital-based rehabilitation staff. If the physiotherapist also lives in the local area, this networking may extend and develop to form a rich tapestry of information and contacts, which may enhance and support the physiotherapist's professional work.

> In human-related professions there is a gradual recognition of the flow of experience between various roles that people take on in their daily lives. (Denshire 2000, cited in Higgs & Titchen 2001, p 269)

Although many community-based physiotherapists work as part of multidisciplinary, interdisciplinary or perhaps transdisciplinary teams, many work for most of their day in professional isolation. Such isolation requires the ability to be truly autonomous and resourceful and to problem-solve, as there is no one to quickly turn to for help, as might be the case in the hospital environment.

The practicalities

Community-based physiotherapists often work from their car, rather than a traditional office. As well as portable treatment equipment, their tools may include a mobile phone and a laptop computer. These tools, together with sound local knowledge and a network of contacts, enable them to access a wide variety of resources, including equipment and local medical and community services. The timely coordination of treatment, equipment and services is a necessary but complex skill that develops with experience and effort, and contributes to efficient time management. Time management is important for community work, where good planning is needed to allow adequate travelling time for safety, balanced with adequate cost and time efficiency. Despite such pressures, many community-based physiotherapists enjoy the freedom that working in the community allows them.

The development of technology has provided community-based physiotherapists with a wide array of potential resources. These resources can range from the provision of home programs on audiotape, videotape or DVD to the use of virtual reality, video capture (or webcam), entertainment (such as play-stations) and web-based systems. Video-conferencing allows physiotherapists to interact in real time with patients in remote rural areas. Voice-over-internet protocols, email and SMS messaging afford quick methods of communicating with patients, such as reminding a patient to do exercises.

Community-based physiotherapists are part of a community of practice and the wider social community. Individually, using the words of Gibbon (1738), they need to rely on 'a heart to resolve, a head to contrive and hands to execute'.

Evaluating effectiveness

It can be argued persuasively that community-based work has an important place in physiotherapy practice and that conceptually, in certain contexts, it would seem to be the best choice of service delivery. But where does it sit in the spectrum of evidence-based practice? In a discussion paper on primary health care and physiotherapy, Soever (2006) categorised types of physiotherapy-related outcomes, and this would appear to be a logical method to use for such a diverse model of health care:

- *Systems level* – Community-based physiotherapy could be evaluated at a system level, where outcomes such as decreased waiting times and waiting lists, cost-effectiveness, reduced referral rates to specialists, and increased service efficiency could be appraised.
- *Provider level* – At the provider level the outcome may be improved levels of satisfaction among other members of the health team, a decreased level of inappropriate referrals to specialists and increased communication between health professionals.
- *Client level* – At the client level there may be enhanced client satisfaction with the service and improved clinical outcomes. Byrne and Hardy (2005) surveyed family satisfaction in a community-based physiotherapy service for children with cystic fibrosis. A patient satisfaction questionnaire was posted to all involved families. An overwhelming majority of families were satisfied with the service, and just over a quarter of families requested more home visits as they found them more beneficial than clinic visits. The multifaceted nature of community-based physiotherapy suggests that evaluating the outcome of intervention is complex, and no single standardised method of evaluation will apply to all clients. However, one potential method of evaluating outcome is Goal Attainment Scaling (Malec et al 1991), in which patient-centred goals can be scored prior to and after intervention, and this provides a means of measuring individual goals.
- *Condition-specific level* – Finally there are a number of outcomes that can be measured at a condition-specific level, for example, reduced back pain, reduced number of falls, and improved cardiovascular function in specific population groups, such as Parkinson's disease or older adults. The Community Outcome Scale (Stilwell et al 1998) is an example of a measure that was specifically designed to evaluate long-term outcome following traumatic brain injury. It measures a number of constructs considered important for improved community participation: mobility, occupation, social integration and engagement.

However, health promotion activities also target behaviour change and empowerment of communities. These activities may not be so easy to evaluate (Naidoo & Wills 1994). Identifying the cause of changes in community behaviours is a difficult task, and outcomes of empowerment and networking are typically long-term and may be vague and difficult to specify (Naidoo & Wills 1994). For example, the benefits of working with parents of disabled children to improve local disabilities services may take time to eventuate. In the current climate of increasing accountability, strategies involving measurable outcomes may be preferred over strategies involving empowering and enabling, particularly where grant application and justification of funding is required. However, even when required to demonstrate measurable outcomes, community-based physiotherapists can still incorporate health promoting strategies in all provision of service. For instance, a physiotherapist running a 'falls prevention class' for well-elderly could allow time for socialising and networking among team members, provide opportunities for the group to review obstacles in their local area and encourage them to take action to remove these.

Given that community-based physiotherapy is embedded within the broader framework of the social model of health care, it is debatable whether the traditional sources of evidence-based medicine, such as randomised controlled trials, apply. Perhaps alternative sources of evidence of efficacy are more appropriate, including the use of qualitative methodology (Kuipers & Hartley 2006).

SUMMARY

Community-based practice provides scope for an exciting physiotherapy career, a career that is predicted to expand exponentially in the foreseeable future as the world grapples with increasing populations, ageing populations, the burden of chronic disease and dwindling natural resources. Physiotherapy education is responsible for preparing graduates as competent beginning practitioners. This education should also provide graduates with the skills and attributes necessary to explore new avenues of practice and to work in the community *by and with people,* collaboratively finding possible solutions to the challenges of the 21st century.

Reflective questions

- What attributes and skills do I currently possess that would enable me to practise as a community-based physiotherapist?
- What attributes and skills could I develop that would enable me to practise as a community-based physiotherapist?
- What are the possibilities for incorporating health promotion strategies into my physiotherapy practice?
- What opportunities for community-based physiotherapists exist in my community?

Further reading

Crompton A, Ashworth M 2000 Community care for health professionals. Butterworth Heinemann, Oxford

Leavitt R L (ed) 1999 Cross-cultural rehabilitation: an international perspective. W B Saunders, London

References

AIHW 2004 Australia's health 2004: the ninth biennial health report of the Australian Institute of Health and Welfare. AIHW, Canberra

APA 2004 Role definition in physiotherapy practice. Position statement of the Australian Physiotherapy Association. APA, Melbourne

Byrne N M, Hardy L 2005 Community physiotherapy for children with cystic fibrosis: a family satisfaction survey. Journal of Cystic Fibrosis 4:123–127

Cott C A 2004 Client-centred rehabilitation: client perspectives. Disability and Rehabilitation 26(24):1411–1422

Gibbon E 1738 The decline and fall of the Roman empire. Quote No 4603 in Bartlett J 1919 Familiar quotations. Available: http://www.bartleby.com/100/290.4html 23 Aug 2007

Hale L A, Piggot J 2005 Exploring the content of physiotherapeutic home-based stroke rehabilitation in New Zealand. Archives of Physical Medicine and Rehabilitation 86:1933–1940

Heckman K A, Cott C A 2005 Home-based physiotherapy for the elderly: a different world. Physiotherapy Canada 57:274–283

Heinonen A, Sipilä S 2007 Physical activity and health. Advances in Physiotherapy 9:49

Higgs J, Titchen A 2001 Professional practice: walking alone with others. In: Higgs J, Titchen A (eds) Professional Practice in Health, Education and the Creative Arts. Blackwell Science, Oxford, pp 267–272

ILO United Nations Educational Scientific and Cultural Organization, United Nation's Children's Fund, World Health Organization 2002 Community-based rehabilitation (CBR) for and with people with disabilities. Draft joint position paper. Geneva

Kendall E, Buys N, Larner J 2000 Community-based service delivery in rehabilitation: the promise and the paradox. Disability and Rehabilitation 22(10):435–445

Kuipers P, Hartley S 2006 A process for the systematic review of community-based rehabilitation evaluation reports: formulating evidence for policy and practice. International Journal of Rehabilitation Research 29:27–30

Malec J F, Smigielski J S, DePompolo R W 1991 Goal attainment scaling and outcome measurement in post acute brain injury rehabilitation. Archives of Physical Medicine and Rehabilitation 72: 138–143

Mulligan H, Kett V, Jakowetz K 2007 Participation in a community gym setting for an adolescent with autism: a case study. CD of abstracts, 15th World Confederation of Physical Therapy Congress, Vancouver, WCPT Secretariat, London

Naidoo J, Wills J 1994 Health promotion: foundations for practice. Balliere Tindall, London

Rimmer J H 1999 Health promotion for people with disabilities: the emerging paradigm shift from disability prevention to prevention of secondary complications. Physical Therapy 79(5):495–502

Roberts S 2006 Case study. University of Tasmania. Available: http://www.ruralhealth.u.tas.edu.au/healthcarerscasestudies 4 Aug 2007

Soever L 2006 Primary health care and physical therapists – moving the profession's agenda forward. Discussion paper. The College of Physical Therapists of Alberta, The Alberta Physiotherapy Association, The Canadian Physiotherapy Association, Alberta

Stabbs S 2004 Community-based rehabilitation. Available: http://www.iddc.org.uk/disdev/strategies/cbr.pdf 9 August 2007

Stilwell P, Stilwell H J, Hawley C et al 1998 Measuring outcome in community-based rehabilitation services for people who have suffered traumatic brain injury: the Community Outcome Scale. Clinical Rehabilitation 12:521–531

Stricklin M L V 1997 Community-based care: back to the future. Disability and Rehabilitation, 19(4):158–162

Vuori I 2007 Physical activity and health: metabolic and cardiovascular issues. Advances in Physiotherapy 9:50–64

WHO 1978 Primary health care: report of the International Conference on Primary Health. Alma Ata, USSR. WHO, Geneva

WHO 1986 Ottawa charter for health promotion. WHO, Geneva

WHO 1997 Jakarta declaration on leading health promotion into the 21st century. WHO, Geneva

WHO 2001 The international classification of functioning, disability and health – ICF. WHO, Geneva

WHO 2005 Action on the social determinants of health: learning from previous experiences. WHO, Geneva

WORKING IN RURAL AND REMOTE PHYSIOTHERAPY

Anne Croker, Anne Bent and Stephan Milosavljevic

twelve

Key concepts

- Challenges and opportunities of living and working in rural and remote areas
- Characteristics of physiotherapy practice in rural or remote settings
- Ongoing professional development in rural and remote areas

INTRODUCTION

Practising in rural and remote areas provides potential for a wide range of professional and personal experiences. The initial decision to live and work in a rural or remote community may be based on a combination of different factors, such as the availability and nature of work, lifestyle, or location of a partner's work. Physiotherapy students and physiotherapists who have a sound understanding of opportunities and challenges within rural and remote contexts are well positioned to make informed career choices. Awareness of issues related to working and living in rural and remote areas is also important for physiotherapists based in metropolitan areas. Such awareness assists a smoother continuum of service delivery for rural and remote clients accessing services from metropolitan health facilities and enables metropolitan physiotherapists to appreciate the contexts of their rural and remote colleagues. In this chapter we outline the context of rural and remote health service delivery in Australia and New Zealand and explore issues related to physiotherapy practice in rural and remote areas.

CONTEXT OF RURAL AND REMOTE HEALTH SERVICE DELIVERY

An appreciation of factors influencing life and work in rural and remote areas provides a sound foundation for understanding physiotherapy practice in these areas.

What is rural and what is remote?

In this chapter the term *rural* generally refers to a community that is largely dependent upon primary industry for the bulk of its livelihood and is at least 100 km from a city with a major tertiary referral hospital. The term *remote* is mainly applicable to Australian conditions and refers generally to a location with a population of fewer than 5,000 that is isolated from other similar communities and is more than 500 km from a state capital.

The nature of health service delivery varies widely within the *rural* context, from well resourced and well staffed centres in regional areas to smaller centres that provide limited services. *Remote* areas tend to have small populations distributed over large geographical areas, where health professionals often travel significant distances between communities to see clients. Remote area practice is more likely than rural practice to be associated with professional isolation and situations where the logistics of accessing ongoing professional development can be difficult. However, on the positive side, there tends to be increased breadth of service provision and a greater opportunity to develop new services. Indeed, the opportunities via distance learning media to access continuing education offered by professional bodies and pursue postgraduate qualifications through academic institutions are continuing to increase. For example, the Masters of Public Health program at James Cook University in Queensland provides many coursework subjects through distance learning.

The following scenarios give examples of physiotherapists working in areas with increasing degrees of remoteness.

Scenario 1
Regional or large rural area

Ben works with other physiotherapists in a regional hospital of 160 beds. Although primarily responsible for providing physiotherapy services to the rehabilitation unit, he often assists new graduates with postoperative patients in the wards and helps in the fracture clinic.

Scenario 2
Small rural area

Jan is the sole physiotherapist in a small rural town hospital of 25 beds. Well known in the community, she often talks to school groups and sporting teams, and has opportunities to seek financial assistance for equipment from local service clubs. She relies on a network of physiotherapists in larger centres to provide advice for more complex cases requiring specialised management.

Scenario 3
Remote area

Alice is the sole physiotherapist in a multidisciplinary team that provides outreach health services within a large geographical area to people living in remote communities (including Indigenous communities). Her work requires travelling long distances, often by air, to provide a wide range of services to all age groups.

Remote area practice reflects many of the issues associated with rural practice but entails greater emphasis upon external linkages and networking outside the discipline of physiotherapy. For ease of exploring issues related to rural and remote health service delivery, in the remainder of this chapter we focus predominantly on aspects that are common to rural and remote practice rather than on differences.

Overview of health service delivery in rural and remote locations

The diversity of rural and remote clients and their contexts provides both difficulties and opportunities for those planning and delivering health services. As the health needs of Indigenous communities, mining towns, agricultural areas and tourist centres vary, no one service approach or strategy suits all situations (Australian Health Ministers' Advisory Council (AHMAC) & National Rural Health Alliance (NRHA) 2003). Difficulties are compounded where population density is low, settlements are small and distances are large. In these situations health care providers need to overcome problems of isolation, transient populations and high infrastructure costs (Wakerman et al 2006). However within these difficulties lie opportunities for health professionals to work across a broad scope, be innovative and be collaborative. Health care in rural and remote areas involves both treatment of presenting health conditions and development and implementation of preventative health strategies. When developing preventative health strategies, health professionals work collaboratively with local communities and assist in seeking local solutions for local problems (AHMAC & NRHA 2003). Thus abilities such as problem-solving and incorporating new ideas are important in overcoming the challenges and maximising the opportunities for health services in rural and remote locations, where 'innovation born of both local need and community action is a hallmark of much rural and remote healthcare practice' (Wakerman & Humphreys 2002, p 457).

Health professionals working in rural and remote communities are often familiar with geographic classification systems that embody concepts of remoteness, as these systems commonly determine the resources and support provided to health services and clients. Classification systems are commonly based upon combinations of community size and distance from major towns or cities, with some systems also including a location's access to goods and services. Towns and locations are allocated a remoteness category within these classification systems, based on limited statistical demographic information. New Zealand's classification system is the Urban/Rural Profile Classification system (Statistics New Zealand 2006). In Australia the Accessibility/Remoteness Index of Australia (ARIA), the Rural, Remote and Metropolitan Areas classification system (RRMA) or the Australian Standard Geographical Classification (ASGC) may be used (Australian Institute of Health and Welfare (AIHW) 2004). Due to variations between classification systems, the systems preferred by organisations differ. As well, classification systems cannot capture the varying natures of specific locations and communities, although they can provide an indication of the diversity of contexts for rural and remote areas, as well as a hint of the isolation of some communities.

Living and working in rural and remote locations

Health professionals may overlook the potential for careers in rural and remote areas to be rewarding, especially if they have never experienced the lifestyle and their knowledge is based on comments from the media that tend to emphasise challenges rather than rewards. The rewards primarily relate to the nature of the work and the lifestyle, as well as the opportunities to experience living in a variety of locations and working with different communities (see the box overleaf).

Challenges, on the other hand, commonly relate to the implications of living within small or widely distributed populations, with limited services and infrastructure, and the lack of management support. Low populations and limitations to services and infrastructure may reduce employment opportunities for health professionals and their partners, restrict education choices for their children, and necessitate travelling

Life skills considered necessary in home-based stroke rehabilitation

Quotes from *Opportunities as vast as the landscape: working in rural and remote health*, 2006, by J Dunbar et al, Australian Rural Health Education Network

Nature of the work

My work is varied and flexible. I work with interesting intelligent people, and I enjoy excellent working conditions. (physiotherapist)

As a new graduate … I thought the only place I would find an interesting job would be in a metropolitan centre … I never thought I would find an interesting and challenging job in the country that offered so much variety, but I did. (dietician)

The days are long, the travelling often longer than the time with patients, and the accommodation ranges from luxurious bed and breakfasts to swags in community halls. However the gratitude of our patients is the real reward for working in these areas. (podiatrist)

My present position combines all the elements I love: cultural diversity, gutsy people, teaching, creativity and endless possibilities. (public health practitioner)

What do I like about working here? Variety of work, lovely patients, a place where you can walk your dog without a leash, and swim in a river 15 minutes from town. (general practitioner)

Lifestyle

I love the rivers and channels that intersect the region. Here we experience more drought than flooding rains but the outcome is great weather and clever irrigation that transforms the land into an abundant food production area. (physiotherapist)

Living and practising in the country has offered great rewards, both professional and personal. I have been able to raise three children and spend more time with them than may have been possible living in a busier city. (professor of school of rural health)

We didn't anticipate making a heap of new friends and participating in social sport or town events … One minute we were introducing ourselves to strangers, the next thing we knew I was roped into a social touch-football team, of which [my partner] is the new coach! … We look forward to the start of the social netball season … events such as a fun run, opera under the stars and a wine and food festival, plus a local show which features a swanky black tie ball. (general practitioner)

Chance to experience different locations and communities

Travel to remote Aboriginal communities, small mining communities, station homesteads and small townships. We travel by four-wheel drive or small aircraft only, because there is no way ordinary vehicles could make the journey. The scenery changes with the seasons: dry river beds in summer and green flood plains carpeted with beautiful wild flowers in winter. Amazing Aboriginal and pastoral history surrounds us as we traverse these outback roads. (podiatrist)

I've been knocked into shape by outback folk, colleagues and the Aboriginal people I've worked with along the way, challenged by postgraduate studies in tropical health and the Australian rural leadership program, eaten some of the world's best meals in very isolated places, met amazing people who have become great friends and inspirational colleagues. (remote area nurse)

large distances to visit family and friends, access specialised health services and attend major cultural and sporting events. However, strategies to address a number of these constraints are continually being developed. One such strategy is the provision of tertiary education facilities in rural areas in the form of rural clinical schools and university departments of rural health. Not only does this strategy provide rural students with access to tertiary education facilities without the need to move to metropolitan areas, it also expands the potential for professional development for health professionals. New health degree programs have also been implemented in universities in rural areas. For example, 7 of the 15 physiotherapy programs in Australia and New Zealand are now delivered in non-metropolitan universities.

Factors that provide challenges can also provide opportunities. For example, although lack of management support in rural areas can be a challenge for recruitment and retention of allied health professionals (Bent 1999, Struber 2004), it also provides opportunities for taking on management responsibilities at an earlier stage in one's career path as well as developing stronger management skills while retaining a patient caseload. Thus health professionals in rural and remote areas often have a rich knowledge base and a wide range of experience, as their role invariably includes advocacy and policy and management decisions, as well as clinical decisions.

Views of life in rural and remote areas may be based on perceptions rather than reality. A number of these perceptions may be disproportionately negative and even erroneous, as illustrated in a survey of undergraduate physiotherapists undertaken by Mitchell (1996). Students identified a number of deterrents to seeking work in rural areas, including perceptions related to lack of entertainment, rural life being too slow, decreased professional contact and more varied employment in the city. The extent to which these perceptions reflect the reality of rural life could well be disputed by many health professionals who have experienced living and working in rural and remote areas. The following quotes from Dunbar et al (2006) challenge the perception that rural and remote practice decreases professional contact and lacks variety:

> By breaking down the barriers between researchers and clinicians, and increasing the knowledge each has of the others' skills, it becomes easier to incorporate research evidence into clinical practice and for research to become more relevant to the needs of rural communities. (general practitioner)

> Through a Masters in Remote Health Practice I get to meet a lot of remote allied health professionals from all over the country who are very inspiring in their commitment to their work and their desire to overcome the many challenges they face. (allied health academic)

Thus the degree to which challenges become opportunities may be dependent on the individual situations, perceptions and abilities that underpin the experiences of health professionals.

Recruitment and retention of health professionals

Strategies to recruit and retain health professionals in rural and remote areas are aimed at both health professionals in training and those who are fully qualified. Strengthening the health education infrastructure within rural areas enables more students to experience a lifestyle and work environment beyond that of the metropolitan area, thus removing some of the mystique and myths about rural and remote areas. Another strategy, based on the link between rural origin and rural practice orientation (Orpin & Gabriel 2005), is to encourage students from rural and remote areas to study in health-related fields by offering incentives such as scholarships and alternative entry pathways. Specific support is also provided by some universities for Indigenous students from rural and remote communities to enter health professional programs. Strategies have also been developed to encourage qualified health professionals to work in rural and remote areas. These strategies include support to find suitable employment in rural and remote areas, professional development assistance, and incentive packages such as relocation allowances that include travel and removal costs and short-term subsidised accommodation, as well as mentoring schemes.

Many health professionals are amenable to the notion of working in different environments and locations at some stage during their career (Orpin & Gabriel 2005), and the high turnover rate in rural and remote areas may be linked to the variety of employment experiences sought by many health professionals or their partners. The *easy entry, graceful exit* strategy recognises that some health professionals may not want to commit to a life of working in rural and remote areas or, alternatively, they may want to experience life in different rural and remote areas. Kamien (2004, p 319) has suggested that this strategy facilitates a 'guilt free "walk-in, walk-out" approach by concentrating on continuity of the practice rather than continuity of doctor'.

Those who stay in the same location may be frequently required to farewell departing colleagues and welcome new ones. Such mobility may be advantageous to the development of new ideas and ways of working, but can be disadvantageous for continuity of practice. In areas experiencing chronic recruitment difficulties continuity of practice may not be a reality. For example, in Australia the 'tyranny of distance' can lead to chronic recruitment difficulties, and in New Zealand the rugged terrain can be a disincentive to working and travelling in some geographically isolated communities. In such situations the community either learns to cope without a particular health service or travels to an available service centre, or other health professionals work together to bridge the gap where possible.

PHYSIOTHERAPY PRACTICE IN RURAL AND REMOTE AREAS

Physiotherapists working in rural and remote settings have a range of clinical experience; some are relatively new graduates and others have substantial experience. Many find opportunities to expand professional boundaries, to be innovative in clinical management and to work in close collaboration with others. This section explores aspects of physiotherapy service delivery and professional development relevant to rural and remote areas.

Physiotherapists' attributes and elements of physiotherapy practice

Attributes required for successful physiotherapy practice in the rural and remote setting are not unique to this context. However, certain attributes are particularly emphasised and valued. Similarly, certain elements of physiotherapy practice are particularly relevant for rural and remote physiotherapy practice. These attributes and components are outlined in the box opposite and may provide an ongoing professional development guide for rural and remote physiotherapists.

Examples of how these attributes and elements may be used in rural and remote physiotherapy practice are provided in the following scenarios.

Valued attributes and important elements of physiotherapy practice in rural and remote areas

Based on Sheppard and Nielsen (2005)

Attributes valued in rural and remote physiotherapy practice:

- clinical capability
- confidence in self and practice
- resourcefulness and innovation
- flexibility
- adaptable communication skills
- ability to promote and engage in interdisciplinary collaboration
- capacity to negotiate and network

Important elements of physiotherapy practice:

- community involvement to determine population needs
- strategies that are responsive to community needs
- networks of referrals
- evaluation of practice and sharing of success stories
- implementation of research into practice

Scenario 4

Developing and implementing a perceptual motor program

On a visit to a small rural primary school Jan, a physiotherapist, Cara, an occupational therapist, and Tom, a teacher, were discussing the limited opportunities for children to participate in organised sport due to the town's small population. Tom had noticed that a number of his first and second grade students seemed to have poor motor skills and he was keen to implement a perceptual motor program (PMP). Jan and Cara agreed with his suggestion. After conducting a literature search and consulting with specialist physiotherapy services in the nearest capital city, Jan and Cara worked together to develop a 20-week program to fit in with two school terms. They also planned a simple pre-participation test of gross and fine motor skills. As Jan and Cara could visit only once or twice per term the proposed running of the program was explained to staff at an in-service meeting. The program went ahead with enthusiasm and all involved were delighted that improvements in skill levels, balance and coordination were demonstrated when the students were retested at the end of the term. The staff reported that there had also been positive academic outcomes, including significant improvement in children's concentration in the morning session. Attendance figures showed improvement as the children were keen to come to school knowing that the day started with a PMP session. Jan, Cara and Tom shared the success of this project by presenting a poster at a conference for rural and remote health practitioners.

Scenario 4 demonstrates community involvement and interdisciplinary collaboration to develop strategies that are responsive to community needs through innovation, followed by evaluating practice and sharing success stories.

Scenario 5

Follow-up management regime for a burns patient

Alice, a physiotherapist providing outreach services from a large regional centre, received a referral for Cole, a child in a remote community who had sustained burns to his upper limb and hand 12 months earlier. Cole was now scheduled for follow-up surgery in a tertiary referral hospital to release the scar tissue and to provide skin grafts. In preparation for her involvement in Cole's care, Alice visited the treating metropolitan hospital to update her knowledge of the management of burns injuries and to be clear about the exact nature of the proposed follow-up management regime for home and school. A plane trip to Cole's school with the visiting special education teacher enabled Alice to liaise with the family and school staff (the class teacher and the teacher aide who would be providing support within the classroom and playground) to plan clinical and educational support for Cole. The follow-up regime enabled Cole to remain in his community without frequent trips back to the city. In her role as treating physiotherapist and case manager, Alice visited Cole's community twice over the next 12 months and maintained ongoing communication with him, his family and school by phone and email. Alice also continued to liaise with the specialist burns physiotherapist to report on Cole's progress until his next review at the metropolitan hospital.

Scenario 5 demonstrates clinical capability, confidence in self and practice, networking and adaptable communication skills.

Working with others

Physiotherapists in remote areas and smaller rural areas are commonly the sole representative of their discipline within the health service facility. However, rather than being isolated in practice, rural and remote physiotherapists commonly work with other professionals and community groups (education, aged care, industry, disability and welfare) to provide comprehensive integrated care (NRHA 2004). Working in conjunction with others can be an enjoyable component of physiotherapy practice, as illustrated in this communication from a long-term rural physiotherapist: '...great teams, usually with minimal hierarchy – cleaners, nurses, allied health professionals and doctors all have morning tea together. There is easy communication [between staff] and people are approachable ...' (C Welsh, personal communication 2006).

There are comparatively more physiotherapists than other allied health professionals (including occupational therapists, speech pathologists, social workers and podiatrists) practising in rural and remote Australia (O'Kane & Curry 2003) as well as in provincial and rural areas in New Zealand. As clients may not have access to a full range of allied health services, it is important for physiotherapists to be able to work in an interprofessional manner and to demonstrate competency in service provision while still keeping within their scope of practice. For example, a physiotherapist may perform a screening test such as a diabetic foot screen test for a person with an amputation or a visual perceptual assessment for a child with handwriting difficulties. If necessary the physiotherapist can then refer the client to the nearest (appropriate) professional service and provide the ongoing support and management options recommended.

Rural and remote physiotherapists often work with others to enable clients to access out-of-region services for investigations (such as medical imaging) and treatment of health conditions. Effective referral and collaboration with other practitioners requires physiotherapists

- to maintain an overview of available regional and metropolitan health services
- to know when and how to refer
- to utilise distance communication strategies (e.g. telehealth)
- to develop skills in effective teamwork
- to facilitate arrangements for clients to access resources (e.g. schemes providing assistance with travel and accommodation) that support them in multiple locations (e.g. when accessing health care services while away from home).

As well, there may be opportunities to work with specialist services that visit the region. For example, every few months paediatric rehabilitation teams and spinal injury teams may hold clinics that complement and support ongoing local services in rural locations.

Physiotherapists as part of the community

The smaller circles of communication in rural and remote areas may afford opportunities for physiotherapists to provide a broad range of services, for example:

> There are great opportunities to influence and make a difference in a community. You are an important person in the health service and the community. You will contribute to management of the service, staff education and workplace health and safety. You will be asked for your opinion and input – not just within the public health system but also for NGOs [non-government organisations] such as community nursing organisations and nursing homes; you will have close contact with GPs who will ask for your opinion and help. You will often have requests from the community generally – invitations to address groups such as the Australian Breastfeeding Association, men's groups and women's groups, on [a range of topics including] back care, ergonomics, postnatal care, etc. Rural physiotherapy clinical practice is often focused on explanation, education and self-management. (C Welsh, personal communication 2006)

As members of a rural or remote community, physiotherapists may also be drawn into health discussions with current or potential clients in supermarket queues or at social events. In such situations physiotherapists may need to be mindful of quarantining their work environment to prevent their work impinging unacceptably on their personal lives. Maintaining clients' confidentiality, which is fundamental to ethical practice, is an important aspect of professionalism as physiotherapists are often privy to medical information about community members with whom they mix socially.

Physiotherapists practising in areas where there are workforce shortages need to be particularly aware of the importance of balancing professional and personal life to support sustainable practice. See Chapter 22, which outlines strategies to this end.

Clients

Clients in rural practice are noted as being stoical and self-sufficient (Dean et al 2007, Pal et al 2007, van Erp 2002). Positive attitudes for dealing with injury are considered important within the rural and remote workforce, and have the potential to contribute to high levels of job satisfaction for rural and remote physiotherapists. Van Erp (2002) noted that many patients in rural settings had significant impairment but were highly motivated to maintain their functionality and livelihood in order to live in the location of their choice and return to optimal participation as quickly as possible. The high level of camaraderie often displayed by people within the rural workforce provides the basis for valuable social interaction in physically demanding jobs such as shearing (Pal et al 2007) and is often a strong and positive attribute that facilitates rehabilitation and a return to work in injured rural workers. Such positive and independent attitudes have also been identified in rural communities in Sweden (Holmberg et al 2004). These concepts of self-sufficiency and an ability to cope are the drivers for current research in New Zealand to determine the unique occupational, personal and psychosocial characteristics that exist within the rural workforce that often enable these people to continue working despite the presence of injury or disorder (Dean et al 2007). An understanding of this independent character and attitude in their rural clients is invaluable for physiotherapists and other health professionals when considering service strategies that will best meet the health care needs of the rural sector.

Cross-cultural service delivery in both Australia (to Aboriginal or Torres Strait Islander Indigenous communities) and New Zealand (to Māori communities) requires knowledge and understanding of the culture and sometimes the language of clients in order to provide appropriate health support services. These issues are further explored in Chapter 13.

Outreach services

Outreach services are used for areas with low population density where the services from one location are periodically supplied to another location lacking in such services. Follow-up care may be provided between outreach visits by health workers and therapy assistants. Here, a remote physiotherapist describes her experience with outreach services:

> [As visiting health professionals] we travel by four-wheel drive over dirt roads and fly in light aircraft to remote isolated Aboriginal communities and homelands, to deliver services to people who have a different language, culture and lifestyle to our own. [Our region] covers an area of close to half a million square kilometres. We have every spectrum of our professions to cover, all age groups and all clinical conditions. We provide a consultative clinical service, a community health service, education for Aboriginal health workers and nurses, and undertake research and community development activities. (Barker 1995, p 94)

Personnel providing outreach services often use videoconferencing and other means of telecommunication to provide ongoing support for clients and health professionals. Potential barriers to effective use of telecommunication support include cost, concerns about confidentiality of client information, difficulty of internet access in remote areas and lack of client acceptance (Wakerman et al 2006).

The *hub and spoke* model is a health service delivery model often used in rural communities in which less complex health services are linked to those of higher complexity, through a service delivery network adaptable to local needs. The North and West Queensland Primary Health Service is an example of an allied health outreach service. This service, covering a geographical area of approximately 300,000 square km, provides outreach services on a 6-weekly rotational basis to 11 culturally diverse remote communities (NRHA 2004). The three separate multidisciplinary teams (each one including physiotherapy) fly to the communities and are supported by a network of local community-based therapy assistants (NRHA 2004).

Career development in rural and remote areas

Although there may not be clear predetermined career pathways for rural and remote physiotherapists, there may be scope for determining career direction according to personal interests and opportunities created or encountered. Major areas for career development tend to lie within research, clinical supervision, education of health professionals and management. However, university departments of rural health also offer career directions in providing opportunities for rural research as well as student education in physiotherapy and other health professions. For many rural and remote physiotherapists, the need to be manager as well as clinician fosters the development of management skills, which may provide further opportunity for increased managerial responsibilities.

The Australian Physiotherapy Association is examining the case to recognise the 'specialist generalist' role of physiotherapists who work in rural and remote practice.

> For those rural and remote physiotherapists seeking to be recognised as specialists formally within their own profession, a process of identification of key competencies is required. The challenge for rural and remote physiotherapy specialisation is to translate a model of practice that is predominantly characterised by location and scope into a process largely designed to recognise clinical specialties. (Sheppard & Nielsen 2005, p 135)

Rural and remote physiotherapists can contribute to this discussion and to the development of the specialisation process.

Accessing professional development

Distance and cost are common barriers to accessing face-to-face professional development, which may require advance planning to arrange funding, travel and a locum physiotherapist. Communication technology often plays a key role in supporting ongoing professional education and preventing professional isolation for rural and remote physiotherapists. Physiotherapists can participate in seminars via telephone links and videoconferencing, or by accessing online distance education courses and internet resources. An innovative educational strategy for rural and remote health practitioners is the Rural Health Education Foundation's (RHEF) interactive satellite broadcasts and audio podcast productions that include a wide range of health topics (RHEF 2007). Rural and remote physiotherapists also have access to support through organisations such as Services for Australian Rural and Remote Allied Health (SARRAH), which provides services such as conferences and scholarships to allied health professionals living and working in rural and remote areas of Australia. Such services support health practitioners in carrying out their professional duties confidently and competently (SARRAH 2007).

Creating supportive networks

Informal networks comprising physiotherapists or a mix of health professionals also provide valuable support for rural and remote physiotherapists. Rural and remote physiotherapists are encouraged to seek mentoring from more experienced colleagues to assist them in clinical management decisions as well as in dealing with the challenges of rural and remote life, and to enable them to maximise opportunities provided. Ongoing developments in communication technology increase the potential for accessing networks and mentors.

SUMMARY

Physiotherapy practice in rural and remote areas is framed by a diversity of health care services and community environments. Such diversity provides opportunities for physiotherapists to develop a broad range of contextual service delivery skills. Interdisciplinary collaboration, a blurring of professional boundaries and innovative approaches underpin successful and rewarding physiotherapy practice in rural and remote areas.

Reflective questions

- Which aspects of living and working in rural or remote areas appeal to me?
- Considering my work and lifestyle preferences, in which locations could I work?
- How would I ensure an appropriate balance between my professional and personal life?
- Which professional attributes and skills might I need to develop further to work in rural and remote physiotherapy?
- How might I develop these skills and attributes?

Further reading

Smith J D 2004 Australia's rural and remote health: a social justice perspective. Tertiary Press, Melbourne, VIC

Liaw S T, Kilpatrick S (eds) 2008 A textbook of Australian rural health. Australian Rural Health Education Network, Canberra. Avaliable: http://www.arhen.org.au/a_text_book_of_australian_rural_health_arhen_april_2008.pdf

References

AHMAC & NRHA 2003 Healthy horizons outlook 2003–2007: a framework for improving the health of rural, regional and remote Australians. Available: http://nrha.ruralhealth.org.au/publications 31 Oct 2007

AIHW 2004 Rural, regional and remote health – a guide to remoteness classifications. Australian Institute of Health and Welfare, Canberra

Barker R 1995 The origins of the 'Very Remote Allied Health Professional Group'. In: Room to move: proceedings from the Second National Rural and Remote Allied Health Professionals conference, Perth, pp 94–95

Bent A 1999 Allied health in central Australia: challenges and rewards in remote area practice. Australian Journal of Physiotherapy 45(3):203–212

Dean S G, Hudson S, Hay-Smith J et al 2007 Rural workers' experiences of low back pain: exploring why they continue to work. Paper presented at Rehabilitation and Disability Research Colloquium, School of Physiotherapy, University of Otago, November

Dunbar J, Newbury J, Pashen D 2006 Opportunities as vast as the landscape: working in rural and remote health. Australian Rural Health Education Network, Canberra

Holmberg S, Thelin A, Stiernstrom E L et al 2004 Psychosocial factors and low back pain, consultations, and sick leave among farmers and rural referents: a population-based study. Journal of Occupational and Environmental Medicine 46(9):993–998

Kamien M 2004 The viability of general practice in rural Australia. Medical Journal of Australia 180(7):318–319

Mitchell R 1996 Perceived inhibitors to rural practice among physiotherapy students. Australian Journal of Physiotherapy 42(1):47–52

NRHA 2004 Position paper: Under pressure and under-valued: allied health professionals in rural and remote areas. National Rural Health Alliance, Canberra

O'Kane A, Curry R 2003 Unveiling the secrets of the allied health workforce in Australia. In: Proceedings, 7th National Rural Health Conference, Hobart. National Rural Health Alliance. Available: http://nrha.ruralhealth.org.au/conferences/docs/7thNRHC/Papers/general%20papers/sunday%20symposium%20a.pdf 31 Oct 2007

Orpin P, Gabriel M 2005 Recruiting undergraduates to rural practice: what students can tell us. Rural and Remote Health 5(412). Available: http://rrh.deakin.edu.au 31 Oct 2007

Pal P, Gregory D, Milosavljevic S et al 2007 Wool harvesting in New Zealand and Australia – a review of industry risk. Physiotherapy 93(Suppl 1):S775

RHEF 2007 Rural Health Education Foundation. Available:http://www.rhef.com.au/ 31 Oct 2007

SARRAH 2007 Services for Australian rural and remote allied health. Available: http://www.sarrah.org.au 31 Oct 2007

Sheppard L, Nielsen I 2005 Guest editorial: Rural and remote physiotherapy: its own discipline. Australian Journal of Rural Health 13(3):135–136

Statistics New Zealand 2006 New Zealand: an urban/rural profile. Available: http://www.stats.govt.nz/urban-rural-profiles/default.htm 31Oct 2007

Struber J 2004 Recruiting and retaining allied health professionals in rural Australia: why is it so difficult? The Internet Journal of Allied Health Services and Practice. Available: http://ijahsp.nova.edu/articles/Vol2num2/struber_rural.htm 8 Sep 2007

van Erp A 2002 A life changing experience – a rural perspective on living with disability. Dissertation for doctoral thesis, University of Southern Queensland, Toowoomba

Wakerman J, Humphreys J 2002 Rural health: why it matters. Medical Journal of Australia 176(10):457–458

Wakerman J, Humphreys J, Wells R et al 2006 A systematic review of primary healthcare delivery models in rural and remote Australia 1993–2006. Australian Primary Health Care Research Institute, The Australian National University, Canberra

PHYSIOTHERAPY AND INDIGENOUS HEALTH

Shaun Ewen and Dale Jones

thirteen

Key content

- Indigenous people's identity
- Indigenous health status in Australia
- Factors that influence Indigenous people's health

INTRODUCTION

What is it that makes Indigenous people's case for health care special, or at least different from other groups discussed in this book? How are Indigenous people different from other cultural groups, such as recent migrants or people living in rural or remote areas or non-Indigenous women? Shouldn't physiotherapists be educated to provide the best possible care to *all* who seek or need their help, irrespective of differences related to culture or gender? In many ways, Indigenous people are no different from other groups if we limit our focus to their health problems: asthma is asthma, and a debilitating stroke is a debilitating stroke. But it is the socioeconomic circumstances faced by Indigenous peoples, together with a history of colonisation, which create a different context for clinicians. The history of colonisation has resulted in Indigenous people's distrust of and alienation from institutions and people who are perceived to be in a position of power. The 'caring professions' haven't always been so caring of Indigenous people in Australia.

In this chapter we outline definitions of Indigenous identity and demographics, and show some of the appalling health statistics relevant to Indigenous people in Australia, with a discussion about some of the underlying reasons for those statistics. We conclude by illustrating some models of health care in Indigenous contexts, and suggest some ways forward in Indigenous health.

This chapter focuses on Australian Indigenous people, reflecting the authors' scope of knowledge. We acknowledge the need for health practitioners to demonstrate a respect for peoples of different cultures (see also Ch 10), particularly Indigenous peoples. We acknowledge that distinct differences may apply to Indigenous cultures of other countries, such as Aotearoa New Zealand, and we do not intend the content of this chapter to be applied to these other cultures. Readers working with other Indigenous peoples may find commonalities of experience in Australia and their own region. At the end of the chapter we list some resources relevant to New Zealand.

WHO IS INDIGENOUS?

It is estimated that Indigenous people lived, farmed and thrived on the Australian continent many tens of thousands of years before the arrival of the Europeans in the 17th century. Although there is some debate about the exact timeline, most evidence now points to migration of humans from north of Australia about 70,000 years ago, spreading across and down the continent and reaching into what is now the island of Tasmania over the following millennia. European influence on Indigenous people began when several Dutch explorers mapped parts of the Australian continent in the 1600s, but the most profound effect on the modern day Australian population was the arrival of the British at Botany Bay, Sydney, and their consequent colonisation of Australia from 1788.

Indigenous identity today encompasses both the 70,000 years of isolated development on an island continent and the more recent (and much shorter) several hundred years of shared occupation. Indigenous identity is, like many identities, multilayered and complex, from the national level to the individual. The Australian Government recognises two different Indigenous groups, Aboriginal and Torres Strait Islander people.

The working definition for Indigenous identity is:

An Aboriginal or Torres Strait Islander is a person of Aboriginal or Torres Strait Islander descent who identifies as an Aboriginal or Torres Strait Islander and is accepted as such by the community in which he (she) lives.

This definition was adopted following recommendations by the Department of Aboriginal Affairs (Department of Aboriginal Affairs 1981). (Further discussion of the definition of Aboriginality is available at Department of Parliamentary Library, Research Note Number 18, 2000–2001, http://www.aph.gov.au/LIBRARY/pubs/rn/2000-01/01rn18.pdf.)

The three-part definition of Indigenous identity is generally used for determining eligibility for Indigenous targeted services and programs. However, there is great diversity within and between Indigenous communities in Australia, depending upon people's personal histories, socioeconomic circumstances and world views. Many Aboriginal people, such as the Yorta Yorta people from along parts of the Goulburn and Murray Rivers, identify with their clan or tribal ancestry. In other circumstances, a person may identify as a *Murri* (Aboriginal person from Queensland) or a *Koori* (from Victoria or New South Wales). For example, Melbourne is situated on the land of the Kulin nations, consisting of five Aboriginal language groups. (See http://www.aiatsis.gov.au/aboriginal_studies_press/aboriginal_wall_map/map_page for a map of Aboriginal Australia illustrating the vast number of these groupings.) There are many biographies and autobiographies of Indigenous Australians, both written and on film, celebrating their struggles and achievements, which give insight into the factors that make up Aboriginal people's identities.

INDIGENOUS HEALTH IN AUSTRALIA – A NATIONAL DISGRACE?

The health status of Indigenous Australians has been described as a national disgrace (Anderson & Loff 2004). The most striking indicator of the poor health status of Indigenous Australians is that in 2007 life expectancy at birth for Indigenous Australians was about 17 years less than that of all Australians. This means that the life expectancy of an Indigenous male is less than 60 years. But he would not be eligible for the aged pension until the age of 65.

The primary causes of death for Indigenous people are similar to those for the total Australian population, with diseases of the cardiovascular system heading the list (cancer heads the list for all Australians, with cardiovascular system diseases second). Although life expectancy is considerably lower, the burden of disease that Indigenous people experience is considerably higher. Using disability adjusted life years as a measure, a study in the Northern Territory in 2004 showed that Aboriginal people in the Territory had 2.5 times the burden of disease and injury compared to all Australians, with cardiovascular disease being the leading cause (Zhao et al 2004).

There have been some improvements in Indigenous infant mortality in recent years, but it remains two to three times higher than the all-Australian rate. The figures for low birth weight babies show that less developed and less wealthy countries than Australia, such as Ethiopia, Senegal, Zimbabwe and Mexico, have better child birth weight outcomes than Indigenous Australians (Aboriginal and Torres Strait Islander Social Justice Commissioner 2003).

Many hours of physiotherapy intervention are directed towards addressing disability and the effects of chronic disease. Indigenous people are three times more likely to have diabetes, and up to 10 times more likely to have kidney disease, than non-Indigenous Australians. The Australian Institute for Health and Welfare (AIHW 2005) reported that Indigenous Australians were at least twice as likely to have a profound or severe limitation of their daily living activities as non-Indigenous Australians. It is important when considering this data to note that the differences between urban, rural and remote populations are not great.

Indigenous people carry a higher burden of disease, and highly effective clinical skills need to be directed towards treating these conditions. The social and economic context in which many Aboriginal people live needs consideration in terms of planning health-related intervention at the individual clinical level and also at the community level and from the perspective of population health. This context is discussed in the following section.

THE DEMOGRAPHICS OF INDIGENOUS AUSTRALIA

What are some of the demographics that may help us to contextualise and understand the poor health status of Indigenous Australia?

The Australian Bureau of Statistics experimental estimate of the Indigenous Australian population at 30 June 2006 was 517,174 people (ABS 2007). This represented 2.5% of the total Australian population. The 2006 census also showed that most Aboriginal people did not live in remote regions of Australia. In fact, about one-quarter of the Indigenous population lived in remote or very remote areas, with the other three-quarters living in regional towns or major cities. As shown in Table 13.1, over half of Indigenous people live in the two states of New South Wales and Queensland, although they make up only a small percentage of the total population of those states. On the other hand, the Northern Territory's Indigenous population constitutes nearly one-third of the Territory's total population.

Table 13.1 Population distribution, Aboriginal and Torres Strait Islander Australians. Adapted from Population Distribution, Aboriginal and Torres Strait Islander Australians, 2006, ABS, 4705.0, p 5

State/Territory	Population, '000	Proportion of total Indigenous population, %	Proportion of state/ territory population
New South Wales	148.2	28.7	2.2
Victoria	30.8	6.0	0.6
Queensland	146.4	28.3	3.6
South Australia	26.0	5.0	1.7
Western Australia	77.9	15.1	3.8
Tasmania	16.9	3.3	3.4
Northern Territory	66.6	12.9	31.6
Australian Capital Territory	4.0	.8	1.2

Between the two census counts of 2001 and 2006 the Indigenous population increased by 13%, compared to 6% for the total Australian population. This higher growth rate is accounted for by several factors, including higher fertility rates as well as more people being counted as Indigenous for the first time (perhaps by identifying as Indigenous for the first time). The Indigenous population is much younger than the total Australian population, with a median age of 21, compared with 36 for the non-Indigenous population (ABS 2004).

SOCIAL DETERMINANTS OF HEALTH

When we consider the social determinants of health, factors such as education, housing, early life opportunity and employment are all significant contributors to health status. The oft-used public health analogies of *downstream* and *upstream* factors affecting health are relevant in the realm of Indigenous health. Although it is critical that optimum treatment is provided for clinical conditions as they present, the background (or upstream) causes of ill health need to be considered, both in terms of treatment of a condition and prevention of further incidence.

Take housing and overcrowded living conditions as an example. Aboriginal and Torres Strait Islander people are more likely to live in overcrowded conditions, with lower levels of infrastructure (i.e., running water and adequate sewerage systems) than non-Indigenous Australians. Overcrowding and poor housing increase the risks of disease and injury, and negatively affect people's social and emotional wellbeing. As well as contributing to disease and injury, these factors also adversely affect the recovery or rehabilitation process. Hospital discharge planning is often difficult enough, but to successfully manage discharge into an overcrowded environment adds multiple layers of complexity. Consider Case study 1, which illustrates the potential complexity of providing health care services for Indigenous Australians. Can you imagine the difficulty for someone like Albert, who is recovering from a stroke, trying to manage safely in an overcrowded environment?

Case study 1

Albert, a 52-year-old Aboriginal man, is a patient of yours in the rehabilitation ward. He has had a stroke, which has affected his ability to use his right side. He can no longer walk without assistance, and has trouble controlling the movement of his arm. Albert is nearly ready to go home, and the Aboriginal Hospital Liaison Officer has mentioned to you that his discharge and follow-up appointments may be complicated and need careful management.

You arrange a home visit with the Aboriginal Hospital Liaison Officer to check what needs to be done before Albert can safely be discharged home. The visit surprises you, as there seems to be a steady stream of Albert's relatives coming in and out during the hour that you are at his house. You wonder how Albert, who is somewhat irritable since his stroke, will manage with all the activity.

You also ask about the family's ability to get Albert back for the regular physiotherapy appointments he will need. You notice that where he lives is poorly serviced by public transport, and he will be reliant on family to help. His family assures you that someone will be around to give him a lift. His wife wonders why he can't go to the local Aboriginal health service for his physiotherapy appointments, but the Liaison Officer says that they are having trouble getting the position filled.

As you work through Albert's discharge plan, you realise that he has had a stroke like many other people, but that his social and economic environment provides some specific challenges for you to deal with.

Indigenous Australians as a population group have much lower standards of formal education than non-Indigenous Australians. This has obvious repercussions in terms of employment, life opportunity and life course in general. However, one of the key determinants of infant health is the level of education of the mother. Lower birth weight babies have been linked to higher rates of diabetes in older age (National Health and Medical Research Council 2000). Lower levels of formal education are related to poor maternal health, which in turn is linked to lower birth weight for children. It is easy to see a cycle of poverty and disadvantage becoming entrenched unless the social determinants of health are addressed while at the same time optimal clinical care is provided for conditions as they present.

ABORIGINAL COMMUNITY CONTROL

Aboriginal health is not just the physical wellbeing of an individual but is the social, emotional and cultural wellbeing of the whole community in which each individual is able to achieve their full potential thereby bringing about the total wellbeing of their community. It is a whole-of-life view and includes the cyclical concept of life–death–life. (National Aboriginal Health Strategy 1989)

The National Aboriginal Community Controlled Health Organisation (NACCHO, see http://www.naccho.org.au) is the national peak Aboriginal health body, which represents at national and international levels the member Aboriginal Community Controlled Health Services throughout Australia. The above definition of health, developed and adopted from the National Aboriginal Health Strategy in 1989, provides an insight into the holistic approach that Aboriginal health services providers should consider. It also links the individual with the community, acknowledging that achieving wellbeing means incorporating the relationship between individuals and their communities. The philosophy underpinning Aboriginal Community Controlled Health Services is *self-determination*. Self-determination in this context means that Aboriginal communities determine the priorities and functioning of their own health service.

Health services work best when the people that they are meant to serve have input into the type of service that is to be provided. Indigenous people are no different, which is why the first Aboriginal Medical Service was established in 1972 in Redfern, an inner Sydney suburb. That Redfern service was established to overcome the difficulties experienced by Aboriginal people in accessing appropriate health care. Since then, over 130 Aboriginal health services have been created across the country, from large centres with multidisciplinary health care teams to small clinics run by Aboriginal health workers.

In many mainstream hospitals there are professionals called Aboriginal Hospital Liaison Officers. The responsibilities of these officers vary from hospital to hospital, but their core responsibility is to help optimise the outcomes for Indigenous patients who come into the hospital. There are many ways this may be done, from facilitating cultural awareness training for hospital staff, to ensuring patient identification processes are in place, to helping patients with particular requests such as transport, to helping clinical staff with discharge planning. For physiotherapists working in a hospital environment, Aboriginal Hospital Liaison Officer personnel should be kept in mind when thinking about how best to provide care for Indigenous patients, or when developing health promotion programs that may include Indigenous people.

HEALTH AND THE RELATIONSHIP BETWEEN INDIGENOUS AND NON-INDIGENOUS AUSTRALIA

To fully grasp the complexity of the causes of Indigenous ill health, an understanding of the history of the relationship between Indigenous and non-Indigenous Australia is important. In 1995 the Attorney-General of Australia requested the Human Rights and Equal Opportunity Commission to enquire into the 'separation of Aboriginal and Torres Strait Islander children from their families by compulsion, duress or undue influence, and the effects of those laws, practices and policies' (Report of the National Inquiry into the Separation of Aboriginal and Torres Strait Islander Children from Their Families April 1997). The resulting report, known as the *Bringing Them Home* report, presented the policies of past Australian state and federal governments, and the impact on Indigenous families and communities of forced removal of Indigenous children from their families. In short, among the contemporary implications of these policies, apart from the pain and dislocation many Indigenous people feel from their families and communities, is a distrust of institutions such as hospitals from where their relatives may have been removed.

Wednesday 13th February 2008 marked a pivotal moment in Australian history when the Prime Minister said sorry to Indigenous Australians on behalf of successive Parliaments and governments. His apology in part contained the following: 'We apologise for the laws and policies of successive Parliaments and governments that have inflicted profound grief, suffering and loss on these our fellow Australians ... A future where we harness the determination of all Australians, Indigenous and non-Indigenous, to close the gap that lies between us in life expectancy, educational achievement and economic opportunity.' (See Parliament of Australia House of Representatives Hansard for a full transcript of the apology, http://www.aph.gov.au/hansard/hansreps.htm#2008.) The apology signifies the difference between knowledge and acknowledgement, and was an important step in bridging the gap between many Indigenous and non-Indigenous Australians.

Beginning in 1989, the Royal Commission on Aboriginal Deaths in Custody sought to investigate why so many Indigenous people were dying while in custody. In the preface to the report, the commissioners stated that a major reason for the deaths in custody was 'the grossly disproportionate rates at which Aboriginal people are taken into custody, of the order of more than twenty times the rate for non-Aboriginals'. The preface further stated that 'the indigenous people of Australia … were cruelly dispossessed of their land and until recent times denied respect as human beings and the opportunity to re-establish themselves on an equal basis' (Royal Commission on Aboriginal Deaths in Custody Vol 1, Preface 1989).

Both of these key investigations pointed to the ongoing impact of the processes of colonisation on Indigenous people in Australia. The health status of Indigenous Australia cannot be understood without first considering this colonial relationship and its effects. The Report of the National Inquiry into the Separation of Aboriginal and Torres Strait Islander Children from Their Families (the *Bringing Them Home* report) and the Royal Commission on Aboriginal Deaths in Custody made recommendations that Indigenous content and perspectives be taught to all health professionals in Australia at undergraduate, postgraduate and professional development levels. In particular, the *Bringing Them Home* report recommended 'that more and/or better quality training be provided in a range of areas taking note of the following:

- many non-Aboriginal health professionals at all levels are poorly informed about Aboriginal people, their cultural differences, their specific socio-economic circumstances and their history within Australian society'

and

- 'that all professionals who work with Indigenous children, families and communities receive in-service training about the history and effects of forcible removal, and that all under-graduates and trainees in relevant professions receive, as part of their core curriculum, education about the history and effects of forcible removal' (Report of the National Inquiry into the Separation of Aboriginal and Torres Strait Islander Children from Their Families 1997).

COMMUNICATION – SHOULD I LOOK HIM IN THE EYE?

The literature describing cross-cultural communication, cultural competency, cultural safety and cultural security in relation to clinicians communicating and providing treatment for their patients is significant. (Chapter 10 in this book addresses many of these issues from the perspective of physiotherapy.) Although some of the literature is informative and helps describe some of the challenges of communicating with patients of different cultural backgrounds to the clinician, much of it can miss the point if simplistically applied. At the clinical encounter, the patient is an individual seeking treatment for a condition. Making generalisations at a population level to describe discrete cultural characteristics and their manifestation at an individual level is a recipe for potential disaster. Consider this example. An Aboriginal Elder living in Melbourne visited a physiotherapist for treatment for his sore back. After his initial consultation and treatment, the Elder's wife asked how the consultation went. The Elder replied, 'I don't know what sort of training they get these days, but that physio wouldn't even look me in the eye! Maybe he was shy.'

There is a lot of information in books, articles and courses on cross-cultural communication with Indigenous people that says you shouldn't look them in the eye when talking to them. Although this may indeed be true for some groups of Indigenous people, it also highlights the diversity within Indigenous Australia. Suggesting one mode of communication and providing prescriptions for how to communicate with Indigenous Australians doesn't work with everyone. However, it is important to have a broad understanding of what may shape a person's lived experience. For Indigenous people, it is important that their clinicians know about the history of colonisation and its effects. At a regional and local level, it is important to ask about local cultural groups, important places and local customs as they may relate to providing optimal treatment, which means effective communication. In some parts of Australia, it *is* appropriate to look Indigenous people directly in the eye and ask direct questions; to do the same in other contexts is poor communication.

For communication to be successful it is also critical to understand the concept of a 'world view' – yours and that of the person with whom you are working. The non-Indigenous health world view is based on a clear medical model of understanding how the body works and the historical and practised use of expert medical care from health providers. An Indigenous Australian's understanding of health is often linked to very different ideas: curses causing ill health and death, strong links to land, traditional understanding of how the body works and appropriate treatments. The health care professional needs to carefully consider this disparity when explaining medical conditions and the recommended interventions. Much more time and effort may be required to explain a topic that may be quite straightforward in another culture. What to some people may be misconstrued as poor intelligence can be a failure to recognise the knowledge gap between cultures.

There is no prescription for communication with Indigenous people as we are all different. Similarly, a prescription for communicating with non-Indigenous Australians in general would be of little use. The key principles of effective communication are just as important in this context.

AN EXAMPLE OF PROVIDING PHYSIOTHERAPY SERVICES TO AN INDIGENOUS COMMUNITY

In the remainder of this chapter we present a case study that embodies many of the issues discussed above and considers the implications for physiotherapists.

Case study 2

Kela suffered hypoxia at birth resulting in cerebral palsy and global developmental delay with marked hypotonia. His family lived in an Aboriginal community six hours from Katherine.

The town of Katherine in the Northern Territory is classified as a remote location. It is situated 300 km south of Darwin and provides regional services to an area of over 360 000 km². Over 50% of the people of Katherine are Indigenous. Health services in Katherine are unique in that they

171

are provided not only by the Northern Territory government but also through three independent Aboriginal Health Boards.

The team involved in Kela's care consisted of allied health personnel (physiotherapists, occupational therapists, speech pathologists) and nurses and disability personnel who worked for Katherine Aged and Disability Services. This service is part of the Northern Territory Department of Health and Community Services. Personnel provide all age groups with services, including school therapy and rehabilitation, aged care assessments and case management. Services are targeted at maintaining frail aged and people with disabilities in their communities.

The Katherine Aged and Disability Services operate under a transdisciplinary model of service delivery that supports the delivery of comprehensive health care and provides extended services for people living in remote communities. The transdisciplinary model allows staff to take a holistic approach to both assessment and service delivery when working with individuals. It allows staff to develop networks and informal relationships within their targeted communities, and to have a single contact person. It also allows for the establishment of innovative community partnerships, with the opportunity to develop the appropriate infrastructure to support and deliver services in remote communities.

The child health nurse at the community clinic referred Kela to the single point of contact within the transdisciplinary team, or key contact person, for assessment and intervention. The key contact spent several visits developing a relationship with the family and getting to know Kela while observing his abilities. A physiotherapist was initially unable to visit the community. At first the family was not concerned about Kela's difficulties. They were happy to carry him around and to continue to concentrate on breastfeeding rather than progressing to more difficult solids. Between the community visits the key contact would discuss Kela's presentation with the physiotherapist and gather further suggestions to offer to the family. A relationship continued to develop with the family, particularly the grandmothers, who provided much of the primary care and assisted to improve Kela's milestones. Traditional 'bush medicine' practices were used and discussed with the therapist as part of the intervention process. The family moved to Katherine when Kela was 18 months old and he was referred again to the service through the town's Aboriginal Health Board. The key contact had lost contact with the family during the move to Katherine. Indigenous families in remote communities tend to be transient between communities, thus complicating the provision of health care and highlighting the need to develop good rapport with all involved service providers.

Once contact was re-established the physiotherapist began visiting the family at their home. A visit would involve sitting outside with Mum and Grandmother and Kela, chatting and observing and sitting in silence. This approach was important to establish a relationship that empowered the family to gain the most effective two-way communication. After gaining the confidence of Kela and the family, the physiotherapist modelled 'therapy through play' in various positions, bringing highly motivating toys to encourage interaction. This provided a practical demonstration of appropriate toys and ways to stimulate Kela's independence. Kela's enjoyment of the play ensured that Mum and Grandmother consented to the regular 'treatments'. Soon the family was invited to attend treatment sessions at the centre, where there were many more 'toys to play with'. So as not to overwhelm the family, the physiotherapist provided the intervention mostly alone, even though goals of speech pathology and occupational therapy were also highlighted through the transdisciplinary practice. Liaison with these therapists ensured the correct foci for treatment. Combining the goals for the three therapies facilitated a smooth and comfortable intervention process. It also enabled the physiotherapist to use modelling for incorporating sign language into family life.

Grandmothers often brought Kela for the treatment and enjoyed watching his achievements. One of the differences between Indigenous and non-Indigenous understanding lies in the concept of family. To a non-Indigenous Australian, the nuclear family usually involves Mum, Dad and children. To an Indigenous Australian, the nuclear family includes grandparents, aunties, uncles and cousins in a complex system of kinship. Many family members have key roles in the decision-making process for medical intervention. Thus the roles of carer and provider are not always straightforward from the viewpoint of non-Indigenous structure and understanding.

A relationship of trust was firmly developed so that the physiotherapist became the liaison for medical tests from the health clinic, explaining the results of the tests, attending specialist appointments and ensuring clear explanations of the discussions, and organising respite opportunities for the family. Family members now regularly drop in to the centre with questions, or just for smiles and a cuddle. Kela can now walk unassisted, and is spontaneously using signs to assist his communication. Next year he will be eligible for early entry to pre-school, which will provide further opportunities to improve his developmental skills. This progress has been facilitated by the physiotherapist organising appointments and giving much opportunity for the family to discuss any concerns and personal goals.

SUMMARY

The Indigenous population of Australia carries a heavy burden of disease, a high mortality rate and a life expectancy that is 17 years less than other Australians. To successfully work in Indigenous health contexts, one must be an excellent clinician. But it takes more than that. It requires an understanding of the historical relationship between coloniser and colonised, and the implications in a contemporary setting. It also requires an understanding of the impact of the social determinants of health specific to Indigenous people and an understanding of the concept of self-determination, both for individuals to have a part in determining their course of treatment and for communities to be able to control the priorities for their own health care. This chapter has provided a starting point for that journey of understanding.

Reflective questions

- What strategies would you adopt to promote effective communication with a client from an Indigenous background?
- What particular physiotherapy knowledge and skills might contribute to reducing the heavy burden of disease and the high mortality among Indigenous Australians?

Further reading relating to the Māori, the Indigenous people of New Zealand

Main C, McCallin A, Smith N 2006 Cultural safety and cultural competence: what does this mean for physiotherapists? New Zealand Journal of Physiotherapy 34(3):160–166

New Zealand Society of Physiotherapists Inc. Tae Ora Tinana. Available: http://www.nzsp.org.nz 14 Feb 2008

Ratima M, Waetford C, Wikaire E 2006 Cultural competence for physiotherapists: reducing inequalities in health between Māori and non-Māori. New Zealand Journal of Physiotherapy 34(3):153–159

Takoa, Te Aka Kumara o Aotearoa – a directory of Māori organisations and resource people. Available: http://www.takoa.co.nz/iwi_maps.htm 14 February 2008

Tatau Kahukura: Māori Health Chart Book. Available: http://www.moh.govt.nz/moh.nsf/pagesmh/3395/$File/maori-health-chart.pdf 14 February 2008

References

Aboriginal and Torres Strait Islander Social Justice Commissioner 2003 Social Justice Report Human Rights and Equal Opportunity Commission. Available: http://www.hreoc.gov.au/social_justice/sj_report/sjreport03/index.html 14 Jan 2008

ABS 2004 3238.0 - Experimental estimates and projections, Aboriginal and Torres Strait Islander Australians, 1991 to 2009. Available: http://www.abs.gov.au/AUSSTATS/abs@.nsf/ProductsbyReleaseDate/4EF9B192CB67360CCA256F1B0082C453?OpenDocument 14 Jan 2008

ABS 2006 4715.0 - National Aboriginal and Torres Strait Islander Health Survey, 2004–05. Available: http://www.abs.gov.au/ausstats/abs@.nsf/productsbytitle/C36E019CD56EDE1FCA256C76007A9D36?OpenDocument 14 Jan 2008

ABS 2007 3101.0 - Australian Demographic Statistics, June Quarter 2007. Available: http://www.ausstats.abs.gov.au/Ausstats/subscriber.nsf/0/26E2ADC6E07B7A12CA2573A6001351D2/$File/31010_jun%202007.pdf 14 Jan 2008

AIHW 2005 The health and welfare of Australia's Aboriginal and Torres Strait Islander peoples. Available: http://www.aihw.gov.au/publications/index.cfm/title/10172 14 Jan 2008

Anderson I, Loff B 2004 Voices lost: Indigenous health and human rights in Australia. Lancet 364(9441):1281–1282

Department of Aboriginal Affairs 1981 Report on a review of the administration of the working definition of Aboriginal and Torres Strait Islander. Constitutional Section, Department of Aboriginal Affairs, Canberra

National Aboriginal Health Strategy 1989. Available: http://www.health.gov.au/internet/wcms/publishing.nsf/Content/health-oatsih-pubs-healthstrategy.htm 14 Jan 2008

National Health and Medical Research Council 2000 Nutrition in Aboriginal and Torres Strait Islander people: an information paper. Available: http://www.nhmrc.gov.au/publications/synopses/n26syn.htm 16 Jan 2008

Report of the National Inquiry into the Separation of Aboriginal and Torres Strait Islander Children from Their Families April 1997. Available: http://www.austlii.edu.au/au/special/rsjproject/rsjlibrary/hreoc/stolen/ 14 Jan 2008

Royal Commission on Aboriginal Deaths in Custody 1989 National Report Vol 1. Available: http://www.austlii.edu.au/au/special/rsjproject/rsjlibrary/rciadic/national/vol1/ 14 Jan 2008

Zhao Y, Guthridge S, Magnus A et al 2004 Burden of disease and injury in Aboriginal and non-Aboriginal populations in the Northern Territory. Medical Journal of Australia 180(10):498–502

STANDARDS AND EVIDENCE FOR PRACTICE

ETHICS, PRACTICE REGULATION AND PHYSIOTHERAPY

Lynley Anderson and Elizabeth Ellis

fourteen

Key concepts

- The philosophical underpinning of ethical physiotherapy practice
- Application of this knowledge to everyday clinical scenarios
- Analysis of clinical circumstances for their ethical components

INTRODUCTION

Ethical reasoning informs a physiotherapist's everyday clinical practice. The way physiotherapists relate to and interact with patients and their families and the styles of care they choose all have an underlying ethical basis. Recognising the ethical dimensions of clinical practice is important in meeting the needs of patients and also in meeting the professional standards laid down by physiotherapy regulating and professional bodies. In this chapter we elaborate upon the philosophy underpinning ethical practice and then explore it through clinical scenarios.

PHILOSOPHICAL UNDERPINNINGS IN PHYSIOTHERAPY

Physiotherapists will come across a number of complex ethical issues during their professional lives. Some of these might cause them to stop and think about what is the right course of action to take in a particular situation, whereas they might be very clear about the correct course of action in others. How physiotherapists respond to complex ethical issues depends on the ethical factors and the values reflected that they believe are the most relevant to the issue.

The application of these values is not necessarily a simple task. For example, there might be problems if physiotherapists' ethical values conflict with those of the person being cared for or the institution they may be working in, or if the ethical values they were raised with conflict with those of the profession. Thus physiotherapists need to consider how to think through such ethical issues.

When thinking about ethical concerns many people have an initial intuitive response to some issues. These responses might be a good indicator that there is indeed an issue there, as these intuitions may be based more on our distaste or level of discomfort about a situation. Being able to recognise ethical issues in clinical practice is a good start, while also getting to the heart of why such issues might be troubling and beginning to unravel them require a more systematic response. For that we begin by turning to the academic discipline of bioethics.

The application of principles derived from normative ethics to difficult questions is called applied ethics (Kagan 1998), of which bioethics is just one area. Strictly speaking, the term bioethics is used to refer to moral concerns in all areas of life, including human, animal, plant and environmental areas. However, in this chapter we limit the term to refer to the ethical analysis of physiotherapy practice only. In the physiotherapy context, bioethical approaches can be used to provide reasoned analysis for an array of ethical concerns. Ethical analysis can assist a physiotherapist to untangle the issues involved in a particular situation, help to identify and clarify exactly what the moral concerns are, and at times help to find a resolution to the problem. We can explore an ethical problem using a variety of approaches.

MORAL IDEAS FROM EVERYDAY LIFE

All of us are familiar with moral concepts (although they might not have been identified as such) from our upbringing. As children we are taught a range of important moral ideas. We learn, for example, about the importance of telling the truth, of not hurting others, the significance of keeping our promises and respecting the views of others. These concepts are reinforced by our experiences of what it feels like when we are caught out telling lies or when others hurt us.

Much of the time these ideas work well: we keep our promises and others keep their promises to us, or we are kind to others and they reciprocate. However, problems arise when we discover that in order to follow one concept we are no longer able to comply with another. For example, if a friend who is overweight asks, 'Do I look fat in these clothes?' we might begin to question whether honesty is indeed the best policy. So, although honesty is an important concept for a child to learn, later we might learn that complete honesty can cause harm to the feelings of others and that it may be better to say nothing or to modify our statements rather than to tell the complete truth. With friends, people may withhold facts or opinions to maintain the friendship. However, as an individual moves into professional practice it is important to know when to apply which moral idea. For example, honesty may not be the best policy when giving clothing advice to an overweight friend, but honesty is required when talking to patients in order for them to make informed decisions. This is because the moral obligations arising from patient–therapist relationships emphasise respect for a patient's autonomy.

LAW AND ETHICS

Expectations about the quality and standards of all health professionals in their interactions with those they care for may also be expressed in legislation. For example, getting permission to treat, or gaining informed consent, from a patient prior to undertaking any treatment or care is now a legal requirement. For patients to be able to make decisions about care they must receive information about why something is being suggested and what it might mean to make each choice. They also need to know the risks and benefits. Thus, honesty is one of those moral ideas from early life that is developed and clarified in physiotherapy practice, professional codes of practice and related laws.

However, ethical reasoning is not simply an application of legal expectations in professional life. Law and ethics share much common ground, yet they are distinct disciplines. What might be ethically acceptable may differ significantly from what is legally acceptable. For example, some laws might be ethically unacceptable. There may also be times when some activity is not illegal but is certainly considered ethically dubious. Imagine a woman who agrees to take her lonely friend out to the movies but in the meantime gets invited to a party with some people she has been trying to impress for some time. To break the arrangement so that she can go to the party the woman calls her friend, saying she is sick. Although she hasn't done anything illegal, her standard of social ethics could be questioned. An example of this is that physiotherapists are expected to meet the expectations of duty of care for all of their patients, which commonly involves prioritising treatments in relation to health needs rather than personality issues.

A reason sometimes given by health professionals for complying with legislation put in place to protect those they care for is fear of legal reprisals for failure to care. An example of this might be when getting informed consent from a patient. It may be said that this is only done to avoid breaking the law. But the motivation for taking action for fear of legal punishment shows failure by the health professional to comprehend the ethical values of informing patients and respecting their ability to make decisions for themselves. In other words, ethics provides a positive framework for action, whereas the law provides a framework for limiting certain actions.

THE HISTORY AND DEVELOPMENT OF BIOETHICS

Bioethics emerged during the last half of the 20th century, partly in response to the revelation of unethical and unchecked action by doctors and scientists, but also in response to the exceptional clinical developments that began to occur in health care around that time. At the end of World War II the trials of Nazi doctors at Nuremberg revealed horrific experiments carried out on prisoners of war and others. Although many attributed these actions to the horrors of war and the Nazi regime, the fact that doctors could be involved in such atrocities in the name of research was a major concern. Events such as the Nuremberg Trials triggered the process now in place for improving the protections for research participants (Evans & Evans 1996).

However, unethical research was not totally eliminated after the events at Nuremberg. In 1966 Henry Beecher wrote his famous article 'Ethics and clinical research'. Beecher uncovered 22 research studies going on in hospitals in the USA that he claimed were unethical. A desire to improve clinical care led many researchers to disregard the health and wellbeing of research participants, many of whom were vulnerable and/or of a lower social class (McNeill 1993). That article demonstrated that events revealed at the Nuremberg Trials could not simply be attributed to wartime or the activities of an evil regime and that neglect of the welfare of research subjects was more widespread than first thought.

Developments in clinical medicine were burgeoning around this time and these also contributed to the development of ethics and prioritisation of resources. One example, which provided an opportunity for lives to be extended, was the development in 1961 of regular kidney dialysis (Jonson 1998). A shortage of machines for the number of people requiring dialysis meant that decisions had to be made about who should get this precious resource. The social environment of the latter half of the 20th century in which these events occurred (particularly in the USA, but also in Australia and New Zealand) was one of emerging civil rights and liberation movements (Jonson,

1998). These movements helped pave the way for individuals to have greater input into decisions about health care that affected them.

APPROACHES TO ETHICS

The four-principle approach to health care ethics

The framework most commonly seen within the bioethics literature is that of the four principles developed by Beauchamp and Childress (2001). These principles are autonomy, beneficence, non-maleficence and justice. Although originally developed with medicine in mind, many of these concepts are valuable for other health professionals including physiotherapists.

Autonomy

The term autonomy literally means self-rule or self-determination. Autonomy is based on the concept that people should be free to make decisions in line with how they wish their lives to be. We each have our own experiences, identities and significant features in our life; therefore it is thought that we will have the ability to judge what the best decision is for us.

In health care the concept of autonomy involves respecting the ability of a person to make choices about treatment and for those choices to be respected. It implies that individuals have the necessary competence to make decisions for themselves and also that they should not be coerced or forced into making decisions.

The development of autonomy as an important central principle in bioethics is reflected in this principle underpinning many of the ethical obligations of health professionals. This has come about due to a rise in individualism and a growing desire of people to have increasing involvement in decisions about their care. The rise in interest in and expectations of respect inherent in individual autonomy has meant a shift in the locus of health care decision making from being solely the domain of the health care professional to being more patient-centred. This includes respect for the information that patients provide within treatment encounters, or respect for patient confidentiality.

Beneficence

The principle of beneficence determines that we act in such a way as to provide benefit or improve the wellbeing of those we provide care for. This could be understood as one of the fundamental principles underlying the provision of health care. The very purpose of health care in all its forms is to improve the health and wellbeing of its recipients.

However, there are many accounts of what might constitute a benefit or an improvement in wellbeing. We know that people are different from each other. Some like a life that is full of challenge and risk, while others prefer life to be more sedentary. Because we all differ, deciding on what is a benefit for others is a particularly difficult and potentially dangerous task. This suggests that we should respect the autonomous choices of individual recipients and allow them to decide on the benefits, unless they are unable to do so.

Non-maleficence

Non-maleficence can be understood simply as 'do no harm'. This principle requires that we do nothing that will harm or injure a person in our care. When we consider what might constitute harm, we realise that what one person thinks is harmful may not be so for someone else. For example, a sportsperson may consider that placing strapping around a recent fracture may be sufficient to allow play without doing harm whereas a physiotherapist may consider that to assist in such a practice would be harmful. Given that we all differ in our preferences, the difficulty lies in how to determine where the threshold for harm lies.

Justice

Within health care, the principle of justice dictates that health care services should be distributed fairly. We might wish to ask questions about whether everyone has equal access to health care. Here we need to take care that we are not discriminating against people because of their age, race, religion, sexual orientation, marital status, and so on. According to the principle of justice all patients are to be given good quality care. However, that does not mean that we have to give out exactly the same care to each patient. Each will have different requirements based on individual needs.

The principle of justice also relates to the allocation of increasingly scarce resources in health care. At times we might consider allocation of resources at a micro level; for example, perhaps there is only one physiotherapist and too many patients requiring care. In this situation which patients should receive care? At other times we might have to take a much wider viewpoint and ask whether limited funding should be spent on elderly care or on paediatric services, or in cardiac surgery or preventive health care. When considering the wider issues we need to be careful that some groups are not disadvantaged or perhaps taking a greater burden because of existing social inequalities and associated poorer health statistics.

Some criticisms of a principles approach

Some authors have identified problems associated with a principles approach to ethical issues in health care (Clouser & Gert 1990). One of the most commonly identified problems is that, while the principles do not solve our problems for us and while they might highlight particular issues and supply a framework for thinking about the issues, there may be no instruction about how to balance or rank the principles when they do conflict.

Clouser & Gert (1990) considered that the principles do not represent a single theory but are the result of taking a bit from one theory and a bit from another. For example, autonomy is said to be a concept borrowed from a Kantian idea of respect for persons, and beneficence derives from the writings of John Stuart Mill (a utilitarian). Because these concepts come from what are actually conflicting moral theories, the principles may be criticised on the grounds that they lack internal consistency and should therefore be rejected.

PHYSIOTHERAPY CODES OF ETHICS

Two of the key indicators of recognition as a profession are self-governance and having expected professional standards set out via a code of ethics. A code of ethics is the establishment of a morality internal to the profession (Paul 2000). Codes of ethics are usually developed by professional associations but might also be developed by registering authorities. Sometimes the standards are identical, such as the absolute rule prohibiting sexual relationships between practitioners and their clients. At other times, the differences between the codes of associations and registering authorities appear subtle and can reflect the fact that professional associations have a stronger emphasis on the interests of the profession and the authorities have a stronger emphasis on protecting the safety of the public.

ETHICS IN PRACTICE

Having explored one ethical theory and looked at codes of ethics we move on to examine how the ethical frameworks work in practice for physiotherapists. The following are real-life scenarios that physiotherapists typically deal with in their everyday work. Read through the scenarios and use the following information to work out how physiotherapists might deal with such matters when they arise in clinical practice.

Scenario 1a

Kim is asked to provide active treatment for a woman who has respiratory distress after a motor vehicle accident that involved rib fractures and concussion. She has a history of chronic bronchitis and is a heavy smoker, and is currently having difficulty maintaining an adequate PaO_2 and her $PaCO_2$ is rising as the day progresses. Without thorough respiratory care she will almost certainly need to be intubated and ventilated. When Kim goes to talk about treatment options with her, the woman says quite emphatically that she has had physiotherapy in the past and definitely doesn't want physiotherapy now that her ribs are so sore. She says that she would have to be at death's door before she would agree and that she has been worse before and will be all right. The woman then tells Kim that she would like to go home because she really doesn't like hospitals.

If a health care professional treats a person without that person's consent they could potentially be charged with assault within most jurisdictions. For a refusal to be valid it must satisfy the same criteria as valid consent; i.e., that it is informed, voluntary, and the person must be competent.

Gaining informed consent from a patient is one of the key circumstances in which we can see the principle of autonomy in action. Informed consent obviously has two main components – (a) providing information to the patient and (b) allowing the patient to either consent or refuse the suggested course of action. These two components can be broken down further into:

- information
- comprehension
- competence
- voluntariness.

Take the example of a patient being presented with the option of having acupuncture. The physiotherapist would need to provide *information* to the patient, describing: what acupuncture is and what it does; what the procedure entails; what risks and benefits are associated with the needling (including short- and long-term benefits and risks); how much pain could be expected due to the needling; any possible effective alternatives;

what, if any, costs the patient might be expected to incur, and so on. The information needs to be provided in such a way that the patient can understand it. That is not to say that the patient should be spoken down to, but the information should be given at a level that is *comprehensible* to the patient, and is jargon-free. Physiotherapists sometimes wonder how much information to give about a particular treatment. For example, should the physiotherapist give out information about very rare complications related to treatment with acupuncture? There are common concerns expressed, which this kind of information could put people off a procedure like acupuncture, which might otherwise be helpful. To answer this we need to return to the concept of autonomy. To be truly respectful of autonomy, the information needs to be given. Failure to give all the information relating to a treatment and its risks has been a topic under scrutiny in recent times, particularly in the law courts.

As explained earlier, the 'consent' part of informed consent involves considering the *competence* of the patient to give informed consent and the *voluntariness* of that decision. In New Zealand, for example, every person is legally presumed competent to consent unless proven otherwise. For some it may take more explanation and the use of diagrams and other methods, but the presumption should be that adults are able to give consent. Questioning the competence of a patient simply because he or she is making a choice that the physiotherapist disagrees with is not acceptable and not in line with a respect for autonomy.

Consent should also be *voluntary*, meaning that it should not be coerced. An example of coercion would be if a physiotherapist carrying out research tells a patient that some element of care will be withdrawn if the patient does not agree to take part in the research. The patient who consents under these circumstances could be said to have been coerced. Informed consent should be viewed as an ongoing conversation between physiotherapist and patient, not a one-off event. In this way physiotherapists are always checking with patients that care is proceeding along lines with which they are comfortable.

If competence is in question the person needs to be assessed by a suitable professional, such as a psychiatrist. However, as a rough rule if the person is oriented in time and place and has been informed of and can understand the risks and benefits of the treatment and the treatment alternatives, the person should be assumed to be competent. If a patient makes a decision that the physiotherapist does not consider is in that patient's best interest, there can be a risk that incompetence of the patient is presumed. However, a person's right to choose includes the right to choose even if the consequences are negative for health and wellbeing.

Sometimes people can make a decision (decisional autonomy) but cannot actually carry out the effects of that decision (operational autonomy). In Scenario 1a the patient might have been competent to make the decision to go home, but if she left her bed and tried to go home without adequate support she may have experienced an adverse event such as a respiratory arrest.

Scenario 1b

Follow-up

Kim documents the patient's valid refusal and then the woman slips into unconsciousness. Again Kim is asked to treat her – has the situation changed?

There are some who are unable to make autonomous decisions, including those with a severe and acute psychiatric illness or severe brain injury. In these situations we might rightly question the person's competence. There may also be times when people who are normally competent temporarily lose such ability, as with the patient in the follow-up Scenario 1b. Before losing consciousness the patient made her wishes known, but her refusal was qualified by the phrase 'unless I was at death's door'.

There is a defence under the doctrine of necessity of treating without consent. This implies that treatment can be given in order to prevent serious threat to life or health when there is a high probability of retrospective consent. Given the woman's current clinical condition and the qualification on her refusal, it could be argued that it would be the physiotherapist's duty of care to treat her.

People who have strong feelings about how they should be treated when they lose the capacity to make decisions for themselves can make advanced directives or establish an enduring power of attorney. In an advanced directive people can describe how they want to be treated under a range of different circumstances. In some jurisdictions there are special forms that are recognised by the courts; in others it is less formal and they might be less binding on a patient's carers. For a stronger level of authority, people can make a formal arrangement, or enduring power of attorney, to hand over responsibility for their health care decisions to another person, should they be incapacitated. It is then the responsibility of that person to make decisions in a way that would conform to the wishes of the person now incapacitated.

Scenario 2

Catherine is asked to provide physiotherapy for a 16-year-old male with intellectual impairment but he refuses treatment. Catherine believes that it is in the young man's best interests to participate in her exercise program. The young man is adamant that he does not want to but his parents agree to allow the treatment to be given.

Ordinarily the consent of a parent or guardian is sufficient consent for a minor under the age of 18 years. However, adolescents between the age of 14 and 18 have a developing competence that is known as 'Gillick competence' (Wallace 1995), and may be in a position to make a decision for themselves. This principle can apply to those with impaired intellect. Decision making can be enhanced within a supportive environment and by providing time for more effective explanations. As long as the person has sufficient insight and capacity to understand the risks and benefits of the proposed treatment their autonomy should be respected.

Scenario 3

Michael is the sole physiotherapist in a rural area. The nearest physiotherapist is at a base hospital that can only be reached by driving for an hour and a half on a dirt road. Michael's spouse develops severe back pain that is worse when she sits. Michael is competent to treat this type of condition.

Generally speaking, treatment of family members is not ideal, and most health care professions advise against it. One of the main reasons is the potential for a lack of objectivity in the clinician. Our relationships with family members can cloud our judgement and potentially result in poor quality care. Aside from a lack of objectivity there are also other good reasons for not treating family members. For example, it can be difficult to establish a therapeutic relationship when a mother/child or husband/wife relationship already exists, and there is a potential for care to be provided in a less than professional manner, often without appropriate safeguards, such as by providing care in a non-private setting or after a couple of drinks. Also, there is often an assumption that we know the medical history of a family member but this may not be the case. We should consider too whether we are providing them with the choices we would provide to others. How easy would it be for them to ask for a second opinion or (in the case of children) for them to ask not to continue to be treated? Having appropriate professional boundaries is important in providing care, as a physiotherapist may be too accessible to family.

In saying this, there are times when treatment of family members is appropriate. A prime example is the situation in Scenario 3. Here Michael's spouse is in pain and unable to readily access any alternative care. In this case it is appropriate for the physiotherapist to treat his spouse, at least until she can reasonably access alternative care.

Scenario 4

Sarah is single and has become aware that there is a mutual attraction between her and Jake (one of the athletes in a team for which she has been employed as physiotherapist). Sarah has been working with the team for only a month and as yet has not treated Jake. While the team is on tour Jake approaches Sarah to ask her out.

In most jurisdictions and within most codes of ethics, entering into any type of sexual relationship or having any type of sexual activity with a current client is considered improper and an unacceptable breach of professional standards. The definition of 'current patient' includes anyone who is in a therapeutic relationship with a physiotherapist, including people who are treated by a team therapist, whether on tour or not. In the above scenario it could be argued that Jake is not yet a patient of Sarah's, but she is responsible for the team of which he is a part.

The basis for a zero tolerance approach to any sexual activity or contact in the therapeutic relationship is due to the practitioner having a degree of power over the patient or group which places them in a more vulnerable position. Power relationships still occur between the physiotherapist and team members, especially if the physiotherapist has to give clearance for team members to play. If a relationship were to develop in Scenario 4, it could influence professional decision making and thus make it difficult for Sarah to remain impartial. Also it is likely that the team would find out about the relationship so the potential exists for Sarah to lose her professional status with the team.

In general, a person should be considered to be a current client until that person ceases to receive professional advice, treatment or support from the physiotherapist. Even after treatment has ended a relationship between a physiotherapist and a patient may still not be appropriate. It is the nature and length of the professional consultation, as well as the degree of dependency of the patient on the physiotherapist, that determine whether any future relationship is appropriate. Therapeutic relationships that are long-standing involve high levels of dependency of the patient on the therapist, where a great deal of personal disclosure has occurred, or where there has been close physical contact as a genuine part of the therapy should indicate to the physiotherapist that there is potential for abuse of the vulnerable patient. Even a sexual encounter that has been initiated by the patient or where the patient is a willing participant will not excuse the actions of the physiotherapist. A therapeutic relationship is ultimately one of trust. As communities place enormous trust in health care professionals, breaches of that trust are treated seriously by registration and professional authorities.

The physical closeness of the patient–therapist relationship places both patient and therapist in a vulnerable position. Physiotherapists do not have to be subject to or tolerate any unwelcome sexual advances or sexual harassment from their clients or colleagues.

Scenario 5

David has a busy practice with a wide variety of client groups. David is the principal of the practice and employs a number of younger physiotherapists. On the second visit Harry (one of David's patients) brings an expensive gift for David because, Harry explains, he felt much better after his previous treatment and is grateful to David for the treatment.

Gifts given by patients to their physiotherapist are a common occurrence. Although not generally expected, gifts are often gratefully received and enjoyed. Usually it is thought that, if the gift is low in value, such as a few chocolates, garden flowers, home baked biscuits or a card, there is no problem in accepting it. If the gift is of higher value many recipients feel a little more uneasy. However, it is not simply the monetary value of the gift that is at issue. We need to reflect upon what makes a gift acceptable or not. Generally it is the level of obligation that is generated in the recipient that determines appropriateness. Sometimes gifts make us feel as if we should provide something more for that person; this can occur at a subconscious level. We may feel subtle pressure to provide better care, more attention, or make an appointment more quickly than for others, and that may in fact have been the intention of the giver. When we do provide care that is somehow better than that given to others, it runs contrary to the ethical concept of fairness. Gifts given prior to the completion of treatment or gifts of high monetary value have the greatest potential to create a sense of obligation. In Scenario 5 Harry may be giving David an expensive gift with the expectation that he continues to treat Harry and not pass him on to one of the younger physiotherapists to manage. In other words, the gift comes with strings attached. Accepting the gift may limit what David can do or who can treat Harry. A small gift of low value that is given at the conclusion of treatment is probably the least problematic ethically, but even that has the potential to create a sense of obligation if the patient returns at a later date. The above discussion should not prohibit physiotherapists from receiving gifts, but implies that David, for example, should be careful and reflective about the kinds of obligations that receiving such a gift from Harry might generate.

Sometimes gifts have particular cultural significance. If a physiotherapist is not aware of the significance of a gift from someone of a particular culture, it is recommended that the giver be asked about it rather than acting insensitively through ignorance.

Scenario 6

Andy has a patient who is responding to physiotherapy but somewhat more slowly than expected. Andy gets to the point where the funding agency will not pay for any more treatments for this condition. The patient says that she cannot afford to pay for further treatment but has heard of instances where practitioners have started invoicing one family member's treatment to another family member. The patient asks if Andy could do this so that she can continue to receive treatment.

On one hand the clinician may want to provide the optimal number of treatments for the patient (beneficence) but, on the other hand, he would be dishonest if he complied with the client's request. Fraud of this kind is serious and is considered professional misconduct and not in the public interest. Health insurance fraud reduces social trust in the profession and increases insurance costs to the community at large. In Scenario 6 other solutions for payment need to be found, such as delayed payment plans or finding other sources of funding.

SUMMARY

It might be argued that the application of an ethical framework round clinical issues creates unnecessary complexity. Clinical scenarios always have ethical considerations, but they may not be obvious without the ethical lens. Without the clarity that ethical consideration brings to clinical decision making, physiotherapists are more likely to stumble into situations and potentially harm those they are trying to help.

Consistent high standards of clinical practice require ongoing ethical reflection. A strong sense of awareness in physiotherapists of the ethical dimensions of clinical practice is necessary in order to meet the needs of patients and the profession as well as the expectations of society.

Further reading

Anderson L, Pelvin B 2006 Ethical frameworks for practice. In: Pairman S, Pincombe J, Thorogood C et al (eds) Midwifery preparation for practice. Elsevier, Sydney, pp 191–207

Cambell A, Gillett G, Jones G 2001 Medical ethics, 3rd edn. Oxford University Press, Melbourne

Kerridge I, Lowe M, McPhee J 2005 Ethics and law for the health professions, 2nd edn. Federation Press, Leichhardt, NSW

NSW Policy: 2005 Consent to medical treatment – patient information. Available: http://www.health. nsw.gov.au/policies/ib/2005/pdf/IB2005_054.pdf 11 Nov 2007

Examples of codes of conduct

New Zealand

http://www.nzsp.org.nz/Index02/index_Welcome.htm
http://www.physioboard.org.nz

Australia

http://apa.advsol.com.au/independent/documents/download/APACodeOfConduct.pdf
http://www.physioreg.health.nsw.gov.au/hprb/physio_web/pdf/rights.pdf
http://www.physioreg.health.nsw.gov.au/hprb/physio_web/pdf/profconductmay07.pdf

References

Beauchamp T, Childress J 2001 Principles of biomedical ethics, 5th edn. Oxford University Press, Oxford

Clouser K D, Gert B 1990 A critique of principlism. The Journal of Medicine and Philosophy 15: 219–236

Evans D, Evans M 1996 A decent proposal. Wiley, New York

Jonson A 1998 The birth of bioethics. Oxford University Press, New York

Kagan S 1998 Normative ethics. Westview Press, Boulder, CO

McNeill P 1993 The ethics and politics of human experimentation. Cambridge University Press, Melbourne

Paul C 2000 Internal and external morality of medicine: lessons from New Zealand. BMJ 320: 499–503

Wallace M 1995 Health care and the law, 2nd edn. The Law Book Company, Sydney

PHYSIOTHERAPY AND EVIDENCE-BASED PRACTICE

Peter Bragge and Kathryn Refshauge

fifteen

Key content

- What is evidence-based practice?
- What is research evidence?
- Finding evidence

INTRODUCTION

This chapter presents an overview of evidence-based practice (EBP) as applied to physiotherapy. First, the key concepts and principles that underpin EBP are introduced. Next the steps involved in turning a clinical question into a search strategy are described. Finally, the principles of research evaluation are outlined.

Have you contemplated skipping this chapter? Common reactions to the term 'evidence-based practice' include 'that stuff that researchers do while I'm doing *real* physiotherapy' and 'I've heard that EBP is important but I haven't got time to read journal papers because I'm too busy treating patients'. Although there's an element of truth to both of these statements, they imply that EBP is a discrete concept, separate from clinical practice.

However, the fundamental concept of EBP is that there *is no boundary* between research and clinical practice. For those learning or practising physiotherapy this may be somewhat daunting because it implies that they will be drawn away from patient care to 'do research' or that all treatments have to be proven effective in 4,578 randomised controlled trials. These statements are a distortion of the purpose of EBP. The aim of this chapter is to describe the true, practical value of EBP to the clinical physiotherapist.

WHAT IS EBP?

Evidence-based medicine has been defined as 'the integration of best research evidence with clinical experience and patient values' (Sackett et al 2000, p 1). Similarly, Herbert et al (2005, p 2) stated that 'the practice of evidence-based physiotherapy should be informed by relevant, high quality clinical research, patients' preferences and physiotherapists' practice knowledge'. These definitions encompass the three elements that are the foundation of EBP – *patient perspectives*, *clinical experience* and *research evidence*.

Although physiotherapists have always known the importance of these elements, the strength of EBP lies in the idea that these elements cannot exist in isolation:

- Involving patients in treatment decisions is a key component of ethical practice and in the internet era patients are better informed than ever before. But if treatment were driven solely by patient preference, physiotherapists could spend much time doing relaxation massage without prescribing exercises.
- Clinical experience, knowledge continually gained through both patient contact and observation of effective and ineffective practices, is an unmeasurable but often pivotal element of patient care. However, practice driven solely by clinical experience would inevitably deny patients access to the many proven treatments that a physiotherapist has not practised or observed.
- Research cannot exist in a vacuum. Unless clinical questions relevant to the experiences of patients and physiotherapists are addressed, research results are difficult to transfer into physiotherapy practice (Bialocerkowski et al 2004).

PURPOSE, LIMITATIONS AND STRENGTHS OF EBP

The purpose of EBP is to:

- improve quality, effectiveness and appropriateness of clinical practice
- share decision making with patients
- substantiate the care provided to patients
- reduce variations in practice patterns resulting from geographical difference or gaps in current knowledge
- close the gap between evidence in the literature and the use of this evidence in practice
- evaluate large volumes of literature and summarise the high-quality evidence (systematic reviews) (Cormack 2002, Herbert et al 2005).

Ideally, every physiotherapy treatment would be the perfect marriage of patient preferences, clinical experience and research evidence. In reality, like all concepts, EBP has limitations, including:

- organisational limitations – existing practice/clinic/hospital culture, changing workforce profiles, pressures on patient throughput limiting the ability to apply evidence to patient care (Straus & McAlister 2000), bureaucratic hurdles
- individual limitations – limits of time and resources for finding and evaluating research evidence, shortage of coherent, consistent scientific evidence, difficulty applying evidence to the care of individual patients (Straus & McAlister 2000), lack of interest, learning fatigue.

These limitations need to be weighed against the critical importance of EBP to three areas of physiotherapy practice (Herbert et al 2005). First, patients have an expectation of and a right to safe and effective interventions based on the most up-to-date knowledge. Second, physiotherapists, as autonomous health professionals, have an obligation to provide physiotherapy that is based upon the best available evidence. Finally, funders of physiotherapy services (individuals, health insurance companies, policymakers) need to have confidence that the physiotherapy services they are funding are safe and effective. Evidence is critical in framing decisions about funding priorities for health services (Gray 2001), and physiotherapy is no exception.

Balancing physiotherapists' obligations to practise EBP against the aforementioned limitations can be challenging, but the rewards are substantial. For example, spend a minute or two reflecting on your worst and your best experience as a patient. Negative patient experiences are often distinguished by a sense that

- things are being rushed
- you don't feel part of the process
- the physiotherapist/doctor/health professional is unsure of him/herself
- the treatment seems inconsistent with your understanding of your condition's management.

Conversely, many people describe positive patient experiences as those in which their health professional

- took time to listen to their concerns and involved them in the assessment and treatment process, conveying an understanding of how to take an appropriate history for the presenting problem
- seemed to know appropriate treatment for the presenting problem
- was competent in administering this treatment.

This encapsulation of the three elements of EBP is a powerful reminder of its purpose.

HOW IS EBP UNDERTAKEN?

There are six steps in the EBP process:

1. Convert a patient problem into a specific question.
2. Search the literature for evidence related to the question.
3. Critically appraise the pertinent literature.
4. Integrate the appraisal of the literature with the clinician's expertise and the patient's circumstances and values (informed and shared decision making) to make a decision about clinical care.
5. Incorporate the information and decision into clinical practice.
6. Re-evaluate the outcome, and ask another question if needed (Cormack 2002, p 484).

In the remainder of this chapter we focus on steps 1 to 3.

FINDING EVIDENCE

Step 1 Converting a patient problem into a specific question

The EBP process always starts with a patient problem, or *clinical question*. In physiotherapy, clinical questions often pertain to treatment effect, for example:

Is ultrasound or manual therapy more effective for reducing acute low back pain?
Does EMG (biofeedback) improve muscle strength in urinary incontinence?

A brief discussion with a colleague, looking up departmental clinical guidelines and consulting a textbook are all useful ways of addressing a clinical question. However, the latest evidence relevant to clinical questions is found on electronic databases such as Medline®, The Physiotherapy Evidence Database or PEDro (Centre for Evidence-Based Physiotherapy 2005) and The Cochrane Collaboration (2007).

Unfortunately, unlike professional colleagues, databases do not speak our language; they use a special syntax based upon key words and phrases. Understandably, many time-poor clinicians and students simply search databases using a few key words and phrases to address their clinical question. This is not the most effective strategy because a random selection of words and phrases might not be understood by the database. (It's a bit like getting a blank response when asking in English where the train station is when you are in Germany.)

Efficient database searches require a structured search strategy, written in a 'database' language. This process of translation (analogous to using an English–German phrasebook) creates a *searchable question*. The 'PICO' approach (Stone 2002) is a useful way of making this translation:

- Patient, Population or Problem
- Intervention
- Comparison
- Outcomes.

Clinical questions can be rephrased according to these component parts:

In [Population], what is the effect of [Intervention] on [Outcome], compared with [Comparison]?

That is,

In [acute low back pain], what is the effect of [ultrasound] on [pain], compared with [manual therapy]?

When one intervention is not being compared to another, the Comparison component of PICO is simply omitted:

In [urinary incontinence], what is the effect of [EMG] on [muscle strength]?

Step 2 Searching the literature for evidence related to the question

The elements of a clinical question identified using the PICO approach are then used to develop the *search strategy*, the final result of translating the searchable question into a language understood by electronic databases.

Basics of search strategy development: a worked example

Development of an optimal search strategy involves identifying as many synonyms as possible for each key component identified using the PICO approach. Consider the question:

In [urinary incontinence], what is the effect of [EMG] on [muscle strength]?

Synonyms can be identified by:

1. *Using existing knowledge and resources such as known articles or textbooks (great sources of the specialised terms of physiotherapy practice)* – synonyms for 'urinary incontinence' may include 'urinary stress incontinence' or simply 'incontinence'. It is also helpful to spell out abbreviations, such as 'electromyography' for 'EMG'. Synonyms can range from specific to general; for example, as EMG is commonly a part of physiotherapy management, some 'physiotherapy' synonyms could be considered.
2. *Searching the medical subject headings (MeSH®) thesaurus where available* – this thesaurus is the 'English–German' phrasebook of electronic literature searching

– a database of medical terms developed by the United States National Library of Medicine (National Library of Medicine 2007). The terms are used to index, catalogue and search health-related resources on MeSH®-compatible databases such as Medline®. The process of searching MeSH, known as *subject mapping*, can only be done in a database that is MeSH-compatible; however, MeSH terms can be used in a non-MeSH database such as PEDro.

Refining terms

If you have a large physiotherapy vocabulary and access to a MeSH thesaurus, chances are your simple clinical question will have grown to a large (and possibly daunting) list of synonyms and MeSH terms. The final list of terms used in the search strategy will be a combination of PICO headings, your own synonyms and synonyms identified by subject mapping. A simple method of identifying duplicate terms and deciding which ones to use in the search strategy is to tabulate them as shown in Table 15.1.

Table 15.1 Example of search strategy development for the question: In [urinary incontinence], what is the effect of [EMG] on [muscle strength]?

PICO term	Your synonyms	MeSH® synonyms	Final list of search terms
P = urinary stress incontinence	incontinence urinary incontinence urinary stress incontinence	urinary incontinence stress	incontinence urinary incontinence urinary incontinence stress
I = EMG	EMG biofeedback physiotherapy physical therapy rehabilitation	electromyography physical therapy modalities exercise therapy	EMG biofeedback physiotherapy physical therapy rehabilitation electromyography physical therapy modalities exercise therapy
O = muscle strength	strength muscle strength	muscle weakness	strength muscle strength muscle weakness

Combining terms

The above terms are combined in electronic database searches using the Boolean operators 'OR' and 'AND':

- 'OR' is used to combine synonyms for an individual PICO element, for example all the words for 'incontinence'. This is an *expanding* combiner, because it asks the database to find an article with *any one* of the listed synonyms (incontinence OR urinary incontinence OR urinary stress incontinence).
- 'AND' is used to link PICO elements together, for example 'incontinence' AND 'EMG'. Therefore it is a *limiting* combiner, because an article must contain words under *all* of the separate elements to be retrieved.

Using these principles, the search strategy in our example is:

(incontinence OR urinary incontinence OR urinary incontinence, stress)

AND

(EMG OR biofeedback OR physiotherapy OR physical therapy OR rehabilitation OR electromyography OR physical therapy modalities OR exercise therapy)

AND

(strength OR muscle strength OR muscle weakness)

Non-MeSH and other simple databases

Some databases do not allow long search strings and combinations of terms, but nevertheless are critical sources of physiotherapy literature, for example the PEDro database (Centre for Evidence-Based Physiotherapy 2005). In these situations, a simplified version of the 'ideal' search strategy is created by selecting fewer terms, using dropdown menus or employing other database-specific search methods.

Refining search results

There is no ideal number of citations from a literature search. Because the number of citations required varies according to available time and other factors, there is often a need to refine the search to either increase or decrease citation yield. Citation yield can be *increased* by:

- adding synonyms for each PICO element
- removing a PICO element, for example searching only for 'P AND I' instead of 'P AND I AND O'.

Citation yield can be *decreased* by:

- removing synonyms
- applying further limiters such as 'humans only', 'English language only'
- seeking a specific study design such as a randomised controlled trial.

It is important to realise that relevant articles can be lost when reducing citation yield.

EVALUATING RESEARCH EVIDENCE

Now that you know how to search the relevant databases it is important that you are able to evaluate the research evidence. Entire books are devoted to the topic of evaluating research evidence, in addition to numerous tools, schemes and checklists. Here we introduce two key concepts underlying research evaluation; further reading resources are listed at the end of this chapter.

Step 3 Critically appraising the pertinent literature

Regardless of the type of research and the method of appraisal, there are two fundamental questions of research evaluation:

1. What was done?
2. How was it done?

What was done? Types of research evidence

The first step in research evaluation is to determine what type of research has been conducted. Broadly speaking, journal articles will fit into one of the following categories:

- literature review
- primary study
- editorial / opinion paper.

Literature reviews are secondary studies in which a body of research evidence pertaining to a specific clinical question is retrieved and evaluated. Literature reviews can be *systematic* or *narrative*. In a *systematic* review:

- an exhaustive search strategy is employed, with the aim of gathering all the studies relevant to the clinical question
- inclusion and exclusion criteria for the review are predetermined
- study quality is rigorously evaluated using a standardised critical appraisal tool
- information about study characteristics and quality is synthesised, either mathematically (using meta-analysis) or descriptively
- inferences from this process are usually evidence-based (Agency for Healthcare Research and Quality 2002).

A *narrative* literature review also presents research evidence pertaining to a clinical question. However, search strategies and study selection are often not specified and appraisal techniques are variable (Jones & Evans 2000). Systematic reviews are therefore less prone to bias than narrative reviews (Agency of Healthcare Research and Quality 2002). Systematic reviews are often retrieved from standard medical databases. There are also specialised systematic review databases, including:

- The Cochrane Database of Systematic Reviews (The Cochrane Collaboration 2007)
- The Physiotherapy Evidence database (Centre for Evidence-Based Physiotherapy 2005)
- The Joanna Briggs Institute (The Joanna Briggs Institute 2007).

The **primary study** is the cornerstone of research evidence, as it is the source of all secondary studies such as systematic reviews.

Quantitative vs qualitative research

A *quantitative* study is broadly defined as one in which *numerical* data are collected and analysed. Examples of quantitative data include range of motion, pain measured on a scale of 1–10, computer-generated data such as electromyography (EMG) and functional scales such as the Functional Independence Measure (FIM). The majority of biomedical research is quantitative in nature.

However, for some research questions the answers cannot be measured in numbers. These include important subjective elements of physiotherapy assessment and management, such as patients' emotional responses to pain and disability, or their attitudes towards certain treatments. For these questions, *qualitative* research is more appropriate.

The aim of qualitative research is to understand and explain social phenomena (Giacomini & Cook 2000, McReynolds et al 2001) by investigating aspects of human behaviour such as beliefs, attitudes and motivations (Holman 1993, Malterud 1993). The emphasis on description in qualitative research, rather than numerical measurement of variables (Thomas 2003), results in a rich and deep understanding of the topic under study (Giacomini & Cook 2000). The qualitative research paradigm is based upon a different set of methodological principles to quantitative research, for example:

- Due to the emphasis on description, participants are purposefully chosen based on their ability to contribute specific knowledge or experience of the phenomenon of interest (Coyne 1997, Sandelowski 1986). In contrast, random (probability) sampling is generally used in quantitative research.
- Quantitative studies generally test a specific predetermined hypothesis (Greenhalgh & Taylor 1997); qualitative research utilises an inductive approach in which hypotheses regarding the phenomenon of interest are generated and refined as the data are analysed (McReynolds et al 2001, Pope et al 2000, Sandelowski 1993).

As with quantitative studies, qualitative research employs numerous approaches to data collection and analysis, including participant observation, in-depth interviews and focus groups (Greenhalgh & Taylor 1997). There is also a plethora of associated qualitative analytical theories and frameworks, including:

- ethnography, the description and interpretation of cultural behaviour (Law et al 1998a)
- case study, in-depth investigation of a specific individual, group, organisation or setting (Patton 2002)
- phenomenology, which emphasises a description and understanding of people's subjective experience (Law et al 1998a, Schwandt 2001).

Just as quantitative study designs are scrutinised to ascertain their suitability for addressing a specific clinical question, it is important to ascertain whether the qualitative approach used in a study is appropriate.

Editorials, opinion papers and correspondence pertaining to previously published research that does not involve either primary or secondary research are highly prone to bias because such papers are predominantly based upon the opinions and experience of their authors. For these reasons, such papers are limited in their ability to address clinical questions.

Ranking study designs

One method of classifying types of research evidence is to use a *hierarchy of evidence*, for example that of the Australian National Health and Medical Research Council (NHMRC 2005). Most hierarchies of evidence, including that of the NHMRC, rank quantitative study designs. For example, the NHMRC ranks quantitative intervention study designs, as shown in Table 15.2.

Note that editorial and opinion papers are not ranked at all on the NHMRC hierarchy, reflecting their limited value in addressing clinical questions. Similar hierarchical rankings for studies addressing diagnosis, prognosis, aetiology and screening are also contained in the NHMRC (2005) framework.

There are many hierarchies of evidence other than the NHMRC hierarchy, containing various types of studies, levels, terms and systems of classification. The principle underlying all hierarchies is that the methodological design of a given type of study (for example intervention, epidemiology) is ranked according to its inherent level of bias (NHMRC 2000). *Bias* is defined as an inaccuracy that is different in its size or direction in one of the groups in a study compared to another group. Bias favours (influences the results of) one group over the other (Law et al 1998b), distorting the

Table 15.2 NHMRC levels of evidence. From NHMRC additional levels of evidence and grades for recommendations for developers of guidelines: Pilot program 2005–2007, 2005, p 4

Level	Intervention[a]
I[b]	A systematic review of level II studies
II	A randomised controlled trial
III-1	A pseudorandomised controlled trial (i.e. alternate allocation or some other method)
III-2	A comparative study with concurrent controls: Non-randomised experimental trial[c] Cohort study Case-control study Interrupted time series with a control group
III-3	A comparative study without concurrent controls: Historical control study Two or more single arm studies[d]
IV	Case series with either post-test or pre-test/post-test outcomes

[a] Definitions of these study designs are provided on pp 7–8 of *How to use the evidence: assessment and application of scientific evidence* (NHMRC 2000).

[b] A systematic review will only be assigned a level of evidence as high as the studies it contains, excepting where those studies are of level II evidence.

[c] This also includes controlled before-and-after (pre-test/post-test) studies, as well as indirect comparisons (i.e. utilise A vs B and B vs C to determine A vs C).

[d] Comparing single arm studies, i.e. case series from two studies.

results of a study and, potentially, the subsequent conclusions. There are many types of bias, some of which are specific to certain research designs. Examples of bias include:

- *sample* bias – may result in the sample being unrepresentative of the population of interest
- *measurement* bias – errors in how an outcome was measured
- *intervention* bias – resulting from errors in how the treatment was carried out (Law et al 1998b).

How was it done? Methodological quality

The second step in the appraisal of research evidence is to evaluate how it was done. The *quality* of a study is defined as 'the methods used by the investigators … to minimize bias and control confounding within a study type' (NHMRC 2000, p 14).

A *critical appraisal tool* evaluates how a given study has performed against a set of methodological quality criteria. Because sources of bias differ according to study design (NHMRC 2000), the method of quality appraisal also varies. For example, inadequate randomisation is a potential source of bias in a randomised controlled trial, but is not relevant to study designs such as a case series. A different set of quality criteria again apply to the evaluation of systematic reviews. Despite the plethora of critical appraisal tools, there is no accepted 'gold standard' (Katrak et al 2004). Important characteristics to consider in selecting a critical appraisal tool are:

- published evidence regarding the tool's construction, validity and reliability
- published guidelines for use to ensure consistency in the application of the criteria (Katrak et al 2004).

The key consideration in the selection of a critical appraisal tool is its appropriateness to the research design. Below is a brief overview of some generic and research design-specific critical appraisal tools.

Evaluating primary quantitative studies

The Critical Review Form – Quantitative Studies (Law et al 1998b) is a generic tool developed for evaluating occupational therapy literature and, therefore, has relevance to physiotherapy research. It comprises a combination of 'yes/no' and descriptive criteria under several broad headings, including:

- study purpose
- sample (description, sampling methods and justification)
- outcomes (reliability, validity and frequency of outcome measures used)
- intervention (description, contamination, co-intervention, replication)
- results (statistical significance, appropriateness of analysis methods, reporting of clinical significance, drop-outs).

The guidelines include an overview of quantitative study designs and types of bias.

An example of a research design-specific tool is that of the Centre for Evidence-Based Physiotherapy, available at the Physiotherapy Evidence Database (PEDro) website. This was designed to evaluate the quality of randomised controlled trials on the PEDro database (Maher et al 2003). It comprises 11 items pertaining to the conduct of randomised controlled trials, including group allocation, blinding, dropouts and statistical procedures (Centre for Evidence-Based Physiotherapy 2005).

Evaluating primary qualitative studies

Because of the substantial methodological differences between qualitative and quantitative research, it is inappropriate to apply criteria for establishing reliability and validity in quantitative studies to qualitative research (Cutcliffe & McKenna 1999, Powell & Davies 2001). Critical appraisal of qualitative research therefore involves evaluation of different quality criteria.

1. *Credibility*, or *truthfulness* (Slevin & Sines 1999) is the qualitative equivalent of *internal validity* in quantitative research (Lincoln & Guba 1985). A qualitative study establishes credibility by rendering a description of the phenomenon under investigation that is recognisable to the people who experience that phenomenon (Hills 2000).
2. *Triangulation* is the use of multiple methods of inquiry to facilitate a comprehensive and in-depth understanding of a phenomenon (Bechtel et al 2000, McReynolds et al 2001), for example by interviewing both patients and clinicians regarding a phenomenon and analysing the key themes that emerge. Triangulation enhances the credibility of qualitative data (McReynolds et al 2001, Slevin & Sines 1999).
3. *Transferability* in qualitative research, or *applicability* (Appleton 1995, Sandelowski 1986), is related to the quantitative concept of *external validity* (Appleton 1995, Lincoln & Guba 1985). Transferability refers to the relevance of qualitative findings to other contexts or settings (Hills 2000, Powell & Davies 2001, Sandelowski 1986) and depends upon the similarity between the contexts of the original research and the setting in question. It is therefore necessary to describe the research in sufficient detail to allow evaluation of transferability (Lincoln & Guba 1985).

4. *Dependability* in qualitative research, or *consistency* and *auditability* (Sandelowski 1986), is analogous to *reliability* in quantitative research (Lincoln & Guba 1985). Dependability refers to the extent to which another investigator can follow the specific approach taken to analyse the qualitative data, otherwise known as the *decision trail* (Sandelowski 1986). The findings of qualitative research are considered dependable if an independent researcher, given the same data, could arrive at a conclusion that is similar to that from the original study (Hills 2000, Sandelowski 1986) or accepts the conclusions of the research based upon examination of the data (Lincoln & Guba 1985).

The Critical Review Form – Qualitative Studies (Law et al 1998a) is the qualitative equivalent of the quantitative tool described above. The format is similar to the quantitative version, but the content reflects the methodological differences between these two research approaches, for example:

- sample (description, qualitative sampling methods and justification)
- data collection (descriptive clarity, procedural rigour, context)
- data analysis (preciseness, auditability, theoretical connections, appropriateness)
- trustworthiness (triangulation, member checking to verify findings).

Due to the numerous qualitative methods and associated underlying theories, it may be necessary to consult introductory qualitative research methods literature prior to conducting a critical appraisal of qualitative research.

Evaluating systematic reviews

Critical appraisal guidelines focus on the evaluation of systematic reviews because of their relative methodological strength compared to narrative reviews. Many of the principles of evaluating systematic reviews – stating methods clearly, avoiding bias – apply to all forms of research. Avoiding bias in study selection and evaluation is of particular importance. Quality criteria for systematic reviews have been developed by Oxman (1994) and Greenhalgh (1997).

Study design versus study quality

A common misconception in EBP is to confuse the two key issues of study design and study quality. In this context there are three important principles to keep in mind:

- No matter how highly ranked in the hierarchy and how well performed, a study that has not employed a design appropriate to the research question is of little value.
- A study ranked high in a hierarchy of evidence, such as a randomised controlled trial, can be poorly executed.
- Conversely, much can be learned from a well-executed study that is ranked lower on a hierarchy of evidence, such as a case series.

If the differences between study design (what was done) and study quality (how it was done) are considered and understood, such misconceptions are less likely.

WHAT NEXT?

Once appropriate research addressing a clinical question has been found and evaluated, there are several further issues to consider. First, having evaluated study design and quality, it is important to examine not just the magnitude and direction of the study's findings but their consistency with similar studies or reviews. This contextualising of the results can have a considerable influence on their interpretation. Systematic reviews have obvious value in this process.

Second, it is important to emphasise that although this chapter has focused on finding and evaluating *research evidence*, this does not diminish the importance of *patient preferences* and *clinical experience* to EBP. For example, if you have found credible research evidence that soft tissue massage is effective in managing elevated muscle tension in patients with cervical spine pain, the extent to which you apply this information in practice in any individual case will depend upon:

- information from the clinical examination, including how the patient has responded to any previous soft tissue massage, and the patient's views and preferences regarding this modality
- your level of experience and expertise in the appropriate soft tissue massage techniques, including recall of the effect of this in previous patients with similar conditions.

Finally, the EBP process is never complete. With thousands of new papers published each day, and increasingly sophisticated electronic means of accessing them, the need to stay abreast of new trends and developments pertaining to your clinical question has never been greater. Search alerts, which run your search strategy on a regular basis and email to you any new citations, are an efficient means of doing this. Such alerts can be requested at the conclusion of a search on major electronic databases. It is also valuable to consider and discuss with colleagues the relevance to clinical practice of a robust, high quality body of research evidence, and whether the overall findings are consistent with any known clinical or other practice guidelines. Networking with colleagues often happens informally, but a regular staff/student journal club presentation or forum is a great way to encourage EBP.

SUMMARY

EBP combines patient perspectives, clinical experience and research evidence to maximise the quality and appropriateness of clinical practice by closing the evidence–practice gap. The obligation to engage with EBP flows from the ethical and professional obligations of physiotherapy practice. Putting EBP into practice involves converting patient problems into searchable questions and developing targeted search strategies for electronic databases. Once relevant research evidence is gathered, the level of bias in the study is examined by:

- establishing the strength and appropriateness of the research design undertaken
- evaluating the methodological quality of the study design using an appropriate critical appraisal tool.

The results of this evaluation should be viewed in the context of related research, the clinical environment and patient preferences. Regular searching and review of emerging research evidence is also critical.

Reflective questions

- Identify three clinical scenarios that provoked a need to enhance knowledge. How would you address these knowledge gaps?
- Identify a clinical question from your recent clinical practice. What sort of study design would be appropriate for addressing this question?
- Reflect on the last piece of research evidence that you found convincing. Why was it convincing? Consider areas of methodological quality, such as study design, sampling methods, reliability, and forms of bias.
- Identify an area of physiotherapy specialty that has recently changed. Consider the role of EBP in this change. For example, why are there now physiotherapists employed in emergency departments?
- Identify a case in which objective signs have resolved, but subjectively the patient has not recovered. As a physiotherapist, what role can you play in the resolution of these subjective issues? What form of research would best address these issues?

Further reading

Evidence-based practice

Melnyk B M, Fineout-Overholt E 2005 Evidence-based practice in nursing and healthcare. Lippincott Williams and Wilkins, Philadelphia

Qualitative research: introduction and methodologies

Gibson B E, Martin D K 2003 Qualitative research and evidence-based physiotherapy practice. Physiotherapy 89:350–358

Pope C, Mays N 1995 Reaching the parts other methods cannot reach: an introduction to qualitative methods in health and health services research. British Medical Journal 311:42–45

Qualitative research: evaluation

Giacomini M K, Cook D J 2000 Users' guides to the medical literature: XXIII. Qualitative research in health care A. Are the results of the study valid? Evidence-Based Medicine Working Group. Journal of the American Medical Association 284:357–362

Mays N, Pope C 1995 Rigour and qualitative research. British Medical Journal 311:109–112

Quantitative research methodologies

Portney L G, Watkins M P 2000 Foundations of clinical research: applications to practice, 2nd ed. Prentice Hall Health, Upper Saddle River, NJ

Quantitative research: evaluation

British Medical Journal (BMJ) 'How to read a paper' series; Journal of the American Medical Association (JAMA) 'Users' guides to the medical literature' series: access by searching these titles in Medline®

References

Agency for Healthcare Research and Quality 2002 Systems to rate the strength of scientific evidence, Evidence Report / Technology Assessment Number 47. Agency for Healthcare Research and Quality, Rockville, MD

Appleton J V 1995 Analysing qualitative interview data: addressing issues of validity and reliability. Journal of Advanced Nursing 22:993–997

Bechtel G A, Davidhizar R, Bunting S 2000 Triangulation research among culturally diverse populations. Journal of Allied Health 29:61–63

Bialocerkowski A E, Grimmer K A, Milanese S F et al 2004 Application of current research evidence to clinical physiotherapy practice. Journal of Allied Health 33:230–237

Centre for Evidence-Based Physiotherapy 2005 Physiotherapy evidence database (PEDro). Available: http://www.pedro.fhs.usyd.edu.au 26 Nov 2007

The Cochrane Collaboration 2007 The Cochrane library: evidence for healthcare decision-making. Available: http://www3.interscience.wiley.com/cgi-bin/mrwhome/106568753/HOME 4 Dec 2007

Cormack J C 2002 Evidence-based practice ... what is it and how do I do it? Journal of Orthopaedic and Sports Physical Therapy 32:484–487

Coyne I T 1997 Sampling in qualitative research: purposeful and theoretical sampling; merging or clear boundaries? Journal of Advanced Nursing 26:623–630

Cutcliffe J R, McKenna H P 1999 Establishing the credibility of qualitative research findings: the plot thickens. Journal of Advanced Nursing 30:374–380

Giacomini M K, Cook D J 2000 Users' guides to the medical literature: XXIII Qualitative research in health care B. What are the results and how do they help me care for my patients? Evidence-Based Medicine Working Group. Journal of the American Medical Association 284:478–482

Gray J A M 2001 Evidence-based healthcare: how to make health policy and management decisions. Churchill Livingstone, Edinburgh, pp 10–13

Greenhalgh T 1997 Papers that summarise other papers (systematic reviews and meta-analyses). British Medical Journal 315:672–675

Greenhalgh T, Taylor R 1997 Papers that go beyond numbers (qualitative research). British Medical Journal 315:740–743

Herbert R, Jamtvedt G, Mead J et al 2005 Practical evidence-based physiotherapy. Elsevier, Edinburgh, pp 2–8

Hills M 2000 Human science research in public health: the contribution and assessment of a qualitative approach. Canadian Journal of Public Health 91:I1–I7

Holman H R 1993 Qualitative inquiry in medical research. Journal of Clinical Epidemiology 46:29–36

The Joanna Briggs Institute 2007 The Joanna Briggs Institute: promoting and supporting best practice. Available: http://www.joannabriggs.edu.au/about/home.php 4 Dec 2007

Jones T, Evans D 2000 Conducting a systematic review. Australian Critical Care 13:66–71

Katrak P, Bialocerkowski A E, Massy-Westropp N et al 2004 A systematic review of the content of critical appraisal tools. BMC Medical Research Methodology 4:22

Law M, Stewart D, Pollack N et al 1998a Critical Review Form – qualitative studies. Available: http://www.srs-mcmaster.ca/Default.aspx?tabid=630 26 Nov 2007

Law M, Stewart D, Pollack N et al 1998b Critical Review Form – quantitative studies. Available: http://www.srs-mcmaster.ca/Default.aspx?tabid=630 26 Nov 2007

Lincoln Y S, Guba E G 1985 Naturalistic inquiry. Sage, Newbury Park, CA

Maher C G, Sherrington C, Herbert R D et al 2003 Reliability of the PEDro scale for rating quality of randomized controlled trials. Physical Therapy 83:713–721

Malterud K 1993 Shared understanding of the qualitative research process: guidelines for the medical researcher. Family Practice 10:201–206

McReynolds C J, Koch L C, Rumrill Jr P D 2001 Qualitative research strategies in rehabilitation. Work 16:57–65

National Library of Medicine 2007. Medical subject headings. Available: http://www.nlm.nih.gov/MeSH®/intro_preface2008.html#pref_rem 4 Dec 2007.

NHMRC 2000 How to use the evidence: assessment and application of scientific evidence. Biotext (Australian Govt), Canberra. Available: http://www.nhmrc.gov.au/publications/synopses/cp69syn.htm 4 Dec 2007

NHMRC 2005 NHMRC additional levels of evidence and grades for recommendations for developers of guidelines: Pilot program 2005–2007. Available: http://www.nhmrc.gov.au/consult/_files/levels_grades05.pdf 7 Dec 2007

Oxman A D 1994 Systematic reviews – checklists for review articles. British Medical Journal 309: 648–651

Patton M Q 2002 Qualitative research and evaluation methods, 3rd edn. Sage, Thousand Oaks, CA, pp 447–452

Pope C, Ziebland S, Mays N 2000 Qualitative research in health care: analysing qualitative data. British Medical Journal 320:114–116

Powell A E, Davies H T 2001 Reading and assessing qualitative research. Hospital Medicine 62: 360–363

Sackett D L, Straus S E, Richardson W S et al 2000 Evidence-based medicine: how to practice and teach EBM, 2nd ed. Churchill Livingstone, Edinburgh, p 1

Sandelowski M 1986 The problem of rigor in qualitative research. Advances in Nursing Science 8: 27–37

Sandelowski M 1993 Theory unmasked: the uses and guises of theory in qualitative research. Research in Nursing and Health 16:213–218

Schwandt T A 2001 Dictionary of qualitative inquiry, 2nd edn. Sage, Thousand Oaks, CA

Slevin E, Sines D 1999 Enhancing the truthfulness, consistency and transferability of a qualitative study: utilising a manifold of approaches. Nurse Researcher 7:79–97

Stone P W 2002 Popping the (PICO) question in research and evidence-based practice. Applied Nursing Research 15:197–198

Straus S E, McAlister F A 2000 Evidence-based medicine: a commentary on common criticisms. Canadian Medical Association Journal 163(7):837–841

Thomas R M 2003 Blending qualitative and quantitative research methods in theses and dissertations. Corwin Press, Thousand Oaks, CA

PHYSIOTHERAPY AND LITIGATION: IMPLICATIONS FOR PRACTICE AND EDUCATION

sixteen

Clare Delany and Debra Griffiths

Key content

- Negligence
- Standard of care
- Material risk
- Scope of advice
- Documentation
- Evidence-based practice
- Communication
- Expert witness

INTRODUCTION

As primary health care practitioners, physiotherapists are positioned within a layered regulatory framework. The first layer, self-regulation, comprises the ethical standards set by the profession itself (e.g. Australian Physiotherapy Association (APA) 2001, New Zealand Society of Physiotherapists Inc (NZSP) 2003), which are based on bio-ethical principles of health care (Beauchamp & Childress 2001). The second layer is professional registration legislation. The overriding purpose of physiotherapy registration Acts is to protect the public by defining minimum standards of professional practice and conduct and setting a process for hearing and determining complaints. The third layer comprises the civil and criminal laws of the legal system. *Health law* refers to laws controlling what health professionals do, what they should refrain from doing, and what health care institutions are expected to do (Forrester & Griffiths 2005). This chapter focuses on this third layer of regulation, providing an overview of health care litigation and highlighting the ways in which physiotherapists can become involved in the process.

Despite the increase in litigation in health care contexts reported, particularly during the 1990s, a growth in the number of court actions has not necessarily meant that there are more negligent health professionals. Rather, there is a range of reasons for litigation, including a greater awareness of patients as consumers and of their right to use the courts (Wodak 1998). Moreover, the greatest proportion of medicolegal litigation involves medical practitioners and hospitals (Skene 2004).

Although the incidence of reported involvement of physiotherapists in litigation is low, as primary practitioners physiotherapists should be aware of their potential for liability in the area of health care litigation. Physiotherapists have advanced and independent roles and responsibilities in the delivery of health care practice (Higgs et al 2001). Within their field of expertise, they are subject to the same standards of care as are applied by the law to all other primary health practitioners (Kerridge et al 2005, Skene 1998). As discussed in other chapters in this book, physiotherapists practise in a wide range of settings. Their patients range from the very old to the very young, from elite sports athletes to the profoundly disabled. This means physiotherapists need to be aware of standards of skill and care across a broad range of treatment areas. They should understand both substantive law and the litigation process for the purposes of risk management and professional accountability in all areas of physiotherapy practice. They should understand their obligations if they are called upon to give independent expert evidence or to give evidence of treatment in a litigious context.

Many aspects of practice have the potential to give rise to litigation involving physiotherapists. Actions in civil law include a breach of contract where the physio-therapist has a duty to comply with conditions agreed with the patient or the duties of confidentiality and privacy. There are possible actions in trespass, such as assault, battery and false imprisonment, when patient consent has not been adequately obtained. Moreover, criminal law may be invoked should the practitioner's communication or behaviour be less than clear with a patient. Actions relating to criminal assault, including sexual assault or rape, could arise from a complaint upheld against a physiotherapist for inappropriately touching a patient (Breen et al 1997).

THE PHYSIOTHERAPIST DEFENDANT: NEGLIGENCE

The most common area of law used by patients wishing to sue health professionals is the tort of negligence. The most obvious way that a physiotherapist might become involved in litigation is as a defendant (the person against whom a claim of negligence in treatment has been made). The physiotherapist sued may be the sole primary health care professional or a member of a treatment team or an employee in a proceeding where others are also defendants. There are two limbs to the duty of care – the duty to treat without negligence and the duty to inform the patient of the risks of treatment and to obtain informed consent to the course of treatment proposed.

The law of negligence in health care practice

The tort of negligence has two main purposes:

- to compensate a person who has suffered a wrong
- to state the standards expected by the community in respect to wrongs.

Claims that a physiotherapist has been negligent require determination, on the balance of probabilities of the following fundamental elements (MacFarlane 1995, p 99):

1. The patient was owed a duty of care by the health professional.
2. There was a breach of that duty in that the health professional's conduct fell below the required standard of care.
3. The conduct caused the damages suffered by the patient.
4. The loss or damage suffered was reasonably foreseeable.

Proving the first element is not generally contentious (Jones 1992) as, once a patient is being treated, health professionals owe a duty of care to that patient. Because the existence of that duty is non-contentious this chapter focuses upon the second element, the *standard* of care required by law. In this chapter we provide a clear and coherent summation of what the law requires. Whether a physiotherapist's breach of the duty of care *caused* a patient's injury (element 3) generally depends upon the facts of the particular case, for example, 'Was the cervical manipulation performed a material cause of paraplegia?' Such factual matters are determined on a case-by-case basis and are not discussed in this chapter. Additional information is contained in the list of suggested further reading.

The tort of negligence

The law of negligence as it relates to health professionals has undergone significant change in the past two decades. Before 1992 the law in Australia was governed, in part, by the 'Bolam principle'. According to this principle, named after the English case of *Bolam v Friern Hospital Management Committee* (1957, p 582), the standard of care required of a health professional was determined by prevailing professional practices. This meant that a health practitioner's actions were not negligent if the practitioner was acting 'in accordance with a practice accepted at the time as proper, by a responsible body of medical opinion' (*Sidaway v Governors of Bethlem Royal Hospital*, 1985, p 881).

The later English case of *Bolitho v City and Hackney Health Authority* (1988, p 243) moderated this principle to some extent:

> In cases of diagnosis and treatment, there are cases where, despite a body of professional opinion sanctioning the defendant's conduct, the defendant can properly be held liable for negligence… In my judgment that is because, in some cases, it cannot be demonstrated to the judge's satisfaction that the body of opinion relied upon is reasonable or responsible.

In Australia, these principles were replaced in 1992 by the decision of the High Court of *Rogers v Whitaker* (1992, p 479). In this landmark case and later cases, the High Court substantially followed North American judicial authority, rejecting the Bolam principle and emphasising the needs and entitlement of the patient to information. In so doing, the court established judicial authority, which has been emphasised in case law, the importance of individual autonomy as a foundational principle in the appreciation of basic human rights and dignity (*Rosenberg v Percival*, 2001 at para 145).

In *Rogers v Whitaker*, the plaintiff, Mrs. Whitaker, underwent surgery to improve the appearance and possibly the sight of one eye. She had been almost totally blind in that eye since the age of nine. Prior to the operation, Mrs Whitaker incessantly questioned her surgeon as to adverse consequences associated with the surgery. The surgeon did not warn her of the risk of developing sympathetic ophthalmia, which had an occurrence rate of 1:14,000, in her good eye following surgery. The surgery itself was performed without negligence. The surgery did not result in sight being restored to the injured eye and the condition of sympathetic ophthalmia led to blindness in the sighted eye. The breach of duty related to obtaining a valid consent. The High Court held the surgeon liable irrespective of whether the patient sought information, deciding that the surgeon owed a positive duty to provide the information as to the risks of treatment before proceeding, whether such information was actively sought by the patient or not.

In *Rogers v Whitaker* (p 489), the High Court distinguished between the provision of a diagnosis or treatment and the provision of information or advice. The court emphasised the important influence of responsible professional opinion in the provision of treatment. Crucially, the High Court stated that, in relation to information and advice, the question of breach and the identification of the relevant standard does not solely depend on professional opinion.

In New Zealand the obligation to obtain informed consent for all health professionals is located in the *Code of Health and Disability Services Consumer Rights Regulations 1996* (the Code). In particular, Right 6 (the right to be fully informed) and Right 7 (the right to make informed choice and give informed consent) establish clients' rights and, thereby, the professional's responsibilities when providing health care. The Code also incorporates relevant professional and ethical standards as guidelines for expected practice.

Recent trends in relation to the law of negligence

In 2002, in response to concerns about increasing costs associated with damages awards arising from personal injury caused through negligence, the Australian Government appointed a panel of eminent persons to review the Australian law of negligence (The Ipp Committee 2002). The Ipp Committee reviewed the decisions in medical negligence cases, including *Bolam* and *Bolitho*. It retreated from the High Court's position in *Rogers v Whitaker* and adopted the *Bolitho* approach (Bennett & Freckelton 2006, p 384):

> A medical practitioner is not negligent if the treatment provided was in accordance with an opinion widely held by a significant number of respected practitioners in the field, unless the court considers that the opinion was irrational.

This recommendation, like others of the Ipp Report, has been adopted and incorporated in statutes across the states and territories of Australia to varying degrees and, in general, does not benefit the plaintiff patient (who is claiming negligence on the part of the health practitioner) (Bennett & Freckelton 2006). In view of the inconsistency between the laws of the various states, practitioners are well advised to proceed on the *Rogers v Whitaker* basis so far as the provision of information as to risk of treatments is concerned.

In New Zealand the approach has been to move to a no-fault accident compensation scheme. The Accident Compensation Corporation (ACC) administers the scheme, which provides personal injury cover for all New Zealand citizens and residents. People do not have the right to sue for personal injury, other than exemplary damages. The pertinent legislation is the *Injury Prevention Rehabilitation and Compensation Act 2001* (NZ), but the scheme first came into effect in 1974. The ACC is responsible for a range of aspects relating to personal injury, including injury prevention services, determining whether claims for injury are covered by the scheme, the provision of medical and rehabilitation services, and paying compensation to injured individuals. The effect of this scheme in relation to litigation is to appreciably restrict the likelihood of clients suing in negligence.

Negligence: what is currently required of physiotherapists?

Here we use both statements of law and factual scenarios considered by the courts to outline the current state of the law of negligence as it applies to Australian physiotherapists. The founding principles of the law of negligence for physiotherapists are that physiotherapists owe a duty of care to their patient, and that this duty of care comprises two separate components: the duty as it relates to informed consent and the duty as it relates to treatment.

The most common complaints made by patients about their physiotherapist relate to (Guild Insurance Ltd & APA 2004, Roddis 2005):

- alleged injury exacerbation
- breaches of confidentiality or privacy
- provision of incorrect or poor advice
- allegations of mismanagement, including failure to refer on to another health practitioner for appropriate screening or testing (e.g. failure to refer a patient for magnetic resonance imaging (MRI) to screen for possible disc damage or other pathology).

The duty: informed consent

Physiotherapists owe a duty to patients when obtaining consent for treatment. In New Zealand the duty is enshrined in legislation, the *Health and Disability Commissioner Act 1994*, which incorporates the Code mentioned above. In Australia this duty requires that physiotherapists take reasonable care to tell patients about material risks inherent in the provision of treatment and to provide other relevant information.

What do the courts consider a 'material risk'?

In *Rogers v Whitaker* it was held that a risk was material if, in the individual circumstances, a reasonable person in the patient's position would attach significance to it in deciding whether or not to undergo the treatment. The High Court established a two-part disclosure test. The first part incorporates the reasonable patient test. It is an objective test that requires physiotherapists to consider whether an average or ordinary person, in the patient's position, would be likely to consider that a particular risk is important or significant. If a physiotherapist concludes that an average or ordinary person would consider the risk important, then it is a material risk and must be disclosed. The second part focuses on the particular patient. This is a subjective test and physiotherapists are required to disclose a risk if they are or should be aware that a particular patient would be likely to consider the risk significant. Referring to this subjective duty, the court stated that a risk would be material if 'the … particular patient … would have been likely seriously to consider and weigh up the risk before reaching a decision on whether to proceed with the treatment' (*Rogers v Whitaker*, p 488).

In the case of Mrs Whitaker, a person already blind in one eye, it was considered that she would have been likely to consider and weigh up the possible risks of blindness in the other eye. It was accepted that Mrs Whitaker might not have asked a precise or specific question relating to sympathetic ophthalmia. Nonetheless, she made her concerns clear that nothing should happen to her good eye.

The Australian High Court has been somewhat indirect regarding what constitutes a material risk in the context of 'objective duty'. However, in general guidance, a *small* risk of incurring greater harm should be communicated, whereas a larger risk of incurring *trivial* harm might not need to be mentioned (*Rosenberg v Percival*, p 77). In all cases, it is vital to consider the individual circumstances of the patient.

Case study 1

A 40-year-old self-employed builder presented to a physiotherapist with acute right-sided low back pain extending into his right buttock (Niere & Short 2007). On the day of presentation the builder had severe pain and was unable to work. The builder had two treatments with the physiotherapist and, within that time, the pain worsened. The physiotherapist suggested to the patient that he attend his local doctor. The patient returned to the physiotherapist following a week's bed rest with less pain but increased neurological deficits. The patient ultimately attended an emergency hospital department of a public hospital and, after an MRI investigation, underwent surgery for an L4–5 disc prolapse. The patient was left with residual neurological injuries, including a foot drop.

If this patient decided to sue the physiotherapist for failure to warn of the material risks and benefits associated with physiotherapy management of his back pain, the court would consider whether this patient (being a self-employed builder anxious to get back to work) had been given sufficient information to decide between, on the one hand, delaying more detailed investigations such as MRI for possible disc injury and, on the other hand, continuing a 'wait and see' conservative treatment approach. It is likely that the possible consequences of delaying investigation in circumstances where a more serious injury could result from delay is information that this patient would consider material.

The scope of advice and information a physiotherapist is expected to give covers (Delany 1996, 2002):

- the nature and likely prognosis of the condition
- the physiotherapy and other care options
- options for additional diagnosis and confirmation
- warnings as to possible adverse outcomes of treatment or no treatment
- estimation as to degree of uncertainty or outcome associated with treatments
- time and cost involved and any aspect of the procedure that is especially costly or protracted.

The duty: treatment

Physiotherapists owe a duty of care to patients to treat them in a manner that could reasonably be expected of a person professing to be an ordinary, skilled physiotherapist. In other words, physiotherapists are measured against the skills of the profession, and may be liable if they fall short of that level.

If the patient discussed in Case study 1 decided to sue the physiotherapist on the basis that treatment was negligent because there was an omission to appropriately test for nerve involvement (neurological testing) and a failure to diagnose, or refer, or communicate with another health colleague, then the court would consider the standard of care in relation to those aspects of the treatment. If a physiotherapist acting in a triage capacity (see Case study 1, Ch 24) made an incorrect diagnosis or failed to refer to another more appropriate colleague, and the patient suffered harm as a result, this would also be a potential breach of duty of care. In assessing any alleged breach, judging the performance of the physiotherapist, and setting the standard of the duty of care, the law would rely upon:

- the standards of care set by the profession (physiotherapy guidelines, position statements, and expert opinion about the particular area of clinical practice)
- the best available evidence supporting physiotherapy assessment, diagnosis and management of lumbar spine pain
- the documentation made by the physiotherapist of the assessment, tests used and test results and treatment, and of the advice, warnings and information given.

Scenario 1

In the case of Burrows v Queensland (2001) a patient alleged that a physiotherapist caused the rupture of a patient's flexor digitorum profundus (FDP) tendon during the physical assessment component of the treatment. In this case, the court relied on three main sources of information:

- The accounts of the treatment given by the plaintiff (the patient) and the defendant (the physiotherapist). These accounts differed as to the sequence and nature of the treatment.
- The physiotherapist's notes recording details of the assessment, findings and treatment.
- Expert evidence from doctors regarding the nature and possible causes of injury to the FDP tendon.

The court preferred the evidence of the physiotherapist, based on her 'detailed contemporaneous records' and her verbal account of the treatment. The court was also influenced by the evidence submitted by the experts that a rupture was not likely to have been caused by the physiotherapy treatment described in the notes or verbally. The physiotherapist was therefore found to be not negligent.

IMPLICATIONS FOR PRACTICE AND EDUCATION

Civil health care law, the third layer of regulation, ideally functions as a facilitator for good practice, rather than as a threat that results in defensive practice. In the many areas of physiotherapy practice, the standards of care established by the law of negligence provide positive markers for good practice and risk management. The overriding message to be taken from negligence law is that physiotherapists:

- owe patients a duty of care
- have a duty to inform patients of all material risks inherent in the treatment. If a patient asks for information, it must not be withheld
- are more likely to avoid liability if they provide treatment to patients in a manner and to a level consistent with the skills of a competent physiotherapist. That is, they must not fall short of the standard generally expected from the profession.

These standards are established and reviewed by the physiotherapy authorities (Australian Physiotherapy Council 2007) and include codes of conduct (APA 2001, NZSP 2003), position statements, clinical guidelines and standards of practice (NZSP 2006). The implications of the law of negligence for both education and ultimately clinical practice may be divided into three domains: documentation, communication and evidence-based clinical practice.

Documentation

In all clinical areas of practice where the role of the physiotherapist is to assess, diagnose, treat and provide advice, the adequacy of the interaction will be judged by what the physiotherapist documents. The patient's record becomes highly significant should the physiotherapist become involved as a defendant in litigation. The patient's record may form part of the court exhibits and therefore be examined and scrutinised by each party. Courts prefer oral evidence that is reinforced by contemporaneous annotations to evidence that relies on an unaided recollection of events. If the oral evidence of the parties conflicts, a clear record made by the physiotherapist, which includes the clinical findings, treatment provided and advice given, carries substantial authority in court. Conversely, poorly written patient notes can be used to reduce the credibility and raise questions as to the professional ability of the physiotherapist (Breen et al 1997). The box below lists the principles to consider when recording information.

Essential requirements regarding client information documented in physiotherapy records

1. Entries are made contemporaneously and are legible
2. Entries must be signed and dated
3. The style and content of notes should be meaningful and consistent
4. Abbreviations should be both accurate and consistent
5. Diagnostic test results must be included
6. Movement of records is tracked
7. No personal or judgemental comments are made or recorded
8. Informed consent is obtained and recorded in a consistent manner (and should include benefits, risks and alternatives to treatment)
9. Information given about treatment effects and potential exacerbation after treatment should be recorded
10. Response to treatment must be recorded

These principles should be considered within physiotherapy education settings, and introduced in learning sessions parallel with practice skills, such as assessment, testing and basic treatments. Ideally, students should have the opportunity to develop competent and concise writing skills, including how to record patient information and how to write summaries of treatments, referral letters and expert reports, from the first year of their undergraduate physiotherapy education.

Evidence-based practice

The treatment techniques and advice given by physiotherapists must reflect the best available research evidence. In recent Australian decisions, courts have demonstrated a reliance on evidence and levels of evidence underpinning practices via the provision of expert evidence and by reference to clinical guidelines (Tibballs 2007). This means that physiotherapists in practice must maintain active participation in continuing professional development and keep abreast of current best practice.

Experience alone or reliance on 'what seems to work' is not enough according to standards of care set by the law. Recent graduates may be more alert to current research than more experienced clinicians, but the onus to be up-to-date and aware of current research is a continuing obligation. Physiotherapy students need to acquire knowledge and skills in understanding, interpreting, evaluating and integrating research evidence into clinical practice during their education and as a component of their clinical work. Educators have a responsibility to ensure that evidence-informed practice underlies the competencies of graduating physiotherapists.

Communication

Explanations to patients about the nature of any treatment intervention, including the risks and benefits of and alternatives to such treatment, should be a standard and integrated component of physiotherapy treatment. Research into physiotherapy practice suggests that physiotherapists tend to communicate information to a patient if they think it will enhance the outcome of the treatment (Delany 2007). Using the law as a guide, physiotherapists need to communicate information (benefits, likely effects of treatment including exacerbations and risks, alternatives, cost, expectations of involvement, evidence supporting treatment) as a standard part of their therapist–patient interactions, regardless of whether the information is needed to enhance the therapeutic outcome.

In practice, this means that physiotherapists need to plan ahead and prepare different types of documentation and written information. Such documentation includes forms to record physiotherapy treatment notes, assessment results and follow-up protocols. For patients, information should include booklets covering common effects of treatment, how to monitor treatment effects, and who to contact if concerned. Physiotherapy educators should encourage students to both research and practise effective communication strategies that enhance and facilitate a collaborative and interactive dialogue. Students should be provided with opportunities to develop skills in imparting both written and oral information to patients that integrates evidence-based knowledge (see e.g. Stewart et al 2007). Physiotherapy students should be given opportunities to learn the skills of promoting and enhancing collaboration within the therapist–patient relationship and with colleagues. Where a patient exhibits a desire to rely on the therapist's expertise only regarding information about the treatment, the therapist has a positive duty of care to engage the patient and provide material information.

The ability to communicate effectively is also important in the provision of written reports or when providing an expert opinion. This is the second main area in which physiotherapists may become involved in the litigation process.

THE PHYSIOTHERAPIST AS THE EXPERT WITNESS

Generally, lay witnesses can give evidence of what has been derived from their senses only: what they saw, heard, touched, smelt or tasted. Expert witnesses are set apart from lay witnesses in that they provide evidence of opinion. They are called when there is a need for the assistance of a person who possesses special knowledge, skill or experience in a specific area (Ross 2005).

Physiotherapists may be called as expert witnesses as a result of varying circumstances. As primary practitioners, physiotherapists are often required to prepare reports at the request of a third party. The request for opinion can be made prior to or during the course of court proceedings. It may be in the course of a patient's claim for worker's compensation or other benefits. It may require a review of the treatment provided by a fellow practitioner, including circumstances where a claim against the practitioner has not yet commenced. Importantly, the expert may be called upon to give evidence to the court on the standard of care expected in his or her particular area of clinical expertise and to provide an opinion as to whether the treatment of the patient departed from an acceptable standard. The physiotherapist may be called upon to give evidence in his or her own defence, if sued. In such a case, unlike the other examples given, the physiotherapist is not an expert witness but a party to the action, required to recount facts relating to the case.

When acting for a third party by preparing a written report or expressing an expert opinion, it is important that the physiotherapist is aware that the primary responsibility of the independent physiotherapy witness is to the court or tribunal, regardless of who is paying for the report (Black 1999). That duty applies when the physiotherapist is called upon to report on the facts of his or her treatment or actions, or act as an independent practitioner providing expert opinion about a set of facts or findings. Moreover, the expert witness is not an advocate for any party and should maintain impartiality throughout.

Expert evidence

Expert evidence is not admissible as the ultimate determinant of the matter before the court. The intention is that the subject matter of the opinion provided by the expert witness forms part of a body of knowledge or experience that is outside the range of knowledge of the court and is sufficiently recognised to be accepted as reliable (Freckelton & Selby 1998). A convenient and authoritative summary in relation to the criteria for admissibility of expert evidence is that found in the reasons for judgment of Heydon JA (*Makita (Aust) Pty Ltd v Sprowles* 2001) and presented in Table 16.1.

When physiotherapists provide a report based on observation of fact, that is, based on what they observed or noted during an assessment and/or treatment of a patient, they should be careful to separate this content from their expert opinion about a patient, or about a colleague's assessment or treatment. Physiotherapists need to be clear about their role and the instructions they receive from a third party requesting their expert opinion, as these instructions should form the basis of and be disclosed by the expert in the report. In summary, physiotherapists need to be aware of the boundaries set around the writing and giving of expert evidence to ensure that:

• their evidence is in admissible form and in accordance with expert witness codes of conduct/guidelines
• their overriding duty to the court is discharged and their independence as an expert is not compromised.

Implications for practice and education

In the case discussed earlier, where the patient required disc surgery following physiotherapy treatment, an independent physiotherapist might have been asked to provide an expert opinion about the nature and adequacy of the assessment performed by the treating physiotherapist. The box on page 215 sets out an example of the overall structure of an expert report for this case.

Table 16.1 Considerations for writing and giving expert evidence. From *Makita (Aust) Pty Ltd v Sprowles* (2001)	
Expert evidence: boundaries for admissibility	**Expert evidence: content**
1. Established field	It must be agreed or demonstrated that there is a field of 'specialised knowledge' or there must be an identified aspect of that field in which the witness demonstrates that, by reason of specified training, study or experience, he or she has become an expert
2. Knowledge base for opinion	The opinion proffered must be 'wholly or substantially based on the witness's expert knowledge', or ■ so far as the opinion is based on facts 'observed' by the expert, they must be identified and admissibly proved by the expert, or ■ so far as the opinion is based on 'assumed' or 'accepted' facts, they must be identified and proved in some other way
3. Factual foundation of opinion	It must be established that the facts on which the opinion is based form a proper foundation for it
4. Rationale for opinion from factual basis	The opinion of an expert requires demonstration or examination of the scientific or other intellectual basis of the conclusions reached: an explanation of how the field of 'specialised knowledge' in which the witness is expert by reason of 'training, study or experience', and on which the opinion is 'wholly or substantially based', applies to the facts assumed or observed so as to produce the opinion propounded

Physiotherapists should be aware of both the procedural requirements and the duties and functions of an expert report. This knowledge provides the necessary structure for developing reports and opinions, and means that such material will be useful within the litigation process. Writing expert reports should be included as a core component of physiotherapy education.

SUMMARY

This chapter has provided an overview of the law of negligence, in particular, the two main ways that physiotherapists might find themselves involved in the litigation process: when a standard of care has been breached and as an expert witness. In countries such as Australia the practice of physiotherapy is considered specialised and should be practised by those who are cognisant of the standards required by law. Those standards are acquired during educational programs and are formulated by relevant professional organisations. When considering actions of negligence, the court also examines and determines the requisite standards of care. The expert witness role of providing evidence of opinion highlights the importance of the profession's engaging with and emphasising current expected standards. To avoid breaching the standard of care and to maintain and advance clinical practice values, physiotherapists must continually maintain a current knowledge base and deliver care in accordance with evidence-informed practice.

Example of the structure of a report formulated from the case of the patient with a disc lesion (Case study 1)

1   I have been asked by X to provide an expert opinion about the nature and adequacy of the assessment and treatment of Y on (date). I have specifically been asked to provide my opinion about (A, B, C).

2.   In discharging the task required, I have been provided with a copy of the expert witness guidelines applicable in the Supreme Court of Victoria. I have adhered to those guidelines and borne in mind my overriding duty to the Court in reporting and expressing my opinions.

3.   I enclose copies of the correspondence between me and X since the initial request. This correspondence has been aimed at clarifying the focus of my opinion.

4.   I have carefully read the physiotherapist's written notes recording and describing the procedure that was followed within the three treatment sessions. I have also been provided with a report detailing the patient's subsequent orthopaedic surgery. Where there is any conflict between the written notes and the factual account in my instructions, I have identified the areas of conflict. I have expressed my opinion separately, assuming:
     (a) the instructions to be correct; alternatively,
     (b) the notes to be correct.

5.   In coming to my opinion, I have relied upon:
     • written instructions as to what is said to have occurred, assuming in all cases what is said in those instructions to have occurred is true and accurate;
     • copies of the treatment notes of the treating physiotherapist;
     • my clinical experience of Y years practising in this clinical area;
     • knowledge of the latest research evidence about the adequacy of neurological testing.

6.   My expert opinion as to the adequacy of the physiotherapist's assessment and treatment based on my understanding and interpretation of what is recorded in his notes, is that the assessment was/was not a comprehensive neurological examination and that it does/does not accord with the best practices of neurological examination given the patient's presenting symptoms.

7.   The opinions provided in this report are my own. They are based on the assumption so far as the notes are concerned that what is written in the physiotherapist's notes (copies of which have been provided to me) are in fact a record of the actual assessment and treatment.

Reflective questions

• If you were asked to be an expert witness what challenges would you face?
• What do you see as your role in maintaining standards of care?

Further reading

Bagaric M, Arenson K 2007 Criminal law in Australia: cases and materials, 2nd edn. Oxford University Press, Melbourne

Balkin R, Davis J 1996 Law of torts. Butterworths, Sydney

Chambers K, Krikorian R 2003 Review of the final IPP report and its impact on health claims. Australian Health Law Bulletin 11(4):37

Ross D 2007 Ross on crime, 3rd edn. Lawbook Company, Pyrmont, NSW

References

APA 2001 Code of Conduct. Available: https://apa.advsol.com.au/scriptcontent/aboutphysio 12 Oct 2005

Australian Physiotherapy Council 2007 Australian standards for physiotherapy. Available: http://www.physiocouncil.com.au/australian_standards_for_physiotherapy/ 12 Oct 2007

Beauchamp T, Childress J 2001 Principles of biomedical ethics, 5th edn. Oxford University Press, Oxford

Bennett B, Freckelton I 2006 Life after the Ipp reforms: medical negligence law. In: Freckelton I, Peterson K (eds), Disputes and dilemmas in health law. The Federation Press, Sydney, pp 381–405

Black M E 1999 Guidelines for expert witnesses in proceedings in the Federal Court of Australia. Litigation Lawyer Newsletter 6(Dec 1988–Jan 1999)

Breen K, Plueckhahn V, Cordner S 1997 Ethics, law and medical practice. Allen & Unwin, St Leonards, NSW

Delany C 1996 Should I warn the patient first? Australian Journal of Physiotherapy 42(3):249–255

Delany C 2002 Cervical manipulation: how might informed consent be obtained before treatment? Journal of Law and Medicine 10(2):174–186

Delany C 2007 In private practice, informed consent is interpreted as providing explanations rather than offering choices: a qualitative study. Australian Journal of Physiotherapy 53:171–177

Forrester K, Griffiths D 2005 Essentials of law for health professionals, Elsevier, Sydney

Freckelton I, Selby H 1998 Expert evidence. Lawbook Company, Sydney

Guild Insurance Ltd & APA 2004 Guildwatch risk management for physiotherapists, Guild Insurance and Australian Physiotherapy Association, Victoria

Higgs J, Refshauge K, Ellis E 2001 Portrait of the physiotherapy profession. Journal of Interprofessional Care 15(1):79–89

Jones M 1992 Medical negligence. In: McHale L, Tingle J (eds), Law and nursing. Butterworth-Heinemann, Oxford

Kerridge I, Lowe M, McPhee J 2005 Ethics and law for the health professions, 2nd edn. Federation Press, Annandale, NSW

MacFarlane P 1995 Health law: commentary and materials. Federation Press, Sydney

NZSP 2003 Guidelines for the NZSP code of ethical principles. Wellington, New Zealand

NZSP 2006 Standards of physiotherapy practice, 3rd edn. Wellington, New Zealand

Niere K, Short D 2007 Managing your risk. Motion, Australian Physiotherapy Association. June:21

Roddis D 2005 Risk management: managing risk in private practice. Paper presented at the International Private Practitioners Association Conference, Melbourne, Vic, Sep

Ross D 2005 Advocacy. Cambridge University Press, Cambridge

Skene L 1998 Law and medical practice. Sydney, Butterworths

Skene L 2004 Law and medical practice, 2nd edn. LexisNexis Butterworths, Sydney

Stewart J, Zedliker K E, Witteborn S 2007 Together: communicating interpersonally: a social construction approach, 6th edn. Oxford University Press, Melbourne

The Ipp Committee 2002 Review of the law of negligence, Second report. Canberra. Available: http://revofneg.treasury.gov.au/content/review2.asp 12 Oct 2007

Tibballs J 2007 Clinical practice guidelines in the witness box: can they replace the medical expert? Journal of Law and Medicine 14(4):479–501

Wodak T 1998 Damage control. The Law Institute Journal 72(4):12

Cases and legislation

Code of Health and Disability Services Consumer Rights Regulations 1996 (NZ)

Bolam v Friern Hospital Management Committee (1957) 1 Weekly Law Reports 582

Bolitho v City and Hackney Health Authority (1998) (UK) Law Reports, Appeal Cases 232

Burrows v Queensland (2001) Queensland Supreme Court 344

Health and Disability Commissioner Act 1994 (NZ)

Injury Prevention Rehabilitation and Compensation Act 2001 (NZ)

Makita (Aust) Pty Ltd v Sprowles (2001) 52 New South Wales Law Reports 705

Rogers v Whitaker (1992) 175 Commonwealth Law Reports 479

Rosenberg v Percival (2001) 205 Commonwealth Law Reports 434

Sidaway v Governors of Bethlem Royal Hospital (1985) AC 871

RESEARCHING PHYSIOTHERAPY

Megan Smith, Gwendolen Jull and Karen Grimmer-Somers

seventeen

Key content
- Identifying research questions relevant to physiotherapy
- Research designs and methods applicable to physiotherapy research questions
- Strategies for ensuring quality physiotherapy research

INTRODUCTION

Researching physiotherapy is an integral aspect of our professional practice. Any consultation between practitioners and their clients can give rise to questions that cannot be answered by reference to the existing body of physiotherapy knowledge. Current physiotherapy practice requires physiotherapists to be educated consumers of research as well as capable physiotherapy researchers. Researching physiotherapy need not be restricted to the activities of academics and research students; rather, researching physiotherapy is integral to the practice of all physiotherapists.

Since its inception the physiotherapy profession has sought recognition for its scientific enquiry. In the profession's early days, basing its practices on science stood the profession apart from the less salubrious massage practices with which it was sometimes confused. This stand ensured that physiotherapy is now recognised as one of the mainstream healing medical sciences. There has been a progressive increase in the amount and quality of physiotherapy research, particularly since education programs have been university-based. Clinical practice requires artistry by practitioners (Paterson & Higgs 2001), yet how research informs the art of delivering health care continues to confound researchers and clinicians when defining good clinical practice. The interaction between therapist and patient in the delivery of an intervention, even with strong research evidence for the intervention, goes a long way to determining its effectiveness for that patient. That acknowledged, however, it is no longer acceptable to practise without reference to relevant research.

In this chapter we have chosen not to provide a 'how to conduct research' guide – there are a number of suitable texts devoted to this topic, both specific to physiotherapy and more generally to health care (see 'Further reading'). Instead we focus on the types of research questions that arise in physiotherapy clinical practice and the strategies used to answer these questions through quality research.

THE SCOPE OF RESEARCHING PHYSIOTHERAPY

The scope of physiotherapy research encompasses a broad range of research activities and methodologies. Recently, in line with an increased emphasis on practice informed by evidence, there has been an increased focus on randomised controlled trials investigating and comparing physiotherapy interventions. However, many of the questions that emerge in our clinical practice are not limited to comparing one intervention with another; research in physiotherapy is inclusive of a much broader range of activity.

Physiotherapy research is now led by physiotherapists themselves, reflecting the maturity and educational capacity within the profession. Nevertheless, physiotherapy practice will always be informed by research undertaken in external fields such as physiology, psychology, sociology and medicine. As well, most of the current successful physiotherapy research teams have a multidisciplinary composition, using the expertise and perspectives of other disciplines to enhance the quality of physiotherapy research.

Throughout the history of physiotherapy research, there have been a number of drivers for the content and type of research that is conducted. These drivers have included the particular health care needs and practices of the time, the prevailing scientific and social conceptions of health care, the available technology and the prevailing political and social influences. Key historical events such as the polio epidemic and World Wars I and II have also influenced research and practice. An illustration of these drivers is found in the use and evaluation of breathing exercises in postoperative patients. Initially, breathing and chest exercises were incorporated in the management of soldiers with chest and lung wounds, and following surgery (MacMahon 1915). As the medical profession undertook increasingly complex types of surgery (such as open-heart surgery and thoracoplasty) from the 1940s to the 1970s, the use of breathing exercises in the postoperative patient increased (Innocenti 1995). These more complex procedures were initially associated with long periods of bed rest and there was increased risk of postoperative respiratory complications. During the 1980s researchers began to investigate optimal strategies for the management of postoperative patients, such as mobilisation (Dull & Dull 1983). In the 1990s, research emerged questioning the role of breathing exercises in these traditional populations (e.g. Stiller et al 1994), with decreasing support for their use. This reappraisal of the need for breathing exercises, together with an increasing emphasis on early mobilisation, coincided with progressive medical developments that resulted in improved pain relief, minimally invasive surgery and re-evaluation of the need for prolonged periods of postoperative bed rest. Concurrently the profession was experiencing political pressures for accountability, with drives for physiotherapy to have a scientific base and to function within a paradigm of evidence-based practice (Ritchie 1999).

As reflected in history, a number of features of current health care practice are driving future physiotherapy research directions. These include, for example, the trend towards models of health care in which consumers are actively involved in their health, and the increasing emphasis on illness prevention and health promotion in addition to the remediation of illness. Topical factors to consider include the changing demographics of populations using physiotherapy services, which reflect the longer lifespan enjoyed by an ageing population.

Recent decades have witnessed growth in interprofessional collaborations in clinical practice and research. Research technology has also advanced to an extraordinary extent, facilitating more sophisticated experimental research. In a review of the history of research in physiotherapy, Crosbie (2000) highlighted the progressions in research methodology that have occurred. In much of the initial physiotherapy research the methods used relied on animal studies and studies with physiotherapy students. Although convenient, these studies often lacked relevance to the population to whom the research was intended to apply. Likewise, early studies of treatment efficacy lacked rigorous research design features, such as inclusion of control groups, which constrained their ability to validly inform physiotherapy practice. There has been increasing emphasis on enhancing physiotherapists' capabilities in research to improve the quality of the research conducted and to promote the identification and interpretation of quality research (Maher et al 2004).

RESEARCH DESIGN

Research designs relevant to physiotherapy come in primary and secondary forms.

Primary research

Primary research usually reports the findings of a single study, in which data have been collected from subjects (human or animal). It is conducted to answer a specific clinical question. The research question determines the research design or methodology most suited to answering it. Examples of research questions leading to research designs are provided in Table 17.1, to highlight the range of opportunities for conducting research.

Ethics approval is required before the research can proceed. Primary research takes a number of recognised forms and can be conceptualised along a continuum. At one end are quality improvement activities. These potentially incur the greatest bias in interpretation and generalisation, because of limitations regarding the patients recruited to provide the data. However, this type of research can assist in clarifying research questions, and can provide important preliminary findings on which subsequent research can be built. At the other end of the continuum is potentially the least biased form of research, the experimental study, in which biases are controlled through methodological rigour by means such as random sampling and blinding of study participants. In between are a range of other design types (methodologies), encompassing basic science research, health measurement research (reliability and validity studies), health policy research, cost–analysis research and epidemiological research (prevalence and cause and effect studies). Qualitative research is increasingly being used in health research. Qualitative methods focus on exploring the human and social world and its context using qualitative (non-numerical) judgements (Herbert & Higgs 2004). Each research design should inform other research conducted on the same topic, as it is rare for one piece of primary research to provide all the answers to a clinical question.

One of the complexities of determining evidence to support all aspects of physiotherapy service delivery is that physiotherapists undertake a range of tasks in their day-to-day work, and each task is potentially informed by a different type of research evidence (Grimmer & Kumar 2005). For instance, to engage each patient in a manner appropriate to the individual, the environment and the health problem (perhaps this could be called the art of therapy), physiotherapists adopt specific and holistic patient–therapist approaches that value patients' cultures, backgrounds, education, anxieties, expectations, symptom type and levels, health status and condition. Choice of appropriate engagement strategies for different patients should be informed by qualitative research (Jones et al 2006a). Physiotherapists then assess

Table 17.1 Sample physiotherapy primary research questions and research designs

Primary research questions	Possible research designs
How good am I at treating low back pain? How many patients with low back pain have been discharged from treatment in this clinic, having consumed an affordable and reasonable number of treatments and achieved a good outcome?	■ A quality improvement study, such as a retrospective record audit, in which criteria for affordable and reasonable number of treatments and good outcome are established first, and then each patient's notes measured against these criteria to establish how good I am at treating low back pain
What is the most appropriate outcome measure for acute low back pain?	■ Qualitative research in which people with experience of acute low back pain reflect on how the condition affected them, and how they dealt with it ■ A comparative outcome measures study, in which people with acute low back pain complete several standard outcome instruments and the answers subjected to statistical modelling, such as factor analysis, to identify the most important measurement characteristics. Standard outcome instruments for acute low back pain could be e.g. the Glasgow Pain Questionnaire (Thomas et al 1996), the Patient-Specific Scale (Stratford et al 1995), the Roland-Morris Questionnaire (Roland & Morris 1983) or the Oswestry Disability Index (Fairbank & Pynsent 2000)
Are long hours of computer use associated with acute low back pain?	■ Epidemiological (or population-based) research that observes usual behaviours and practices, assesses cause and effect (exposure and disease), and determines whether individuals who spend long hours in front of the computer are also those reporting acute low back pain
Does an exercise program for individuals with acute low back pain produce a better outcome than drug therapy?	■ A prospective intervention (experimental) study in which better outcome is first defined, then similar groups of patients provided with either the exercise program or the drug therapy, and their outcomes compared. This type of research is known as a randomised controlled trial
Is physiotherapy treatment of acute low back pain cost effective in terms of days lost from work?	■ A cost–benefit study or health policy research, in which the benefits of treatment are considered in terms of the direct and indirect costs of achieving them

patients' symptoms and signs, and screen patients for risks for poor prognosis, in order to determine appropriate treatment strategies. These assessment and screening activities are supported by epidemiological research, which identifies key assessment criteria and important risk factors. Clinical reasoning research then provides a structured framework within which therapists can put all aspects of the assessment together to determine the most appropriate treatment approach (Jones et al 2006b). To identify the most appropriate measures of outcome to demonstrate whether therapy has been effective for a patient with a particular condition, physiotherapists need to be guided by research into the psychometric properties and clinical utility of outcome instruments (for instance those reported in the developmental literature for instruments used to evaluate therapy outcomes for acute low back pain, as listed in Table 17.1). Effective treatment of individual patients then requires therapeutic decisions based on experimental study findings and patient choice.

For physiotherapists to continue to be well informed across all areas of practice, they would need to read hundreds of primary research reports every month to keep up with the volume of scientific literature being published. As this is not feasible for most therapists, a more efficient way of keeping on top of current knowledge is necessary.

Secondary research

Secondary research has emerged over the past 15 years in response to the volume of published research. Secondary evidence synthesises primary research into summary recommendations (Sackett et al 2000). Its data come from published research reports rather than directly from subjects. Secondary research is the only form of research for which ethical approval is not required. There are different types of secondary evidence that relate to the study type being synthesised and the questions being asked. Meta-analyses and systematic reviews summarise the available information for a clinical question. A *meta-analysis* uses sophisticated statistical techniques that pool and re-analyse raw data from randomised controlled trials with homogeneous subjects, the same intervention or exposures, and the same measures of outcome. The meta-analysis investigates whether, by combining the primary experimental study datasets, the findings of the pooled data remain as strong as the findings of the individual studies. In physiotherapy it is rare to find meta-analyses because of the difficulty of identifying primary studies whose data can be combined. For instance, an intervention such as 'exercise for low back pain' may lead you to believe that it is the one general approach to treatment that lends itself to meta-analysis of datasets. However, not only can 'low back pain' be defined differently in terms of chronicity, injury mechanism, location, duration and severity, and 'pain' be measured by an array of scales and instruments (questionnaires), but 'exercise' can be delivered in an astounding variety of ways including the exercise itself, whether it is performed submaximally or maximally, how frequently it is performed and for how long each session (duration), progression of the exercise program over time, and patients' compliance with the program. Thus, because of the variability in the methods of primary research that purports to examine the same clinical question, it is more common to find secondary evidence in the form of systematic reviews.

Systematic reviews are mostly descriptive or narrative as they synthesise the findings of primary studies with different study designs and different study approaches that address the same clinical question. The primary studies are usually different in terms of subjects, interventions/exposures and outcome measures and, thus, narrative comparisons are the only feasible approach to synthesis. Systematic reviews can report on one study design only (e.g. experimental studies, observational studies), or a review can include a range of study designs. The type of primary study design included in the systematic review can potentially alter the findings. Of note are two reviews of conservative treatment of carpal tunnel syndrome that reported different findings because of different component study designs. Goodyear-Smith and Arrol (2004) included only randomised controlled trials, and found limited evidence for the use of laser–acupuncture, splinting, yoga, nerve gliding and therapeutic ultrasound, whereas Muller et al (2004) included all study designs, and found convincing evidence for these same interventions. Clinicians reading these systematic reviews for guidance regarding the effectiveness of, say, splinting in the management of carpal tunnel syndrome would thus have to make a value judgement based on their knowledge of the hierarchy and quality of the included primary studies.

Clinical guidelines provide a different type of secondary evidence, as they compile the available evidence for the management of patients with a specific condition. In times past, clinical guidelines were often established by one or more 'experts', using their knowledge base as reference. Hence many early guidelines were open to criticism because of perceived bias. Now, clinical guidelines are mostly comprehensive documents developed by teams of researchers and clinicians, who use a structured technical approach to pull together the findings of relevant published research into transparent and defensible recommendations. Clinical guidelines are generally developed with the purposes of reducing variability in practice and improving quality and safety of care (Brooks et al 2005). Well-constructed clinical guidelines can also provide an overview of the strengths and weaknesses of the current body of evidence, and hence inform primary research targeted to fill research gaps. For many conditions treated by physiotherapists there are still research gaps, where there has either been no research at all for a particular clinical question, or limited or poor quality research. In these instances, clinical guidelines in physiotherapy often use 'clinical practice points', which are 'recommended best practice based on clinical experience and expert opinion' (National Stroke Foundation 2007, p 6). These provide guidance for clinicians in the absence of better quality research evidence. An example of a clinical practice point is in the Clinical Guidelines for Acute Stroke Management (2007) endorsed by the Australian National Health and Medical Research Council. Guideline 5.1 for dysphagia states, 'Patients who fail the swallowing screening should be referred to a speech pathologist for a comprehensive assessment' (p 35).

RESEARCH FROM LABORATORY TO CLINICAL PRACTICE

In this section we use the clinical scenario of a client presenting with neck pain to further illustrate primary research and the interplay between clinical practice and research. In particular, we aim to show how a clinical question facilitates the research process and how findings from the laboratory can inform the next stages of clinical research. Examples are given of methods of applied quantitative experimental and qualitative clinical research.

Scenario 1

A patient presents to the physiotherapist with a two-year history of neck pain and requests the prescription of an exercise program to improve her neck pain and function.

The clinical question 'What is the best exercise program to prescribe?' opens a series of broad research questions which could reasonably include:

- What happens to the neck muscle system in association with neck pain?
- What types of exercise strategies best address these impairments?

- Is a program of such exercises effective in reversing the impairments, restoring function and relieving the neck pain?
- How does the client's experience of his/her pain or of performing prescribed exercises impact on pain relief and restoration of function?

Laboratory-based research informs about muscle function in neck pain

Historically the neck muscles, as in the example, have posed particular challenges for research due to their number, inaccessibility, size and depth. The advances in technologies over the past two decades in particular have meant that more precise, rigorous and high quality research can be undertaken in the laboratory to better understand the changes that may occur in the muscle system, which in turn will better inform research into exercise rehabilitation strategies, for ultimate translation into clinical practice.

Several techniques can be used to measure muscle performance. For example, radiological imaging techniques such as ultrasound and magnetic resonance imaging, which are safe and non-invasive, are used to provide precise information about the peripheral adaptations of individual cervical muscles (e.g. muscle degeneration) in the presence of neck pain (Elliott et al 2006, 2008; Rankin et al 2005). Electromyography (EMG) is commonly used to investigate and measure physiological and functional aspects such as changes in the spatial and temporal characteristics of muscle activity. Advances in computer technology, as well as knowledge of and programs for EMG signal analysis, mean that activity can now be measured from representative fibres of a particular muscle down to a single motor unit. For example, and pertinent to the neck pain patient scenario, EMG research into the spatial characteristics of neck muscle activation indicates that in association with neck pain there is reorganisation of the motor strategies of the neck muscles in both cognitive and functional work tasks (Falla, Bilenkij & Jull 2004; Falla, Jull & Hodges 2004b; Szeto et al 2005). Differences have also been demonstrated in temporal characteristics, with neck muscles displaying a deficit in the automatic feedforward control of the cervical spine in patients with neck pain (Falla, Jull & Hodges 2004a; Gurfinkel et al 1988). In addition to EMG, dynamometry devices are used to provide mechanical measures of muscle function in terms of strength and endurance. Several studies using various devices have shown reductions in cervical flexor and extensor muscle strength and endurance with neck pain (O'Leary et al 2007). Such research undertaken in the laboratory provides knowledge about possible morphological, physiological and functional changes that may occur in the muscle system and its neural control in musculoskeletal pain states. Such research lays a scientific foundation for the next stage of applied research into exercise strategies for rehabilitation.

Research informs the types of exercise strategies for neck pain patients

The findings from the laboratory in the examples provided indicate that the changes in muscle activity associated with neck pain are likely to be the result of a combination of altered neural input to muscles and changes in the structure of the muscles themselves. As indicated, the laboratory findings guide the development of the exercise program and the next phase of research. In this case, the findings of such research suggest that therapeutic exercise approaches should address both peripheral and central neuromuscular adaptations.

There are two streams in this phase of the research. Firstly, laboratory-based experiments need to be conducted in collaboration with clinicians to develop and test different exercise strategies. This type of study is undertaken to determine which type of exercise can best ameliorate the specific impairments identified in the muscles and their neural control. There are many ways in which exercise can be undertaken; for the advancement of therapeutic exercise it is important to determine which strategies are most effective to make physiological and functional changes that, most relevantly, improve the patient's pain and functional status. It also needs to be known what dosage of exercise is required. Considering laboratory findings, it would be most likely that different exercise strategies are required within an exercise program to address the peripheral adaptations and changes in neuromotor control in the cervical muscle system identified in patients with neck pain.

The second and important phase for translation of the research into clinical practice is to formally test the effectiveness of the exercise program, developed from the basic research, in a randomised controlled trial. Such a research design can test whether that rehabilitation approach can have a significant impact on patients' levels of neck pain and disability, functional capacity and quality of life. There are many aspects to trial design that must be incorporated to ensure a high quality trial. Trial methodology must stand up to scientific scrutiny so that there are valid outcomes that can contribute to the bank of evidence for physiotherapy practice. The primary question of the trial could be to determine whether the specifically designed exercise intervention was superior to another regime of general exercise or to no exercise (e.g. a 'wait and see' approach). Trials should test the short-term and especially the long-term effectiveness of the interventions. A trial could be designed with a secondary aim, for example, of determining whether there was a specific subset of neck pain patients who were more responsive to the experimental intervention, to assist physiotherapists in selecting the patients most likely to respond to such an intervention. It is also necessary in contemporary clinical trials to include a cost effectiveness analysis.

Research informs understanding of clients' experience of pain and physiotherapy intervention

Other questions may arise in clinical practice that relate to the individual experience and meaning that clients associate with their pain or with the interventions recommended to them. These types of question are often best addressed through qualitative research methods. Qualitative research addresses research questions where attempting to measure or translate the data into numbers is not appropriate. Qualitative research is applicable to seeking answers to research questions where the phenomenon is complex and not reducible to numbers, and where a rich understanding of clients' experience is valued. For example, a program of exercise might be identified as the most effective for the resolution of pain; physiotherapists may then be interested in developing a deep understanding of how clients experience this program. The program may be effective in relieving pain, but is it so onerous to manage in their daily life that they do not adhere to it? Campbell et al (2001) used qualitative methods to understand noncompliance with physiotherapy in clients with osteoarthritis of the knee. They found that, whereas initial compliance related to loyalty to the physiotherapist, ongoing compliance was more complex, involving factors such as clients' willingness and ability to include exercises within their life, the perceived severity of symptoms, attitudes towards arthritis and previous experience of osteoarthritis. Findings such as these are generated through an open stance to clients' experience rather than by imposing researchers' expectations, as may occur if preformed questionnaires or scales are used to measure compliance. Qualitative methods can also indicate interactions between factors that may contribute to how clients experience interventions.

The use of qualitative research has increased considerably in professions such as nursing and occupational therapy, with medicine also evidencing increased interest in its value to practice (Bleakley 2005). There has been less qualitative research in physiotherapy, although the potential value of qualitative methods to physiotherapy practice has been identified (Grant 2005, Johnson & Waterfield 2004) and studies are starting to be published. A particular application of qualitative methods has been in clinical reasoning research, where the complex and contextual nature of physiotherapy decision-making processes is explored (Edwards et al 2004). The more recent emergence of qualitative research in physiotherapy means that practitioners and researchers tend to be less familiar with the research processes and standards for rigour than they might be with experimental research. Yet the potential contribution of knowledge generated through qualitative research to physiotherapy practice should prompt increased involvement by physiotherapists.

RESEARCH QUALITY

Ensuring quality of research is a separate consideration from research design. To ensure quality research, researchers must establish clear and specific research questions and hypotheses to investigate each of the broad research questions, choose appropriate methodologies and valid measurements, identify potential confounders, and establish clear inclusion/exclusion criteria for subjects for the specific projects.

Regardless of the research design, similar questions about external and internal validity issues should be asked during study conceptualisation and conduct. Several hundred checklists exist to assist research readers to assess external and internal validity (Katrak et al 2004). *External validity* relates to how well the study findings can be extrapolated to clinicians' own patients, skill base and settings. The relevance of the research context has been shown to be a key element influencing clinicians' uptake of new evidence (Sackett et al 2000). External validity relates to the detail provided about the primary research, which allows clinicians to decide its relevance to them. This can occur when clinicians read primary studies, or when they read about the studies within secondary research. External validity reflects how well subjects are described in terms of their demographics, their health status/health condition, their responses to the research, and the reasons why some sections of the sample may respond differently from others. When experimental studies are conducted, describing the intervention in detail is particularly important, so that clinicians can decide whether they could also provide this treatment within their current skill base and work setting. *Internal validity* relates to how well the study was conducted, and thus how well biases were avoided. For all study types it reflects rigour in sample selection from a known population, and validity and reliability of chosen study measures. For experimental studies it also reflects rigour in allocating patients to intervention arms. Internal validity also includes the quality of analysing and reporting the findings of a study, for instance reporting measures of variability in study outcomes, and reporting dropouts occurring and loss to follow-up throughout the study.

SUMMARY

Physiotherapy research is integral to our practice. As we have argued in this chapter, the conduct of research that is relevant and of high quality is imperative if the research is to meaningfully inform our practice. Relevant research is achieved by identifying research questions that are important for considering and exploring the multiple aspects of the knowledge that underpins physiotherapy. Quality research is achieved via the rigour in its conduct and by using methods that best answer the research question.

Research drives clinical practice and clinical practice drives research questions. The process of discovery is exciting. Importantly, the outcomes for patients are optimised through a close working relationship between clinicians and researchers. Current research is providing more and more answers, yet as the knowledge base increases more questions are raised to challenge physiotherapists in the future.

Reflective questions

- Keep a diary of questions that arise during your daily practice as a physiotherapist. What type of research design would help answer those questions?
- Involve your colleagues in compiling a list of prospective research questions. Do you have a team who can engage in collaborative research?
- What is your level of knowledge about how to conduct research? What professional development activities could you explore that would help increase your capacity to undertake quality research?
- How can I have a more active role in research as a subject, assistant or researcher?

Further reading

Helewa A, Walker J M 2000 Critical evaluation of research in physical rehabilitation. WB Saunders, Philadelphia

Liamputtong P, Ezzy D 2005 Qualitative research methods, 2nd edn. Oxford University Press, Oxford

Portney L G, Watkins, M P 2000 Foundations of clinical research: application to practice, 2nd edn. Prentice Hall, Upper Saddle River, NJ

References

Bleakley A 2005 Stories as data, data as stories: making sense of narrative inquiry in clinical education. Medical Education 39:534–540

Brooks D, Solway S, MacDermid J et al 2005 Quality of clinical practice guidelines in physical therapy. Physiotherapy Canada 57:123–134

Campbell R, Evans M, Tucker M et al. 2001 Why don't patients do their exercises? Understanding non-compliance with physiotherapy in patients with osteoarthritis of the knee. Journal of Epidemiology and Community Health 55:132–138

Crosbie J 2000 Physiotherapy research: a retrospective look at the future. Australian Journal of Physiotherapy 46:159–164

Dull J, Dull W 1983 Are maximal inspiratory breathing exercises or incentive spirometry better than early mobilization after cardiopulmonary bypass? Physical Therapy 63:655–659

Edwards I, Jones M, Carr J et al 2004 Clinical reasoning strategies in physical therapy. Physical Therapy 84(4):312–335

Elliott J, Jull G, Noteboom J et al 2006 Fatty infiltration in the cervical extensor muscles in persistent whiplash associated disorders (WAD): an MRI analysis. Spine 31:E847–855

Elliott J, Jull G, Noteboom T et al 2008 MRI study of the cross sectional area for the cervical extensor musculature in patients with persistent whiplash associated disorders (WAD). Manual Therapy 13(3):258–265

Fairbank J, Pynsent P 2000 The Oswestry disability index. Spine 25:2940–2953

Falla D, Bilenkij G, Jull G 2004 Chronic neck pain patients demonstrate altered patterns of muscle activation during performance of a functional upper limb task. Spine 29:1436–1440

Falla D, Jull G, Hodges P 2004a Feedforward activity of the cervical flexor muscles during voluntary arm movements is delayed in chronic neck pain. Experimental Brain Research 157:43–48

Falla D, Jull G, Hodges P 2004b Patients with neck pain demonstrate reduced activity of the deep neck flexor muscles during performance of the craniocervical flexion test. Spine 29:2108–2114

Goodyear-Smith F, Arrol B 2004 What can family physicians offer patients with carpal tunnel syndrome other than surgery? A systematic review of non-surgical management. Annals of Family Medicine 2:267–273

Grant A 2005 Editorial: The use of qualitative research methodologies within musculoskeletal physiotherapy practice. Manual Therapy 10:1–3

Grimmer K, Kumar S 2005 Allied health task-related evidence. Journal of Social Work Research and Evaluation 6:143–154

Gurfinkel V S, Lipshits M I, Lestienne F G 1988 Anticipatory neck muscle activity associated with rapid arm movement. Neuroscience Letters 94:104–108

Herbert R D, Higgs J 2004 Editorial: Complementary research paradigms. Australian Journal of Physiotherapy 50:63–64

Innocenti D 1995 An overview of the development of breathing exercises into the specialty of physiotherapy for heart and lung conditions. Physiotherapy 81:681–693

Johnson R, Waterfield J 2004 Making words count: the value of qualitative research. Physiotherapy Research International 9:121–131

Jones M A, Edwards I, Higgs J et al 2006a Challenges in applying best evidence to physiotherapy practice: part 1. Internet Journal of Allied Health Science and Practice July 4(3) http://ijahsp.nova.edu/articles/vol4num3/jones.pdf 26 Sep 2007

Jones M A, Edwards I, Higgs J et al 2006b Challenges in applying best evidence to physiotherapy practice: part 2. Internet Journal of Allied Health Science and Practice Sept 4(4) http://ijahsp.nova.edu/articles/vol4num4/jones.pdf 26 Sep 2007

Katrak P, Bialocerkowski A E, Massy-Westropp N et al 2004 A systematic review of the content of critical appraisal tools. BMC Medical Research Methodology 4:22 http://www.biomedcentral.com/bmcmedresmethodol/ 26 Sep 2007

MacMahon C 1915 Breathing and physical exercises for use in cases of wounds in the pleura, lung and diaphragm. Lancet 2:769–770

Maher C, Sherrington C, Elkins M et al 2004 Challenges for evidence-based physical therapy: accessing and interpreting high-quality evidence on therapy. Physical Therapy 84: 644–654

Muller M, Tsui D, Schnurr R et al 2004 Effectiveness of hand therapy interventions in primary management of carpal tunnel syndrome: a systematic review. Journal of Hand Therapy 17:210–228

National Stroke Foundation 2007 Clinical Guidelines for Acute Stroke Management. Available: www.strokefoundation.com.au/acute-clinical-guidelines-for-Acute-Stroke-Management 15 February 2008

O'Leary S, Jull G, Kim M et al 2007 Cranio-cervical flexor muscle impairment at maximal, moderate, and low loads is a feature of neck pain. Manual Therapy 12:34–39

Paterson M, Higgs J 2001 Professional practice judgement artistry. Occasional paper 3. The University of Sydney: Centre for Professional Education Advancement

Rankin G, Stokes M, Newham D 2005 Size and shape of the posterior neck muscles measured by ultrasound imaging: normal values in males and females of different ages. Manual Therapy 10: 106–115

Ritchie J 1999 Using qualitative research to enhance the evidence-based practice of health care providers. Australian Journal of Physiotherapy 45:251–256

Roland M, Morris R 1983 A study of the natural history of low back pain: part 1. Development of reliable and sensitive measures of disability in low back pain. Spine 8:141–144

Sackett D L, Straus S E, Richardson W S et al 2000 Evidence-based medicine: how to practice and teach EBM, 2nd edn. Churchill Livingstone, Edinburgh

Stiller K, Montarello J, Wallace M et al 1994 Efficacy of breathing and coughing exercises in the prevention of pulmonary complications after coronary artery surgery. Chest 105:741–747

Stratford P, Gill C, Westaway M et al 1995 Assessing disability and change on individuals patients: a report of a patient specific measure. Physiotherapy Canada 47:258–262

Szeto G, Straker L, O'Sullivan P 2005 A comparison of symptomatic and asymptomatic office workers performing monotonous keyboard work – 1: neck and shoulder muscle recruitment patterns. Manual Therapy 10:270–280

Thomas R, McEwen J, Asbury A 1996 The Glasgow pain questionnaire: a new generic measure of pain: development and testing. International Journal of Epidemiology 25:1060–1067

WORKING WITH OTHERS

PHYSIOTHERAPISTS AS COMMUNICATORS AND EDUCATORS

Rola Ajjawi and Narelle Patton

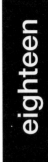

eighteen

Key content

- Global and local trends that emphasise the role of communication in physiotherapy practice
- Strategies that enhance partnerships with clients and their caregivers in the physio-therapeutic process
- Barriers to professional–professional communication that exist in your context
- The effects of effective and inadequate communication on quality client care
- Learning and improving communication, including the ability to educate others

INTRODUCTION

The roles and responsibilities of competent physiotherapists include effective communication with clients, caregivers, peers, colleagues and other health professionals. In this chapter we consider these various relationships and the role of physiotherapists as communicators and educators. We outline some of the local and global trends that have led to an increased emphasis on communication and communication training. As physiotherapists grow and develop from novice through to expert, communication is one of the capabilities that can and should be explicitly learned and improved.

THE INCREASING IMPORTANCE OF COMMUNICATION IN PHYSIOTHERAPY PRACTICE

Several factors have led to a change in the delivery of health care and an emphasis on effective communication. Health is perceived by many as a purchasable commodity rather than a basic human right (French & Sim 2004). In this context, patients or clients expect to be fully informed and to take a more assertive role in decisions related to their own health (Neubauer 1998). Another influencing factor is the growth in information technology, which has led to consumers having greater access to knowledge. Increasingly medically literate consumers frequently expect to be fully informed about their condition, including explanation of information found via the internet (Carlisle & Sefton 1998). These combined factors underline the need for clear and effective communication in all aspects of care.

Another factor impacting on communication is the shift in health care focus from a curative to a preventative model, to address the needs arising from an ageing population, the increased incidence of chronic disease and the concomitant rise in health care costs (Mullavey-O'Byrne 2000). A preventative model increases the importance of health education and client empowerment, and replaces expectations common in the traditional paternalistic model of care that clients adopt a passive role (Owen Hutchinson 2004). Further, clients with chronic diseases and complex disorders require services from a variety of health professionals for their needs to be comprehensively met (Gibbon 1999). Physiotherapists are increasingly working within multidisciplinary teams in both hospital and community contexts. Clear communication, including skills in interpersonal and collaborative communication, is essential for the effective functioning of teams delivering quality client care.

With the rise of consumer power there is greater demand from clients for professionals to be accountable for their actions, and to explain the decisions and reasoning that led to those actions (Fish & Coles 1998). In the current context of increased litigation the need for accountability is further reinforced. Physiotherapists must ensure firstly that they are reasoning correctly and secondly that they are able to defend their reasoning clearly, logically and articulately. Professional accountability is also demanded by health service delivery managers, who need to meet decreasing health care budgets and to address the greater demand for limited resources in an overstretched system. Physiotherapists are increasingly required to present evidence to support their service and to ensure a continued level of funding (Hanekom et al 2007) or to seek additional funds. Sound reasoning and the ability to articulate complex decisions clearly in a language understood by business managers and politicians are therefore important skills for physiotherapists.

WHAT IS COMMUNICATION?

Communication and language are essential to the way human beings understand and transform the realities in which they live. Communication is not just about individuals exchanging information; it is concerned with the negotiation of relationships and with all the complexities inherent in those relationships, such as power, gender and culture (Thompson 2003). Communication is ongoing and continually evolving, in that understanding and interpretation are informed by previous communicative interactions. Meaning is negotiated between individuals, taking into account their respective ideas, feelings and points of view. Effective communication occurs when what was intended to be said has been heard and the persons involved have reached a shared understanding (Higgs et al 2005). Understanding some of the complexities associated with communication is also necessary for effective communication to occur. Context shapes communication in health care settings, where context includes physical (e.g. noise, lighting), personal (e.g. roles of identity, background, experiences, education), cultural (e.g. culture of the organisation), and structural (e.g. power and gender) factors (Thompson 2003). Communication involves different media such as written, oral, nonverbal and electronic forms, all of which are relevant for professional practice.

PHYSIOTHERAPISTS AS COMMUNICATORS
Communicating with clients and caregivers

Effective communication between clients and physiotherapists is integral to achieving successful physiotherapeutic treatment outcomes. Physiotherapists who use communication to develop honest, authentic partnerships with clients and their caregivers are likely to promote positive health outcomes. Paterson (2001) emphasised the difficulty of achieving client empowerment when practitioners rely on objective evidence and mistrust clients' experiential knowledge in clinical decision making processes. Clients and caregivers are *experts* in their particular circumstances; they bring to the consultation different perspectives and ways of thinking that can instil a new dimension in health care practice (Ahuja & Williams 2005). Health professionals are encouraged to value client knowledge, to consider the degree to which clients want to be involved in decision making, and to tailor management, education and communication to meet each client's needs (Gordon et al 2000). Such strategies are likely to lead to the best outcome in a particular situation (Ahuja & Williams 2005).

There is research evidence in medicine and physiotherapy that links increased client involvement in decision making with improved client outcomes. Kaplan and colleagues (1996) demonstrated better self-reported health and better physiological control of illnesses such as diabetes, hypertension and breast cancer when clients were actively involved in the decision-making process. There is also evidence that rehabilitation effectiveness is improved if clients are involved in goal setting (Arnetz et al 2004, Wade 1999). Therefore clients should be asked to contribute their experiences, goals, values and preferences to the decision-making process, and professionals need to be able to elicit clients' narratives in a supportive, non-threatening environment. However, although clients' and caregivers' theories, perceptions and priorities may be explicit, they may also be hidden, implicit and difficult to detect (Eraut 1994). This may explain research findings which demonstrate that physiotherapists infrequently set goals with clients and that client involvement is limited when goals are set (Baker et al 2001, Parry 2004, Talvitie & Reunanen 2002). Health professionals need a high level of competence in interpersonal skills, including the ability to establish rapport, to be able to invoke client values and goals for improved collaboration in the therapeutic process.

Physiotherapists are increasingly working in health settings underpinned by the principles of primary health care, which include community participation and partnership with clients and their families (Litchfield & MacDougall 2002). Little et al (2001) demonstrated that clients in primary care had a strong preference for a client-centred approach in communication, partnership and health promotion, but cautioned against the assumption that all clients desire the same degree of active involvement in their management. This view was supported by Florin et al (2006), who found that registered nurses were not always aware of their clients' perspectives and tended to overestimate clients' willingness to assume an active role in their management. Focusing on individual clients' information needs and responding to their questions (and silences) may be a good starting point. Highly developed communication skills are needed to explore clients' concerns, requirements for information, and preferences for partnership, and to construct individual therapeutic relationships that authentically reflect clients' unique desires and goals.

Partnerships are created to help clients adopt an active role in their care, to empower them in self-management, and to promote participation in and increase satisfaction with the therapeutic process (Doherty & Doherty 2005, Hook 2006). The establishment of a client–therapist partnership is facilitated by communication that is reciprocal, nonjudgemental, honest, flexible, confidential, collaborative, nondirective and clear. Therapists who form successful therapeutic relationships are aware of body language and facial expressions; they are able to take a holistic approach to client management

(Gyllensten et al 1999). A study of physiotherapists' nonverbal communication demonstrated that actions such as looking away and not smiling can communicate distance between physiotherapists and their clients, and may negatively correlate with clients' perceptions and therapeutic outcomes (Ambady et al 2002). Communicators need to be aware of their own and others' nonverbal messages (including body language and paralanguage such as speed, tone, volume, pitch and intonation), as these influence the way the message is interpreted and therefore influence the meaning attributed to the communication.

In comparison to the wealth of literature on client–professional relationships, there is significantly less literature describing family/caregiver–professional relationships (Northouse & Northouse 1998). In a study of family caregivers of clients undergoing a bone marrow transplant, caregivers reported feeling invisible to the health professional, receiving minimal acknowledgement and being excluded from discussions and decision making regarding the client's care (Stetz et al 1996). Caregivers are an important source of care and support for clients and may be a valuable source of encouragement and motivation in ensuring that therapeutic goals are attended to. In a comparison of client outcomes following hip fracture, clients assigned to early discharge home-based therapy (discharged within 48 hours), with increased involvement of caregivers, had comparable outcomes at 12 months to those receiving conventional hospital rehabilitation (Crotty et al 2003). These clients were, previous to their hip fracture, functionally independent and living in the community. Caregivers in the home rehabilitation group also reported less carer burden at 12 months than did caregivers of clients in the control or hospital-based group. Some papers are emerging that focus on family-centred practice in physiotherapy and other disciplines (Hanna & Rodger 2002, King et al 1998, Park et al 2003, Rosenbaum et al 1998).

Clients and family/caregivers have the right to open, honest and effective communication and the right to be fully informed regarding all aspects of care. To ensure successful therapeutic outcomes, physiotherapists must feel confident and comfortable about discussing issues that clients raise, in sharing responsibility with clients and their caregivers, and in being reflective as to how their own behaviour affects these relationships (Potter et al 2003). Guidelines to consider when communicating with clients and caregivers are presented in the box opposite. Diligence in the formation and development of communication skills should be considered as important as the development of technical clinical skills. An important consideration in communication in health care is addressing the varying abilities of clients and caregivers to communicate. For example, physiotherapists need to develop strategies for successful communication with people across the age spectrum, people from linguistically diverse backgrounds and people with hearing, comprehension or articulation difficulties. Communication training, use of interpreters and learning to communicate in different languages and sign language are strategies that could be pursued.

Communicating with colleagues and other health professionals

Communication is necessary in establishing constructive relationships with colleagues, for decision making among multidisciplinary team members and for quality client care. Failure of communication among staff or between departments and hospitals is one of the main causes of adverse events in hospitals (Wong & Beglaryan 2004). Inadequate

Guidelines for effective communication with clients and caregivers

- Actively listen to your clients and identify their needs
- Think consciously of the message you want to communicate
- Attentively focus on and critique your reasoning processes, including the knowledge, values and beliefs informing your judgements
- Consider your clients' background knowledge, experiences, values, culture, and their emotional, cognitive and psychological states
- Tailor communication to the client's level of understanding and make the message relevant to their situation
- Use appropriate language and avoid jargon
- Use pictures, diagrams, demonstration and metaphor to promote effective communication, as relevant and necessary
- Be aware of any perceived power imbalance and attempt to redress it if possible through open and friendly communication
- Be sensitive to clients' cues that indicate their understanding of the message
- Recognise that your goals may not be the same as the client's
- Explain your rationale to your clients using straightforward language and provide more information if they request it
- Actively involve your clients in the decision making process through information exchange, negotiation of meaning and involvement in choices
- Be honest when communicating, e.g. if not sure of the prognosis then say so
- Monitor your communication and the listener's verbal and nonverbal communication for evidence of shared meaning
- Actively seek and be receptive to feedback from others; it is a powerful way to learn
- Be aware of assumed knowledge and shared language in your community that is not appropriate outside that community

communication can lead to fragmentation of care, client frustration (if information is being repeated) and increased risk of litigation. Types of communication breakdown that are common causal factors in serious incidents include (NSW Department of Health 2005):

- failure to pass on information
- incorrect assumptions that information has been understood
- failure to share information among teams
- lack of consultation or involvement with other health care workers
- lack of involvement of the client.

Northouse and Northouse (1998) described three barriers impacting on professional–professional relationships: role stress, lack of interprofessional understanding and autonomy struggles. Role stress (including the notions of role conflict and role overload) can lead to tensions and interfere with the role functioning of others. Work colleagues may withdraw from one another as a means of coping and may shift priorities from process functions to task functions (e.g. focusing on getting the job done rather than how well the team is functioning). Lack of understanding of interprofessional roles and responsibilities presents another barrier to effective professional–professional communication. This barrier is created by the socialisation of health professionals, through daily interactions at university and in the workplace, into the norms and culture of their own profession (reinforcing 'professional silos' (Hall 2005)). New graduates are thus faced with interprofessional challenges that include unfamiliar vocabulary, different approaches to decision making, and a lack of common understanding of values and issues (Hall 2005). Finally, discrepancies in degree of autonomy among professionals, power hierarchy and conflict can also lead to interpersonal tension (Northouse & Northouse 1998).

Loftus (2006) investigated clinical meetings of a multidisciplinary pain clinic where health professionals were required to articulate and justify their reasoning to each other as they negotiated and reached agreement on the nature of clients' problems and management plans. To master team clinical decision making, these health professionals needed to learn specific language tools and skills. The interpretive repertoire of shared language that was learned in order to make decisions included skills with words, categories, metaphors, heuristics, narratives, rituals and rhetoric. The social context (i.e. norms, interactions, behavioural expectations) substantially impacted on both the language skills and tools used by health care practitioners and the way they had to relearn how to perform and communicate their reasoning within the team compared with working in single discipline settings.

According to Clemmer et al (1998), improving collaboration at work requires developing a shared purpose, creating an open safe environment that is inclusive and fair, encouraging diverse viewpoints, and learning how to negotiate agreement. The following guidelines are also recommended for effective communication with colleagues in the workplace setting (Hosley & Molle 2006):

- demonstrating respect for each person's knowledge and skill level
- accepting each person's contribution to the health care team
- maintaining client and staff confidentiality
- avoiding inappropriate jokes or topics
- adhering to the organisation's and profession's code of ethics.

PHYSIOTHERAPISTS AS EDUCATORS

Physiotherapists play a key role in educating and empowering clients and their caregivers, and in educating colleagues within and outside the profession. Educating others follows similar principles to those espoused above, in that education should be based on creating open, honest relationships and respectful, collaborative partnerships. Some broad guiding principles that can be used in any learning encounter include being learner-focused, encouraging active and deep engagement with the learning content and process, acknowledging and building on prior learning experiences, and respecting learners' autonomy.

Increasingly, empowerment is seen as important in client education. Empowering clients occurs through mutual, open and honest exchange, where clients are not required or pressured to change, and they thus become aware of their ability to control discussion and decision making regarding their health, which in turn enhances self-esteem (Kettunen et al 2006). Paterson (2001) reported that several participants in her study admitted lying to health professionals about self-management strategies because they feared the health professionals would disapprove. It is possible that physiotherapists may base management strategies on incorrect presuppositions, with the client feeling disempowered (and guilty) and no change in behaviour being fostered.

Paterson (2001) further cautioned practitioners against assuming the language of empowerment, such as issuing invitations to client participation while behaving in a manner that implies professional dominance. Practitioners can communicate power within the professional–client relationship through the use of professional jargon, which serves as a barrier to communication and underscores their expert status and the subordinate status of their clients (Gravois Lee & Garvin 2003). Other behaviours that contradict the intent to form a collaborative partnership include:

- display of distrust of clients' experiential knowledge that is not supported by objective evidence
- provision of inadequate resources for client decision making
- expectation of client compliance
- directive statements
- blaming the client for negative health outcomes
- excessive client monitoring behaviours
- information or advice that is irrelevant to the client's situation
- tight scheduling of appointments (Paterson 2001).

Most physiotherapists are likely to be involved in the education of novice therapists in the clinical environment at some time during their careers. Effective learning in clinical settings requires effective interpersonal communication between novice practitioners and educators. These interactions encourage novices to integrate theoretical material with practical experiences and provide opportunities for challenge and resolution by discussion (Spouse 2001). Developing a successful novice–educator relationship requires the establishment of a partnership between the practitioner and novice that fosters collaboration, values the contribution of each individual and is based on mutual respect (Atack et al 2000).

Each health care setting has its unique organisational culture; consequently, students attending clinical placements or new graduates starting a new rotation experience considerable anticipatory anxiety surrounding the culture and expectations of the workplace. Novice practitioners value clear communication regarding placement expectations, as it decreases their anxiety and facilitates learning (McKenzie 2002). It is the responsibility of physiotherapy educators to provide novice physiotherapists with clear guidelines, including a description of the workplace culture and expectations. This could be provided verbally during an orientation session or in written format prior to commencement.

Effective communication of feedback to novice practitioners is also crucial to their ongoing professional knowledge and skill development. Educators may be fearful of providing negative feedback to students, particularly if it involves failing a clinical placement. However, clinical educators have the responsibility to act as *professional gatekeepers*, ensuring that professional standards for quality client care are met. The challenge for educators therefore is to provide feedback in a constructive manner that preserves dignity, promotes learning, allows ongoing communication and facilitates behavioural change (McAllister 2005, pp 247–248). According to McAllister, effective feedback is:

- focused on specific clinical behaviours (not personality traits) that are within the novice's ability to change
- provided regularly and as close to the event that it pertains to as possible
- encouraging and inclusive of positive behaviours to build the novice's confidence and self-esteem with suggested strategies for improvement
- provided in an appropriately private area to ensure confidentiality, and at a time that acknowledges the readiness of the novice to receive the feedback
- fostering the self-reflective skills of novices by encouraging their active participation.

Providing and receiving feedback appropriately is part of all physiotherapists' professional responsibility. Physiotherapists are urged to reflect on their feedback style, using the above characteristics as a guide. Novice physiotherapists benefit from seeking feedback on their practice and reflecting on the content and process of feedback they receive, including their emotional reactions or responses to it. Engaging in a genuine two-way conversation, rather than feedback being one-way transmission, is the responsibility of both parties. Being critical and reflective of one's communication patterns in order to learn and continue to improve them should be a component of regular practice for physiotherapists at all stages.

DEVELOPING COMMUNICATION CAPABILITY

An explicit goal of physiotherapy education is the development of interpersonal communication skills by novice physiotherapists. This development occurs at the university and in workplace settings. Learning communication skills in the classroom may involve: participating in practical tutorial sessions that focus on one aspect of the communication process (e.g. history taking, giving a talk); modelling, role play and vivas in which students practise different communication styles; and learning from peer discussion and feedback. Development of communication skills is also greatly enhanced in the workplace, during practicum and following graduation, because of the richness of the environmental cues and opportunities for authentic practice and reflection.

The workplace provides an environment in which learners can engage in purposeful activities and, in the process, learn to use the cultural tools and practices that have been developed to mediate the achievement of the goals of these activities. The jargon used by health professionals is an example of a culturally mediated tool that can and should be learned in the clinical environment. The role of language is instrumental in establishing professional identity by shaping thoughts, values and attitudes (Lingard 2007). Novice physiotherapists benefit from recognising the richness of the clinical environment in providing learning opportunities for professional development, and from actively seeking out these opportunities.

Learning activities that have been reported to be effective for developing communication ability include:

- communicating with clients and their caregivers
- modelling communication style on that of role models and peers whose style appears favourable and appropriate
- receiving and providing feedback about communication from educators, peers, and clients, based on live observation or audio/video recording, including regularly checking to see that messages are understood as intended (Higgs et al 2005)

- observing and listening to experienced professionals as well as gaining access to their accompanying thought processes (Eraut 1994, Ajjawi & Higgs 2007)
- focusing on communication experiences and interpretation of those experiences, i.e. reflecting on experiences (Eraut 1994) and analysing critical incidents (Ajjawi & Higgs 2007, Parker et al 1995) – for example, Parker et al asked nursing students to write about a particular incident of client care in which they were involved and then discuss the incident with their educators, focusing and reflecting on certain communication issues; the students were then asked to write in their reflective journals what they had learned through critical incident analysis
- critical reflection on day-to-day communication to see, for example, how well communication, content and style are received by the audience – this requires practitioners to pay attention and bring communication to the forefront of all interactions; it is particularly relevant because, although communication is an observable action (in speech, written records), the act of communicating (and learning to communicate) is embedded in our daily activities and relationships and is therefore often subconscious (Ajjawi & Higgs 2007)
- participating in continuing education courses or specific communication workshops, e.g. related to teamwork, negotiation, conflict resolution or leadership.

WRITTEN COMMUNICATION

In this chapter we have so far addressed face-to-face communication. However, written communication is also an important skill for physiotherapists. Physiotherapists are obliged by law to keep meticulous, accurate client records, which are an important form of communication with colleagues and other service providers. Written interprofessional communication may take the form of ongoing medical records for inpatient or outpatient services, handover and referral letters, or summaries of care. Maintaining client records is a critical aspect of professional behaviour and evidence-based practice (Turner et al 1999). As a physiotherapist your client notes should:

- be written in a timely and legible manner with all entries signed and dated
- include details of consent for treatment, subjective and physical examination findings, problem lists, therapeutic goals, treatment plans, treatment interventions, and outcome measures that assess the effectiveness of treatment interventions. (In an audit of physiotherapy files, Turner et al (1999) found that, although initial assessment findings were recorded in 86% of cases, problem lists, goals, treatment plans, outcome measures and functional assessments were notably absent.) (See Ch 16 for legal communication.)
- be respectful of the client's dignity and therefore be written in a professional and objective manner, avoiding personal judgements (remember that clients have the right to access and read their records)
- be kept secure when not in use in order to maintain clients' right to confidentiality (e.g. records should not be left on the desk overnight where they could be read by ancillary staff)
- be written in appropriate professional language, using only abbreviations approved by the particular organisation that you work in (this is particularly important when the notes are used by varied disciplines to avoid misinterpretation and confusion that could result in incorrect treatment interventions and reductions in quality of client care)

- be clear, concise and diplomatic (remember that health professionals are busy people; if you want your report read, keep it brief; the quality of your notes and report writing is a criterion by which your professionalism may be judged).

SUMMARY

Physiotherapists work in a health care environment of increasing complexity and rapid change, of fiscal restraints and demands for accountability that also requires the establishment of collaborative partnerships with clients, caregivers, peers, colleagues and other health professionals. Effective practitioners in the current health care context must develop a range of communication skills that will facilitate the development of these varied professional relationships. The development of communication skills, including the ability to educate others, should be a lifelong learning goal for all physiotherapists.

Reflective questions

- Think of a clinical experience that challenged your communication ability. Which factors relating to yourself, your co-communicator(s) and the situation or the circumstances made it challenging? What specific actions would have improved your communication?
- How can you include clients' goals, values and beliefs in your decision making? What actions can you take to include your clients' family or caregivers in the therapeutic process?
- Northouse and Northouse (1998) discussed three barriers that can impact on interprofessional relationships. Do any of those barriers currently exist among members of your health care team? How can you address some of these?
- What specific actions can you take to develop and improve your oral and written communication skills?

Further reading

Higgs J, Ajjawi R, McAllister et al (eds) (2008) Communicating in the health and social sciences, 2nd edn. Oxford University Press, Oxford

References

Ahuja A S, Williams R 2005 Involving patients and their carers in educating and training practitioners. Current Opinion in Psychiatry 18(4):374–380

Ajjawi R, Higgs J 2007 Learning clinical reasoning: a journey of professional socialisation. Advances in Health Sciences Education pp1–18 DOI 10.1007/s10459-006-9032-4

Ambady N, Koo J, Rosenthal R et al 2002 Physical therapists' nonverbal communication predicts geriatric patients' health outcomes. Psychology and Aging 17(3):443–452

Arnetz J E, Almin I, Bergstrom K et al 2004 Active patient involvement in the establishment of physical therapy goals: effects on treatment outcome and quality of care. Advances in Physiotherapy 6(2): 50–69

Atack L, Comacu M, Kenny R et al 2000 Student and staff relationships in a clinical practice model: impact on learning. Journal of Nursing Education 39(9):387–392

Baker S M, Marshak H H, Rice G T et al 2001 Patient participation in physical therapy goal setting. Physical Therapy 81(5):1118–1126

Carlisle S, Sefton A J 1998 Healthcare and the information age: implications for medical education. Medical Journal of Australia 168(7):340–343

Clemmer T P, Spulher V J, Berwick D M et al 1998 Cooperation: the foundation of improvement. Annals of Internal Medicine 128:1004–1009

Crotty M, Whitehead C, Miller M et al 2003 Patient and caregiver outcomes 12 months after home-based therapy for hip fracture: a randomized controlled trial. Archives of Physical Medicine and Rehabilitation 84(8):1237–1239

Doherty C, Doherty W 2005 Patients' preferences for involvement in clinical decision-making within secondary care and the factors that influence their preferences. Journal of Nursing Management 13:119–127

Eraut M 1994 Developing professional knowledge and competence. Falmer Press, London

Fish D, Coles C 1998 Seeing anew: understanding professional practice as artistry. In: Fish D, Coles C (eds) Developing professional judgement in health care. Butterworth-Heinemann, Oxford, pp 28–53

Florin J, Ehrenberg A, Ehnfors M 2006 Patient participation in decision making in clinical nursing: a comparison of nurses' and patients' perspectives. Journal of Clinical Nursing 15:1498–1508

French S, Sim J 2004 Introduction. In: French S, Sim J (eds) Physiotherapy: a psychosocial approach, 3rd edn. Butterworth-Heinemann, Edinburgh, pp 1–4

Gibbon B 1999 An investigation of interprofessional collaboration in stroke rehabilitation team conferences. Journal of Clinical Nursing 8(3):246–252

Gordon J, Hazlett C, ten Cate O et al 2000 Strategic planning in medical education: enhancing the learning environment for students in clinical settings. Medical Education 34(10):841–850

Gravois Lee R, Garvin T 2003 Moving from information transfer to information exchange in health and health care. Social Science and Medicine 56:449–464

Gyllensten A, Gard G, Salford E et al 1999 Interaction between patient and physiotherapist: a qualitative study reflecting the physiotherapist's perspective. Physiotherapy Research International 4(2): 89–109

Hall P 2005 Interprofessional teamwork: professional cultures as barriers. Journal of Interprofessional Care 19(suppl 1):188–196

Hanekom S D, Faure M, Coetzee A 2007 Outcomes research in the ICU: an aid in defining the role of physiotherapy. Physiotherapy Theory and Practice 23(3):125–135

Hanna K, Rodger S 2002 Towards family-centred practice in paediatrics occupational therapy: A review of the literature on parent–therapist collaboration. Australian Occupational Therapy Journal 49: 14–24

Higgs J, McAllister L, Sefton A 2005 Introduction: communicating in the health and social sciences. In: Higgs J, Sefton A, Street A et al (eds) Communicating in the health and social sciences. Oxford University Press, Oxford, pp 3–12

Hook M 2006 Partnering with patients: a concept ready for action. Journal of Advanced Nursing 56(2):133–143

Hosley J, Molle E 2006 A practical guide to therapeutic communication for health professionals. Elsevier, St Louis, MO

Kaplan S H, Greenfield S, Gandek B et al 1996 Characteristics of physicians with participatory decision-making styles. Annals of Internal Medicine 124(5):497–504

Kettunen T, Liimataunen L, Villberg J et al 2006 Developing empowering health counseling measurement: preliminary results. Patient Education and Counseling 64:159–166

King G, Law M, King S et al 1998 Parents and service providers' perceptions of family-centeredness of children's rehabilitation services. Physical and Occupational Therapy in Paediatrics 18(1):21–40

Lingard L 2007 The rhetorical 'turn' in medical education: what have we learned and where are we going? Advances in Health Sciences Education 12(2):121–133

Litchfield R, MacDougall C 2002 Professional issues for physiotherapists in family-centred and community-based settings. Australian Journal of Physiotherapy 48:105–112

Little P, Everitt H, Williamson I et al 2001 Preferences of patients for patient centred approach to consultation in primary care: observational study. British Medical Journal 322:1–7

Loftus S 2006 Language in clinical reasoning: learning and using the language of collective decision making. Unpublished PhD thesis, The University of Sydney

McAllister L 2005 Giving feedback. In: Higgs J, Sefton A, Street, A et al (eds) Communicating in the health and social sciences. Oxford University Press, Oxford, pp 247–253

McKenzie L 2002 Briefing and debriefing of student fieldwork experiences: exploring concerns and reflecting on practice. Australian Occupational Therapy Journal 49(2):82–92

Mullavey-O'Byrne C 2000 Social change, health care and the education of health professionals for practice in the 21st century: are our graduates well positioned or are they falling behind? Available: http://www2.fhs.usyd.edu.au/ugcr//no5.htm 25 June 2007

Neubauer D 1998 Some impacts of globalisation on health and health care policy. Occasional paper, Centre for Professional Education Advancement, The University of Sydney

Northouse L L, Northouse P G 1998 Health communication: strategies for health professionals, 3rd edn. Prentice Hall, Stamford, CT

NSW Department of Health 2005 Patient safety and clinical quality program: first report on incident management in the NSW public health system 2003–2004. Available: http://www.health.nsw.gov.au/pubs/2005/pdf/incident_mgmt.pdf 25 June 2007

Owen Hutchinson J S 2004 The nature of health and illness: health, health education and physiotherapy practice. In: French S, Sim J (eds) Physiotherapy: a psychosocial approach, 3rd edn. Butterworth-Heinemann, Edinburgh, pp 25–43

Park J, Hoffman L, Marquis J et al 2003 Toward assessing family outcomes of service delivery: validation of a family quality of life survey. Journal of Intellectual Disability Research 47:367–384

Parker D L, Webb J, D'Souza B 1995 The value of critical incident analysis as an educational tool and its relationship to experiential learning. Nurse Education Today 15(2):111–116

Parry R H 2004 Communication during goal-setting in physiotherapy treatment sessions. Clinical Rehabilitation, 18(6):668–682

Paterson B 2001 Myth of empowerment in chronic illness. Journal of Advanced Nursing 34(5):574–581

Potter M, Gordon S, Hamer P 2003 The physiotherapy experience in private practice: the patient's perspective. Australian Journal of Physiotherapy 49:195–202

Rosenbaum P, King S, King G et al 1998 Family-centred service: A conceptual framework and research review. Physical and Occupational Therapy in Paediatrics 18(1):1–20

Spouse J 2001 Bridging theory and practice in the supervisory relationship: a sociocultural perspective. Journal of Advanced Nursing 33(4):512–522

Stetz K, McDonald J C, Compton K 1996 Needs and experiences of family caregivers during marrow transplantation. Oncology Nursing Forum 23(9):1422–1427

Talvitie U, Reunanen M 2002. Interaction between physiotherapists and patients in stroke treatment. Physiotherapy 88(2):77–88

Thompson N 2003 Communication and language: a handbook of theory and practice. Palgrave Macmillan, Hampshire

Turner P A, Harby-Owren H, Shackleford F et al 1999. Audits of physiotherapy practice. Physiotherapy Theory and Practice 15(4):261–274

Wade D T 1999 Goal planning in stroke rehabilitation: evidence. Topics in Stroke Rehabilitation 6(1):16–36

Wong J, Beglaryan H 2004 Strategies for hospitals to improve patient safety: a review of the research, Ontario, the Change Foundation. Available: http://www.changefoundation.com/tcf/tcfbul.nsf/eb2d6f6074fe4c9c 052567180004b916/047539287c3d43a585256e3100486df4/$FILE/Patient%20Safety%202004.pdf 18 June 2007

DEVELOPING PERSON-CENTRED RELATIONSHIPS WITH CLIENTS AND FAMILIES

nineteen

Franziska Trede and Abby Haynes

Key content

- Principles and attitudes underpinning person-centred approaches to physiotherapy
- The value of person-centred approaches in physiotherapy
- The dynamic nature of person-centred professional relationships
- Skills necessary to become a person-centred practitioner

INTRODUCTION

The provision of accessible, safe and effective physiotherapy services depends on our ability as physiotherapists to develop positive working relationships with our clients. In this chapter we describe the dimensions of the person-centred approach and explore some of the key skills involved in establishing person-centred relationships. We highlight the values and motivations that underpin a person-centred approach to physiotherapy, and conclude that person-centred professionals offer ethical services that result in greater client satisfaction and better overall outcomes.

WHAT IS A PERSON-CENTRED PERSPECTIVE?

Person-centred perspectives have developed across many disciplines including health, education, psychology, philosophy and community services. Different disciplines use terms such as patient-centred, student-centred, family-centred, learner-centred or client-centred, but in general these terms are simply a more context-specific way of talking about person-centred approaches. Person-centred approaches acknowledge that learning, thinking, understanding and being in the world are influenced by each individual's personal experiences, as well as their cultural and social backgrounds (Trede & Higgs 2007). In this chapter we look at how person-centred perspectives can and should guide the way that physiotherapists communicate with and relate to their clients and their clients' families.

The movement towards person-centred practice has been informed by humanist values, in response to (traditionally) authoritarian or paternalistic approaches across the health care system that can disempower and dehumanise service users. Person-centred perspectives across the spectrum of interdisciplinary development are underpinned by key concepts such as respect and dignity for all, responsive communication, consideration of each individual's needs and wishes, promotion of independence, provision of choice, and recognition that services are most effective when practitioners regard clients as active partners rather than passive recipients (Innes et al 2006).

Traditionally, clinicians such as physiotherapists defined professional in terms of being objective, rational, detached and bound by the formalities of practice; however, contemporary person-centred clinicians recognise the importance of being empathic and compassionate, of working with patients' beliefs, and of building relationships (McCormack & McCane 2006) that involve each client as a whole person who has knowledge, emotions, strengths, preferences and a life context (Stewart 2001). Thus person-centred physiotherapists appreciate the human dimension of their work in all its complexity, and provide services that are responsive to each client's particular needs, attributes and situation (Trede & Higgs 2003). For example, each 'arthritic knee' is not treated the same way because the knee belongs to a person with unique characteristics. This requires treating physiotherapists to consider factors such as the person's age, fitness level, gender, occupation, day-to-day activities, health conditions, pain tolerance, existing knowledge and previous experience of arthritis, as well as personal goals and expectations of treatment. This practice uses physiotherapists' scientific knowledge and technical skills, but is also dependent on their communication skills and relationship-building abilities to ensure treatment is appropriate and meaningful.

Innes et al (2006) reviewed a range of studies of the personal qualities of health professionals that are most valued by clients. The attributes that were deemed most important are listed in the box below. Our experience as diversity health practitioners confirms the findings of Innes et al that clients value and appreciate professionals who master a person-centred repertoire. One of the roles of diversity health practitioners in a large teaching hospital is to promote a person-centred hospital culture. Clients (and their families/carers) are asked about their experiences of health care and what attributes in the professionals who treat or care for them demonstrate that they are person-centred. The second box overleaf shows the results of these discussions in one clinical setting.

Of course, not all clients place equal value on these attributes. People have different needs and expectations, and different circumstances, all of which influence the professional relationship (Salmon & Young 2005, Swenson et al 2006). For example, not all cancer patients appreciate compassion, not everyone values cheerfulness, and not every client with a chronic condition is well informed about self-managing physical activity and exercises. The benefit of person-centred communication is that it allows

---

Personal attributes most valued by clients

From Innes et al (2006)

- Compassion
- Honesty
- Kindness
- Friendliness
- Thoughtfulness
- Maintaining confidentiality
- Cheerfulness
- Warmth
- Empathy
- Understanding

- Helpfulness
- Respect
- Patience
- Flexibility
- Reliability
- Caring
- Gentleness
- Willingness
- Courtesy
- Fortitude

How to be person-centred: the client's view

- Listen respectfully and take me seriously
- Explain what is happening and why
- Make sure I understand what you're saying
- Let me know how long I will have to wait
- Give me time to ask questions and express worries
- Recognise that I value the support of family and friends around me
- Smile, make eye contact and have a friendly demeanour
- Treat me as a person, not just a problem
- Ask about what is important to me
- Show compassion
- Say 'sorry' when you make a mistake
- Keep me informed about test results
- Be trustworthy and reliable – do what you say you will do
- Offer and arrange health care interpreters
- Respect my dignity and maintain my privacy whenever possible

physiotherapists to move beyond generalisations to find out from clients how they wish to be treated. In order to do this, physiotherapists draw upon a repertoire of key skills that enable person-centred relationships to be formed with a diverse range of clients. These skills can be clustered into seven key dimensions, as illustrated in Figure 19.1.

Technical expertise

The technical expertise that physiotherapists bring to the relationship is highly valuable. It defines us as physiotherapists and assigns us our professional role. Clients visit physiotherapists to understand more about their health problems and what they can do to improve them. However, on its own technical expertise is not sufficient to establish an effective helping relationship. Even the most impressive theoretical and technical expertise is useless if physiotherapists cannot work well with people to apply their technical expertise appropriately. Competence in technical knowledge and skills must be accompanied by the person-centred interactive and facilitative skills outlined in this chapter. Clients need to trust their physiotherapists enough to talk openly, to listen to their advice and to spend time putting this advice into action. In most cases, trustworthiness is assessed not by what physiotherapists know, but by how they act and what kind of people they appear to be.

Engagement

The core skill of any person-centred approach is the ability to engage with people, to establish a trusting relationship. Building this kind of rapport requires adaptable communication skills and an attitude that conveys fundamental person-centred values such as respect, empathy and honesty. Genuine engagement provides opportunities for physiotherapists and clients to clarify beliefs, goals and expectations. It encourages clients to become involved in the decision-making process and evaluation of their treatment.

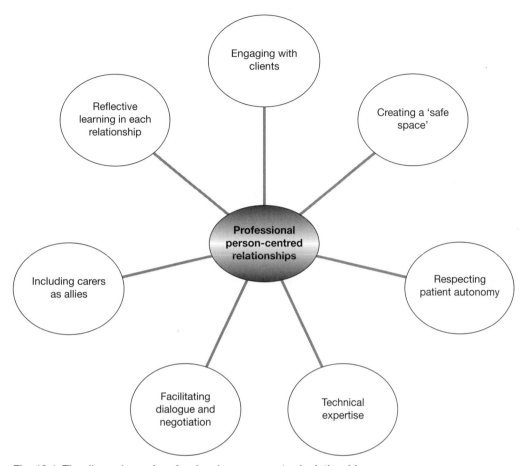

Fig. 19.1 The dimensions of professional person-centred relationships

Creating safe spaces

A safe space is a physical place that provides privacy and the basic comforts and resources necessary for the tasks of physiotherapy; but it is much more than that. In a safe space clients are not afraid to be vulnerable. They can talk about topics that might frighten or embarrass them, they can allow a stranger to touch them, they can admit to emotional frailty, they can show their pain, they can be assertive enough to say when they do not understand something or when treatment interventions hurt them too much, and they can attempt new skills haltingly without fear of judgement. Physiotherapists can create safe spaces by forging professional relationships that demonstrate trustworthiness, empathy and support. These factors are demonstrated through solid technical knowledge, communication skills and responsiveness to clients and their contexts.

Respecting clients' autonomy

Respect for clients' autonomy is underpinned by the understanding that physiotherapists have expertise in their work, but that clients are the experts in their own lives. As physiotherapists we empower clients and respect their right to self-determination when we listen to what they want, offer choices, give information openly so that they can make educated decisions, and negotiate strategies and goals responsively, ensuring that their needs and wishes have been given proper consideration.

Including carers as allies

Families and carers know much more about clients than health care professionals do, and can often provide valuable information about how to work with clients. In many cases, family members are the patient's greatest source of support and encouragement; this is particularly true when they have a caring role. Family members are often the impetus behind a patient's first encounter with health professionals, and provide the strongest advocacy for commitment to therapy regimens. Physiotherapists should regard family members as potential allies and, when appropriate, incorporate them into plans accordingly. For example, when treating older people who require assistance with bed mobility, transfers and ambulation, it is good practice to include carers. Showing family and carers how to assist clients, and at the same time teaching them how to avoid injury themselves, keeps everybody safe.

Reflective learning

Reflective learning is a process of critical awareness in which people question taken-for-granted assumptions, challenge the effectiveness and impact of their actions, consider alternatives and make changes for the better. Reflective practitioners view their work as a source of continual learning. Thus every professional relationship offers opportunities for reflection and improved practice.

Facilitating dialogue and negotiation

Person-centred relationships are built on the principle of collaboration. As physiotherapists we work *with* clients, co-developing strategies that are most effective for them, rather than simply telling them what they should be doing. Distributing fact sheets and brochures with medical advice may provide some guidance and reinforcement, but it does not provide opportunities for clients to engage with and develop their own understanding of the information. Inviting dialogue encourages clients to ask questions, give feedback, raise concerns and participate in their treatment planning. This is not only the most respectful way to work with clients, it is also the most effective. Most clients find it demotivating simply to be given directions and excluded from decision making. Clients are more inclined to take ownership of their treatment and feel a commitment to seeing it through when physiotherapists invite them to discuss options, state what they are prepared to do, and negotiate treatment methods and goals.

To summarise, professional person-centred relationships mean relationships in which the technically skilled professional is open to learning from the client, is trustworthy and respectful and, most importantly, facilitates responsive, empathetic and inclusive dialogue with clients and their families.

WHY FACILITATE PERSON-CENTRED RELATIONSHIPS?

The quality of the relationship we establish with clients influences the quality of the service we provide (Fossum 2003). This can have a dramatic impact on treatment efficacy, patient safety, patient satisfaction and access to equitable services.

Providing more effective services

There is emerging empirical evidence that person-centredness facilitates care that is better tailored to individual needs (Swenson et al 2006), and is ultimately more effective (McCormack & McCane 2006). For example, evidence-based studies of person-centred practice in medicine have shown significant benefits for the management of chronic problems including musculoskeletal conditions, as well as increased adherence to management protocols, reduced morbidity and improved quality of life (Bauman et al 2003).

Enhancing patient safety

Person-centred approaches enable physiotherapists to engage with patients in an open, trusting relationship, and to obtain accurate and thorough patient histories with relevant information that might not be apparent in a biomedically focused and 'clinical' or detached relationship. This increases the appropriateness of treatment plans and reduces misunderstandings that can lead to unsafe practices. For example, clients who are not encouraged to ask questions, or who think it inappropriate to ask, risk doing prescribed exercises at home in a way that does more harm than good. Authoritarian professional relationships can lead to incomplete history-taking, misinterpretation of learning needs, ineffective patient education, silenced and unmotivated clients, frustrated clinicians, unsafe practices, complaints and negligence claims.

Increasing client satisfaction

Person-centred physiotherapists are mindful of each client's wishes and expectations and, when appropriate, incorporate them into treatment planning and management. Clients then feel supported, valued, respected, taken seriously and involved in decision making. This fosters independence, encourages greater responsibility for health, and results in greater satisfaction. Some studies also show that person-centred communication is more satisfying for clinicians as well as for clients (Fossum 2003).

Offering equitable services

Person-centred practice is empowering and acknowledges clients' rights to equitable services (Montgomery 1996). It recognises and respects diversity, and is flexible and responsive enough to ensure that everyone's needs can be heard and met. It is crucial that physiotherapists acknowledge the power imbalances inherent in the client–professional relationship. Power imbalances have implications for the rules of discourse: rules about what should and should not be done, what can be discussed, what is silenced, and whose knowledge is valued. Physiotherapists who are aware of their professional authority embrace practice standards in which 'there is no assault, challenge or denial of [people's] personal identity, of who they are and what they need. It is about shared respect, shared meaning, and shared knowledge and experience, of learning together with dignity, and truly listening' (Williams 1999, p 213–214). Table 19.1 lists practice issues that are enhanced or minimised by person-centred relationships.

Table 19.1 Practice issues that are enhanced/minimised through facilitating person-centred relationships	
Person-centred relationships enhance	**Person-centred relationships minimise**
■ Shared understanding	■ Misunderstandings
■ Inclusive discussions	■ Negative incidents/adverse events
■ Client education	■ Misdiagnosis
■ Flexible and responsive practice	■ Noncompliance
■ Risk reduction	■ Complaints
■ Constructive collaboration	■ Aggression
■ Client and clinician satisfaction	■ Embarrassment
■ Dignity and respect	■ Distress
■ Negotiation	■ Unreflective presumptuous practices
■ Carer participation	■ Power imbalances and misuse
■ Professional learning and development	■ Unilateral decision making
■ Positive health outcomes	■ Sick and stress leave

WHAT ARE THE SKILLS INVOLVED IN FACILITATING PROFESSIONAL PERSON-CENTRED RELATIONSHIPS?

Facilitating professional person-centred relationships requires a diversity of skills. Being person-centred is about building on our strengths and expanding our thinking.

Setting the scene

The impression given in the first minutes of meeting a new client can have a lasting impact on the professional relationship that follows. When time is taken to 'set the scene' thoughtfully, foundations of a person-centred encounter can be laid.

Introductions

It is important for physiotherapists to consider how they introduce themselves. Questions to consider include: What attributes do I convey in those initial moments? Do I make eye contact, or take time to smile? Do I sound genuinely welcoming? Do I give my full attention? When working in a hospital context, do I explain my role?

Asking about previous experiences

It is good practice to enquire about new clients' previous experience with physiotherapy or other interventions intended to treat the presenting problem. Hearing about previous treatments allows clients to tell their story. This gives opportunities for assessing what they know about physiotherapy and what they may need to be told (e.g. to demystify physiotherapy and correct any misconceptions they might have). Most importantly, talking about previous treatment also allows clients to explain what has worked for them and what has not, and to air frustration or disappointment as well as satisfaction. This information often provides clues about how to relate to this person, what to do and what not to do.

Expectations

It is important to elicit from clients their expectations. For example: do they have any concerns about treatment? Any specific goals? Any other useful information? Any questions they would like to ask? Clarifying expectations lessens misunderstandings, helps set realistic goals and establishes open, collaborative ways of working together.

Communication

Effective communication is the foundation of person-centred practice. As physiotherapists we rely on communication skills to engage with clients and their families, and to establish a positive working relationship.

Asking questions

Certain types of questions elicit certain types of answers. Closed questions (e.g. 'Does this hurt?' or 'Were you running at the time?') elicit direct responses that enable the questioner to move rapidly through information. However, if communication partners cannot expand or clarify their answers such questions may miss important material. Although effective for processing certain types of information, closed questions create a one-way communication channel which relies on the questioner asking the right question. In contrast, open questions (e.g. 'How does this feel?' or 'What were you doing at the time?') invite clients to explain their health situation using their own words. Open questions foster a responsive dialogue and provide an opportunity for clients to tell their stories. Such questions also encourage clients to reflect on their way of thinking about and making sense of their health situation, and to be actively involved in their treatment.

Case study 1

Two physiotherapists are trying to understand a client's knee pain.

Physiotherapist A asked, 'Does your knee hurt when you climb the stairs?' to which the client replied, 'Yes'.

Physiotherapist B asked, 'What activities bring on your knee pain?', The client said, 'Going up and down the stairs, getting out of bed in the morning and, more recently, when I cross my legs when I'm sitting down'.

What response did each question elicit?

The closed question obtained a clear, specific answer, whereas the open question provided broader and more contextual information. Both are valuable in different circumstances but need to be used appropriately. When do you think closed questions and open questions are most appropriate?

Closed questions are suitable for eliciting precise and focused information, such as when you need to discount or confirm specific lines of enquiry or distinguish symptoms (e.g. 'Do you do any heavy lifting at work?'). Open questions are preferable for developing rapport, exploring the patient's perspective and gaining a comprehensive understanding of the context (e.g. 'What activities do you particularly want to get back to?'). Table 19.2 summarises some differences between open and closed questions.

Table 19.2 Differences between open and closed questions	
Closed questions	**Open questions**
■ Limit responses ■ Request anticipated information ■ Invite compliance ■ Reinforce current practice ■ Privilege professional authority ■ Support medical discourse	■ Broaden responses ■ Provide opportunities for unexpected information ■ Invite active participation ■ Create ideas for change ■ Encourage collaboration ■ Value multiple perspectives

Understanding as a process

Communication is not a linear, one-way process; we can disseminate information but we cannot transmit understanding. Effective communication requires two people to reach shared meaning through a process of give and take (Ellis & Trede 2008). Willingness to listen, desire to understand the other person's point of view and confirmation of shared meaning are necessary for effective communication.

As physiotherapists we convey significant information to clients (and their families or carers) about consequences and side-effects of treatments, resources required and the role of self-management and self-evaluation. Paraphrasing clients' comments to check that you are understanding them and asking clients to tell in their own words what they understand are important components of communication.

Adaptability

Practising physiotherapists encounter a broad range of clients with diverse needs, preferences, personalities and communication styles. Inevitably, some clients are easier to work with than others, but adaptability assists physiotherapists to work effectively with everyone. It is interesting to note that adaptability/flexibility is one of the most highly rated attributes of caring professionals across a broad spectrum of clients (Innes et al 2006).

Some clients enjoy humour, others value encouragement and reassurance; some want to chat, others prefer a detached business-like relationship; some want to know us as people, others value clear technical information. Nevertheless, all these relationships require a degree of rapport. As we assess our clients' preferred communication styles and respond appropriately we are demonstrating an understanding of their needs and wishes and a willingness and ability to employ responsive communication skills to establish effective working relationships.

Adaptability also means communicating sensitively with people from non-English speaking backgrounds, people with hearing impairments and clients with speech and language difficulties. For example, it may be appropriate to offer a health service interpreter for non-English speaking background clients or an AUSLAN interpreter for those with hearing impairments.

The following summary of helpful hints provides guidance for person-centred communication:

- Listen carefully and check you have understood what others mean.
- Check that they have understood you.
- Don't interrupt.
- Pay attention to nonverbal communication in your interactions.

- Take the time to respond thoughtfully.
- Ask open questions as well as closed questions.
- Offer explanations for your actions and recommendations.
- Invite clients to ask questions and raise concerns. Don't assume you know what is most important to them.
- Be flexible and adapt your communication style responsively to suit each client.
- Use plain English, and explain unfamiliar terms.
- Acknowledge negative emotions as well as positive ones; for example, acknowledge feelings of helplessness, frustration, depression and fear, don't brush them under the carpet.
- Check that clients have understood how to do their exercises safely and correctly.

Empathy

Empathy is the ability to sense and understand someone else's feelings as if they were your own, to understand their point of view. It does not mean feeling sorry for them, but shows that their experience is acknowledged (Halpern 2003). As physiotherapists it is essential that we have a genuinely empathetic appreciation for the impact that injury, disability and pain can have on a person's quality of life and morale. We may not know what it is like to suffer a painful injury or come to terms with reduced mobility, but we can imagine what it is like and learn from our patients what it is like for them. This involves:

- listening to and acknowledging the thoughts and feelings expressed by clients
- being sensitive to and addressing nonverbal emotional undercurrents
- offering encouragement and positive feedback
- giving reassurance when relevant, including normalising people's experiences.

Case study 2

A hospital physiotherapist was taking a new patient up some stairs for the first time after a cardiac attack. The patient began to look fearful and demanded to stop. 'Something's wrong', he said, 'I'm short of breath, even though I'm hardly doing anything!' The physiotherapist replied, 'Of course – you just had a heart attack.' The patient looked shocked and asked to go back to bed.

What could the physiotherapist have done differently to engage this patient?

Could it have made a difference if BEFORE the treatment began she had:

- prepared the patient by talking about the pathophysiology of heart failure?
- told the patient what he might experience during treatment?
- asked him if he had any questions or worries about the treatment?

Could it have made a difference if DURING treatment she had:

- asked him how he was feeling?
- noticed the patient's shortness of breath and normalised it before he raised the issue?
- given an answer that was more empathetic and reassuring?
- replied by explaining the process of what was happening, rather than using the term 'heart attack'?

Physiotherapists familiar with the routine of practice need to maintain awareness of what the experience may be like for new clients; what may be normal and obvious to physiotherapists may be strange and frightening for others. Empathetic skills help to bridge this gap and enable physiotherapists to connect meaningfully with clients to form trusting and effective working relationships.

Empowering clients

Empowering clients is an essential skill in developing person-centred relationships. Empowerment does not mean handing over professional authority and leaving any decision making entirely to clients. Rather, empowerment involves working with clients to build on strengths, knowledge and achievements. This increases motivation, confidence and problem-solving skills, and enables clients increasingly to take control of their health. Health professionals can help to build confidence and self-efficacy by emphasising clients' strengths and using them to develop further plans and goals. For example: does the client take good care of her body? Does he have a good understanding of his limitations? Does she have a positive attitude? Does he have a supportive social environment? Does she ask questions to ensure she understands? Does he find ways to make knowledge his own, such as putting things into his own words, developing metaphors? Has she offered creative suggestions for when/how she can do exercises? Does he have some anatomical knowledge that he can use to help understand his condition? Has she made progress despite encountering obstacles? Has he managed to return to a valued activity? Has she made positive lifestyle changes? Discussing strengths helps reinforce them and enables clients to view themselves as positive, active contributors to the process rather than powerless receivers of expert intervention.

Collaboration

Most physiotherapy interventions require clients to cooperate and be actively involved in their treatment. Working collaboratively with clients and their families towards mutually agreed goals is the cornerstone of person-centred professional relationships. The ability to work collaboratively is also essential in our relationships with colleagues.
Collaboration involves:

- inviting clients to participate actively in planning and evaluating treatment
- re-negotiating strategies and goals on the basis of client feedback
- sharing your skills and knowledge through effective client education
- working with families and carers to help them support the client
- being able to compromise and reconsider your ideas
- having insight into your personal and professional biases
- consulting with appropriate professionals for guidance
- having a commitment to teamwork, which may include colleagues from a range of backgrounds and disciplines.

Dignity and respect

The concept of dignity is extremely important for clients, who often feel stripped of their humanity by health services, particularly during invasive treatments and hospitalisation. Clients' feelings of embarrassment and discomfort can affect their breathing and muscle tonus, as well as their willingness and ability to listen, follow instructions and cooperate with treatment. Physiotherapists need to maximise clients' dignity, and minimise causes for embarrassment, for example:

- Be aware of privacy concerns. Physiotherapists often have to work in environments that make it difficult to maintain privacy (e.g. clients may be in shared hospital rooms or treatment cubicles that are divided only by curtains). However, privacy can be respected by ensuring that discussions are not overheard and that clients cannot be seen by others.
- Try to minimise the impact of clothing removal for clients who find it invasive. Offer appropriate gowns, and explain which body parts need to be exposed for assessment and treatment.
- Be aware that touch can be interpreted in different ways. For some clients, touch can be threatening. For example, consider the impact of touch on a client who has been sexually abused, or for whom it is culturally taboo, or who is frightened due to pain or a previous negative encounter with health professionals. Such circumstances require clients' input to ascertain how to best manage the situation, and consideration of alternatives (e.g. suggesting a friend be invited to attend sessions with the client).
- Be matter-of-fact when discussing potentially embarrassing issues; a physiotherapist's embarrassment can add to a client's feeling of discomfort.
- Provide opportunities to address sensitive questions, e.g. 'Some people worry about X. Is that a concern for you?'
- Offer reassurance and normalisation when possible.

Empathic listening skills and collaborative practice styles demonstrate respect for client self-determination and dignity (Beach et al 2005). Such practice also helps to combat the feelings of helplessness brought on by illness and injury that can contribute to loss of dignity and self-respect.

Context

The people we treat as physiotherapists do not exist in a void. When we take account of clients' contexts we recognise that they are affected by a range of factors in their lives that may either contribute to or hinder therapy (Best et al 2001). Understanding the client's background and context helps physiotherapists make decisions about prioritising treatment goals and establishing evaluation criteria. Working with context includes:

- engaging with family and carers as part of the larger care team involved with decision making and support, but recognising that some clients do not wish to have their families involved and respecting this wish
- if the client is in agreement, asking family or carers if they would like to observe therapy or help with it, to learn how to provide effective ongoing practical support; for example, when treating older dependent clients involve caregivers in procedures of bed mobility and demonstrate how best to support safe ambulation
- educating carers about how to look after themselves; for example, show carers how to protect their backs when helping clients ambulate
- considering clients' circumstances. Factors such as where they live, their work commitments, their financial position and their family environment may have a significant impact on their ability to attend appointments, to commit to exercise

regimens and to feel motivated enough to work through pain when necessary. Talking with clients about their supports and the challenges in their lives can reveal these issues and allow useful discussions about how to take account of them in therapy.

Professional development

A commitment to person-centred practice requires a commitment to ongoing learning. Professional development is considered an important aspect of professionalism. This involves:

- being a reflective practitioner who makes the most of everyday learning opportunities by critically evaluating personal performance, developing alternative methods and putting changes into practice in a person-centred manner
- reassessing personal working methods and interactive styles on the basis of patient feedback
- taking advantage of formal educational opportunities such as workshops, courses and conferences and reading professional journals
- supporting colleagues' learning by sharing knowledge and skills and providing supportive feedback
- engaging in productive discussions about the values that underpin work and, when appropriate, being a champion for these values.

SUMMARY

Developing person-centred relationships is fundamental to providing appropriate, ethical, safe and effective physiotherapy services. Such relationships are fostered not only by technical expertise but also by using responsive communication skills to engage with clients and to create safe spaces for open dialogue that includes family and carers and demonstrates respect for patient autonomy.

Reflective questions

- Think about a time when you were a patient (perhaps a visit to your GP). How did the communication style of the health professional affect your relationship? Did it meet your needs and expectations? What implications might this have for your practice?
- Consider your own style of interaction. Do you favour a directive style or a facilitative and open one? What positives can you build on, and what challenges would you like to address in order to be more person-centred?
- Sometimes clinicians label clients as difficult. What is meant by 'being difficult', and how can a person-centred approach offer solutions to working with these clients?
- Do you know what your clients' biggest concerns about physiotherapy are? If not, how can you find out? How can you make a connection between their concerns/goals and yours?

References

Bauman E A, Fardy H J, Harris P G 2003 Getting it right: why bother with patient-centred care? Medical Journal of Australia 179(5):253–256

Beach M C, Sydarman J, Johnson R L et al 2005 Do patients treated with dignity report higher satisfaction, adherence, and receipt of preventive care? Annals of Family Medicine 3(4):331–338

Best D, Cant R, Ryan S 2001 Exploring relationships in health care practice. In: Higgs J, Titchen A (eds) Professional practice in health, education and the creative arts. Blackwell Science, Oxford, pp 103–114

Ellis E, Trede F 2008 Communicating and the duty of care. In: Higgs J, Ajjawi R, McAllister L et al (eds) Communicating in the health and social sciences, 2nd edn. Oxford University Press, South Melbourne, pp 179–186

Fossum B 2003 Communication in the health service: two examples. Karolinska Institute, Department of Public Health Services, Stockholm

Halpern J 2003 What is clinical empathy? Journal of General Internal Medicine 18:670–674

Innes A, Macpherson S, McCabe L 2006 Promoting person-centred care at the front line, Joseph Rowntree Foundation, York. Available: www.jrf.org.uk/bookshop/eBooks/9781859354520.pdf 21 Oct 2007

McCormack B, McCane T V 2006 Development of a framework for person-centred nursing. Journal of Advanced Nursing 56(5):472–479

Montgomery J 1996 Patients first: the role of rights. In: Fulford K W M, Ersser S, Hope T (eds) Essential practice in patient-centred care. Blackwell Science, Oxford, pp 142–151

Salmon P, Young B 2005 Core assumptions and research opportunities in clinical communication. Patient Education and Counseling 58:225–234

Stewart M 2001 Towards a global definition of patient-centred care. British Medical Journal 322: 444–445

Swenson S L, Zettler P, Lo B 2006 'She gave it her best shot right away': patient experiences of biomedical and person-centred communication. Patient Education and Counseling 61:200–211

Trede F V, Higgs J 2003 Reframing the clinician's role in collaborative clinical decision making: rethinking practice knowledge and the notion of clinician-patient relationships. Learning in Health and Social Care 2(2):66–73

Trede F V, Higgs J 2007 Clinical reasoning and models of practice. In: Higgs J, Jones M, Loftus S et al (eds) Clinical reasoning in the health professions, 3rd edn. Butterworth Heinemann, Oxford, pp 31–41

Williams R 1999 Cultural safety – what does it mean for our work practice? Australian and New Zealand Journal of Public Health, 23(2):213–214

TEAMS AND COLLABORATION IN PHYSIOTHERAPY PRACTICE

twenty

Anne Croker, Julia Coyle and Cheryl Hobbs

Key concepts

- Rationale behind health professionals working together in teams
- Skills that physiotherapists need to collaborate with other health professionals
- Steps that may assist physiotherapists to develop collaborative practices

INTRODUCTION

Physiotherapists commonly work in teams to provide health services to clients. Effective collaboration in teams improves client care, increases levels of job satisfaction and reduces health care costs. Striving for team effectiveness and optimal collaboration is an obvious aim for all health teams; however, teams can be complex and collaboration can be challenging. In this chapter we will discuss issues related to working in health teams and the complexities of working with others, with a particular focus on requirements for effective collaboration between health professionals. We draw upon our research into team practice as the basis for effective teamwork and collaboration.

WORKING IN TEAMS

Due to their varying purposes and contexts, health teams are highly diverse. Health care services increasingly emphasise teams and collaborative practices as a result of the increasing complexity of health care, increased specialisation, an ageing population with co-morbidities, economic rationalisation and a move towards integration of different models of health care. Health teams operate in all parts of the health care system, from acute care to community-based care. Mickan (2005) summarised team effectiveness in terms of the benefits of teams to:

- patients (by enhancing satisfaction and outcomes)
- team members (by providing greater role clarity and enhancing job satisfaction)
- teams (by maximising professional diversity, improving coordination of care and facilitating efficient use of heath care services)
- organisations (by reducing hospitalisation times and unanticipated admissions).

In its broadest sense a health team can be considered to be a collective of individuals, each with a particular role, regularly collaborating for a shared purpose. Broadly, the term *team* can encompass established *formal teams* with regular meetings, temporary *task groups* formed to fulfil a particular goal, and *informal networks* whose members may communicate intermittently.

Readily identifiable differences exist between formal teams, task groups and informal networks. Ideally, formal teams have a clear purpose, leadership, defined membership and established team processes. For example, a brain injury team may use a vision and mission statement to establish shared understanding of the team's purpose, and appoint a team leader to facilitate effective team processes. A temporary task group brings people together for a short period of time for a specific purpose, such as a quality review of client services. Task groups may spend time establishing procedures prior to commencement of the task and may disband after completion (Fried & Rundall 1994). In contrast, an informal network may evolve opportunistically among individuals, and be driven by client caseloads and personal preferences for working with particular people. Although each of these teams differs in structure and processes, all rely on shared purpose, collective responsibility and collaborative practice.

HEALTH TEAM TERMINOLOGY

Increasing emphasis on teams in health has been accompanied by an expansion in terminology used to classify teams. However, the abundance of associated prefixes together with the lack of a shared conceptual framework underpinning their use (Choi & Pak 2006) has the potential to limit the usefulness of such team classifications. Many terms are used in an imprecise, ambiguous manner with different meanings attributed by different authors. In spite of this confusion, three key classifications of teams predominate: *multi-*, *inter-* and *trans-*. Awareness of the meanings commonly attributed to these prefixes can dispel some of the confusion and help physiotherapists to determine the intended meaning.

The prefixes may be used interchangeably to indicate a team composed of different health professional disciplines. When taken to indicate the nature of interactions and roles, these three prefixes tend to form a continuum with *multi-* at one end and *trans-* at the other. Thus multidisciplinary teams involve a group of people representing different disciplines who work sequentially or in parallel within discipline boundaries (Choi & Pak 2006). These teams tend to set their own discipline-specific goals and report or share information. Interdisciplinary teams involve a group of people representing different disciplines who work reciprocally within blurred boundaries to generate new perspectives (Choi & Pak 2006). These teams tend to identify and achieve integrated goals, and may demonstrate components of integrated practice as well as separated practice. Transdisciplinary teams involve a group of people from different disciplines who work in a holistic way and transcend discipline boundaries through role expansion and role release (Choi & Pak 2006). In these teams, one team member may be the client's primary therapist and incorporate aspects of client management/services from other disciplines.

Team descriptors, such as interprofessional (or multiprofessional) and interagency (or multiagency), can also be used to identify *what* is being integrated within the team rather than *how* it is being integrated. For example, the term multiprofessional may be used to indicate the presence of different health professions in the team (such as medical, nursing and allied health). The term multiagency indicates that team members represent different agencies (such as health, education, insurance or legal groups).

CONCEPTUALISING COLLABORATION

Collaboration in health care broadly relates to the process of individuals working with one another to provide client care. The inclusion of different health professional disciplines gives teams wider perspectives on approaches to health care than can be achieved by a single discipline. Collaboration can be conceptualised in terms of three domains: *purpose*, *processes* and *people* (Croker et al 2007a). This conceptualisation provides a framework for physiotherapists to explore the requirements of different collaborative situations.

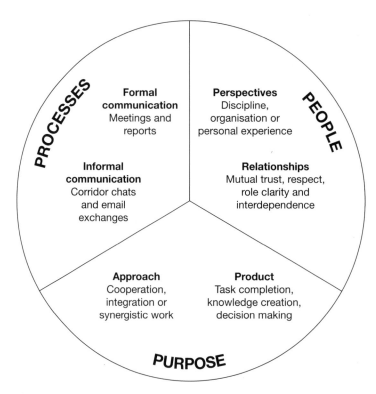

Fig. 20.1 Domains and elements of collaboration. Adapted from Croker et al (2007a)

Collaboration has a *purpose*. The purpose involves creating *products*, such as completing tasks or developing understandings and knowledge to inform decision making, and uses various *approaches* including cooperation, integration and synergistic working. Different products may require different approaches. Coordinating aims and schedules for client treatment may require straightforward cooperation. However, consensus decision making may require complex synergistic interactions in which team members explore issues, contribute their understandings and challenge others' perspectives. Synergistic ways of working enable outcomes to be achieved that are greater than the sum of the individual contributions. Integration is needed when different health professionals are working on overlapping or interrelated areas of patient care. A shared understanding of the purpose of collaboration is important for teams to work together effectively.

Effective collaboration relies on sound communication *processes* that may be *formal* (such as team meetings and written reports) or *informal* (such as corridor chats and email exchanges). Physiotherapists need to be proficient in both formal and informal communication. Whereas formal communication processes are usually easily identifiable and readily accessible, informal communication may be more organic in nature and sensitive to change. The flexibility of informal communication processes can facilitate micro-negotiations between team members and provide opportunities for team members to establish rapport (Ellingson 2003).

People are what collaboration is all about. Although clients and carers are commonly considered part of health teams, this chapter focuses on collaboration between health professionals. Health professionals bring perspectives about the issues under discussion. The development of such perspectives is influenced by a range of factors including: the aims of the organisation; the values, beliefs, attitudes and knowledge of disciplines; and the experience gained from personal and professional life. Collaborative relationships between health professionals are founded on mutual trust and respect, and rely on interdependency and role clarity. Establishing trust and mutual respect is usually associated with positive team experiences and individual team members' confidence in their own abilities and acceptance of other team members' professional competence (Martin-Rodriguez et al 2005).

Sound collaboration in health teams contributes to cohesive client care and involves individuals with various roles interacting with each other to create shared purposes and understandings. These interactions are guided and influenced by formal and informal processes and rely on input from personal and discipline perspectives, together with individual capabilities (Croker et al 2007a). In the following sections we focus on some specific components of collaboration, together with the dimensions of teams and organisations that influence collaboration.

UNDERSTANDING THE COMPLEXITIES OF COLLABORATING IN TEAMS

Collaborative practice is often complex, complicated by human factors (such as personalities, conflicts, different interests and changing team memberships) and organisational factors (such as changing policies). Awareness of such complexities helps physiotherapists to anticipate and minimise collaboration difficulties in team contexts.

Complexities related to roles and relationships

Physiotherapists have client care roles and teamwork roles. Client care roles in teams tend to relate to the team member's discipline and are influenced by the cultural norms of that discipline. Each discipline has a different culture, passed on to new members through a process of socialisation that guides models of care and language (Hall 2005). Different professional cultures can act as barriers to collaboration if team members use discipline-specific jargon or have different priorities and expectations for client care. Professional jealousies and role boundary issues can be barriers to collaboration (Gibbon 1999). Being flexible and adaptive in working relationships, confident in one's professional role and willing to cross boundaries are important for teamwork (Molyneux 2001). Power differences between professions may interfere with effective collaboration (Abramson & Mizahi 2003). Practitioners need to balance their professional autonomy with the interdependence required for collaborative practice (D'Amour et al 2005). Clarity of own roles and responsibilities and respect for the roles of others are important features for interprofessional collaborative practice (Barr 1998).

Team functioning roles are primarily determined by a range of factors including personality, individual abilities, values and motivations, contextual constraints, experience and role learning (Belbin 1993). An appropriate balance of the following team roles contributes to effective team functioning:

- *Co-ordinator* (confident, mature) makes a good chairperson, clarifies goals and promotes decision making.
- *Shaper* (dynamic, motivated, assertive) thrives on pressure and has the drive to overcome obstacles.
- *Plant* (creative, imaginative, unorthodox) solves difficult problems.
- *Resource investigator* (enthusiastic communicator, networker) explores opportunities, develops contacts and finds options.
- *Monitor–evaluator* (strategic, discerning, serious, critical thinker) sees options and makes accurate judgements.
- *Teamworker* (sociable, co-operative, adaptable, diplomat) listens, averts friction and mediates.
- *Implementer* (systematic, reliable, loyal) undertakes practical action and works efficiently.
- *Completer* (conscientious, accurate) looks for errors, has high standards and delivers results on time.
- *Specialist* (dedicated to personal area of expertise) provides particular skills and knowledge (Belbin 1993).

Physiotherapists may find these role categories aid in understanding the interactions in teams and reflecting on their own and others' roles in the team.

Interpersonal relationships between team members often play a supportive role in times of change or challenge. Such support may be needed to deal with problems affecting interpersonal relationships and team functioning. Unusual responses or unexpected reactions to situations may indicate a need for understanding and flexibility or perhaps assistance from supervisors.

Complexities related to communication preferences

Team members often have different preferred ways of interacting. For example, team members may be considered introverts (preferring time to consider issues and preferring written communication to verbal communication), extroverts (energised by others and able to make instant decisions), 'feeling' people (taking time to consider implications for others and valuing harmony in the team) or 'thinking-logical people' (largely unaware of the emotions surrounding issues and relying on logic for decision making) (McKinnon 1998). Awareness of different preferences enables team members to be more flexible with each other.

Conversation styles can also differ (Rehling 2004):

- Overlapping conversational styles can be energetic, spontaneous, sharing, supportive and engaging. This style is well suited to brainstorming situations.
- Turn-taking conversation styles are more suited to polling and establishing consensus. This style is formal, sequential, focused, deliberate and respectful.

If used inappropriately both styles have disadvantages. For example, overlapping styles can be selfish, distracting and dominating, and can lead to incomplete thoughts and frustration, whereas turn-taking can be repetitive and selfish, and lead to serial monologues and withdrawal (Rehling 2004). Awareness and flexibility with regard to different conversation styles enables team members to extend their conversation strategies and use different styles in different situations.

Complexities related to maintaining a collaborative climate

Physiotherapists in the acute sector often work in teams where, for a range of reasons, membership is in a constant state of flux. Professionals may undertake rotations of limited duration as part of their ongoing education; unsynchronised rotations may occur; people may take extended leave; and vacancies may exist, caused by recruitment deficits (Coyle 2008). In situations such as these, changing team membership can create challenges to maintaining a collaborative climate of trust, respect and interdependence. New relationships need to be forged between team members and team processes need to be renegotiated.

Teams commonly progress through various stages of formation: forming (where team members become known to each other, the purpose and rules of the group are established, and roles are assigned), storming (where purpose, roles and team rules are challenged and hidden agendas are revealed), norming (where consensus emerges and the team develops a sense of identity and clarity of roles) and performing (where completion of the previous stages has occurred and the team moves to optimum performance and achievement of purpose) (Tuckman 1965; Tuckman & Jensen 1977). Knowledge of these stages may provide reassurance to team members aiming to establish collaborative practice in new or re-forming teams. Teams undergoing substantial changes in membership may experience different stages of development as the collaborative processes and climate are re-established.

Complexities related to diversity of teams

Health teams have diverse structures and processes, and the nature of collaboration varies between teams. In her doctoral research (Croker et al 2007a), Croker conceptualised such diversity in rehabilitation teams in terms of *arenas for collaboration* (as shown in Fig 20.2). Different arenas of collaboration were identified as *integrated, intersecting* and *hybrid*.

- Individuals in *integrated* arenas work with clear team processes, a specifically appointed team leader and centralised organisational components. Organisational components include an allocated team budget, appointment to a team rather than a discipline department, and a geographical layout providing proximity to other team members. In integrated arenas team leaders tend to take responsibility for managing all team issues including education, team building and social events. Extensive orientation is provided for new members to the team, explaining roles and expectations to help shape their work within the team.
- Health professionals in *intersecting* arenas often have responsibilities to other teams and work without documented team processes or a specifically appointed team leader. These teams do not necessarily have a dedicated budget and are reliant on discipline departments to allocate or rotate representatives to the teams. In intersecting arenas

individuals tend to be oriented to the team by their own discipline, learn team processes 'on the job' and often need to manage competing team and discipline loyalties. Leadership responsibilities are not associated with one individual. For instance, rehabilitation specialists take leadership on clinical issues, whereas leadership for team issues is allocated, shared or claimed when required.

- *Hybrid* arenas combine the characteristics of intersecting and integrated arenas.

The notion of *arenas of collaboration* can be used to assist physiotherapists to recognise the complexity of teams. Such recognition is particularly relevant for navigating entry into new teams and balancing conflicting responsibilities to team and discipline department.

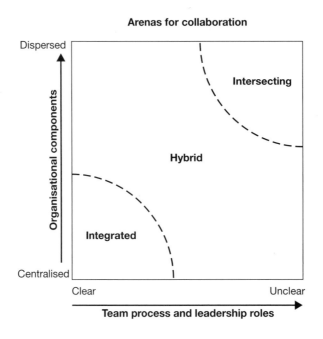

Fig. 20.2 Arenas for collaboration in rehabilitation teams. From Croker et al (2007a)

Complexities related to the dynamic nature of organisations

Collaboration may become even more complex when teams face organisational change and pressures of fiscal accountability. Teams are often required to work within altered organisational structures (such as different lines of management) and comply with new organisational processes (such as new administrative requirements for documenting details of client assessments and care). With increasing reporting requirements, health professionals may need to balance administration's needs for standardised, non-ambiguous, quantifiable information with the team's needs for shared understandings of clients' contexts developed through stories and shared anecdotes. However, teams may also instigate change. Collaborative environments of organisations are not fixed frameworks. Rather, they are frameworks involving people, developed by people, maintained by people and capable of being changed by people (Lawrence & Lorsch 1967). Team members may work with their teams to advocate for changes that are supportive of team collaboration. Teams may seek resources (such as the provision of appropriate time and facilities for team interaction) and opportunities to learn and develop collaborative skills and attributes, and they may pursue horizontal rather than hierarchical organisation structures to facilitate shared decision making (Martin-Rodriguez et al 2005). When advocating for change and negotiating change processes, the combined efforts of the team may be more effective than individual efforts.

TRANSFORMING COLLABORATIVE PRACTICE

The complexities of collaboration present challenges for practitioners transferring between teams with different approaches to collaboration. The ability to transform collaborative practices to suit new situations is an important attribute for health professionals. Croker's research with rehabilitation teams identified a number of *collaborative stepping stones* (Croker et al 2007b) that team members can use to transform collaborative practice to suit changing team membership circumstances. Movement through these steps (see the box below) does not occur in a set sequence and some steps may take longer than others. Steps may also be experienced concurrently.

Collaborative stepping stones

From Croker et al (2007b)

Where I have come from – recognises previous team experiences as the basis for making meaning of the new team

The welcome – involves dealing with the introductions and judgements of new team members

Feeling my way – occurs as understanding of the characteristics of other team members develops and role boundaries are negotiated

Knowing how it works – happens as formal and informal team processes and purposes are identified and understood, and ways of working and interacting are established

Teaming up – involves cultivation of comfortable and constructive relationships with particular members of the team

Moving the mountain – instigates changes to team processes and interactions

---

Awareness of these steps enables new team members to anticipate what may be involved in entering new teams and allows them to be proactive in their interactions with other team members. Current team members may use these steps as a guide for orienting new members, assisting their integration and understanding the perspectives and implementing the processes newcomers may bring to the team. The steps may also provide a guide for reflection on the ability to transform collaborative practice.

EXAMPLES OF EFFECTIVE COLLABORATIVE PRACTICE IN TEAMS

Sam is a first-year physiotherapy graduate who has recently joined a rehabilitation team. She will be working with more experienced physiotherapists, medical practitioners, OTs, speech pathologists, a social worker, nurses and admin staff.

In the following sections we provide examples of insights Sam might gain if she had the opportunity to ask her colleagues about how to collaborate effectively in the team. The quotes used are derived from Croker's (Croker et al 2007a, b) (AC) and Coyle's (2008) (JC) doctoral research, which sought to understand the different dimensions of rehabilitation team practice.

Be secure in your own professional knowledge

You've obviously got to be quite secure in your professional knowledge … it's almost like your foundation isn't it? Then you can afford to let things go, or to experiment or to move boundaries. But if you haven't got that secure base then you won't do that. (AC)

Competence with professional knowledge is important for collaborative practice. When physiotherapists possess sound understanding and confidence in their role it helps other team members to appreciate and value the scope of physiotherapy practice.

Develop an awareness of others' roles

Personally, not having worked well with [other disciplines], not having them on the team, and not really understanding, you get a simplified view of what this profession brings to the team and you think "yeah I can do that …" But once you learn more about it there are a lot of specifics that you weren't aware of. You see it in practice and it makes a huge difference. (JC)

Physiotherapists can develop a deeper awareness of others' roles through working with team members of other disciplines. Without such opportunities there may be a tendency to develop a simplified view of other disciplines' roles.

Respect other's roles

I think people need to be able to step out of their own discipline and think a little bit more about where the other disciplines are coming from. I think that goes a long way in broadening your horizons and approaching the patient as a whole person. (AC)

Understanding others' roles enables physiotherapists to see the scope of what may be brought to client care. It also helps develop a sense of value for the contribution that others make.

See the big picture

Good team players are those who understand more of what's happening, the bigger picture stuff … You know that when they're managing that patient and that patient's getting good overall care. Whereas the less good team players won't see what else should have been done. (JC)

A holistic view provides a better understanding of patient care requirements and the interaction of roles and promotes effective client care.

Be flexibile with discipline role boundaries

I'm quite flexible with boundaries ... I'm quite happy to let [other disciplines] do something that they're able to do, that I could do too. It's all a negotiation process. (AC)

The integration of client care roles between different disciplines often requires practitioners to negotiate blurred discipline boundaries.

Appreciate others' perspectives

It is good to be reminded sometimes that what I see as a good outcome may not necessarily be what the client sees as a good outcome. I need to be aware of what I'm bringing to it, and what others are bringing to it, and what the client wants. So having that diversity actually assists in broadening the perspective. (JC)

Knowledge of others' roles needs to be coupled with understanding of their perspectives. Identifying and understanding the reasons for differing perspectives is the first step in resolving the disagreements.

Be aware of personal communication styles

I'm quite a shy person in a group situation. I'm a bit scared to open my mouth. It probably took me a few months actually to feel comfortable. I guess it still depends on the day what I'm feeling as to whether I feel like opening my mouth. (AC)

Reflection on personal communication styles may help develop effective communication strategies.

Be confident

It is OK to go in and not know everything. That is part of being in the team, having the confidence after a while to say, "I don't know that but I will find out". (JC)

Being able to rely on others is dependent on being able to trust their judgement and advice.

Be aware of the purpose of the communication

Sometimes people can talk about their own discipline for an extensive period of time when we might not need that much information. (AC)

A shared understanding of the purpose of the communication enables team members' input to be appropriate for the situation.

Recognise varying sources of patient information

There are the bare-bones facts of the physio report. And then during discussion there's the colour that fleshes it out, sort of gives it more detail. It is thrown together and gives a more accurate picture. This is important because we're dealing with people in different situations and different environments and it's important for everyone to be aware of the full picture of the patient. I probably pay a bit more attention to the stories than the bare bones. When you hear the stories it's a matter of, "Ahhh, right". (AC)

Stories and anecdotes can convey rich information to other team members.

Communicate in a timely fashion

I'm expecting them to give me a response … It doesn't mean that they have to do it straight away, but I expect that they will let me know when. Generally if I'm not happy with that I can negotiate from there, but I don't want to be sitting around waiting. If it is going to be the end of the week, I would just rather know that it is going to be the end of the week, that's fine. (JC)

Effective team practice depends upon members being able to rely on each other. Communication that supports this reliance is responsive to others' needs, including honesty in relation to the physiotherapist's capacity to meet those needs.

Value interdependence

I think people need to be able to step out of their own discipline and think a little bit more about where the other disciplines are coming from. I think that goes a long way in broadening your horizons and approaching the patient as a whole person. (AC)

Appreciation of others' roles facilitates interdependence. When professional jurisdiction is threatened, health professionals tend to revert to their traditional professional model (Sicotte et al 2002).

Seek opportunities to interact with the team

The tea and coffee loosens up people, so it's like a nice interaction. They share, they cut pieces, they look at each other when you give it to them and say "thank you". So it's like a start of a friendly atmosphere. (AC)

Having regular team events such as morning teas or sharing food during team meetings can help establish rapport among team members. Small teams with fewer people may easily optimise informal opportunities for time together. Large teams with multiple people require additional strategies to increase the time spent together. Aligning rest breaks, seeking opportunities to work with others, and arranging for facilities (e.g. tea rooms) that support interactions among team members are ways of increasing the time that teams spend together.

Keep your eye on the purpose

Someone new can come into the team and they can really grate on you. You think "Oh, I don't like that person", and that can make you not listen to them. I now realise that you can't do that, you have to listen and give that person a chance. I think that's important to respect everyone's role in the team. (AC)

Even when personal relationships between team members are strained, the team should assume a greater importance than personal differences.

Keep it professional

It depends on how personally you take it. I don't get too excited. I'm not always right [laughs], just most of the time [laughs]. Once you have said what you are going to say and you have said it to the right person, if it doesn't change, there is no point getting excited. Over time you realise it is not a personal thing. (JC)

Differences of opinion need not be taken personally, as they are often based on team members' available information and particular points of view rather than personal differences. Exploring differences of opinion often develops increased understandings between team members.

Be flexible and adaptable

With changes of staff and processes and ratios and hours, things changed. We all had to say, "Well just because we did it this way, doesn't mean it's the only way". (AC)

Working within changing parameters can provide opportunities for developing collaborative practice.

Be prepared to suggest appropriate and realistic change

We felt that the medical staff were taking up too much time, and the allied health weren't being given an equal hearing so we did discuss that. Now we go through nursing, all the allied health things and medical is usually last. (AC)

Appropriate feedback and discussions with other team members can facilitate change.

Acknowledge difficulties

We might just pass each other in the corridor and say, "How're you feeling? That was pretty down wasn't it? Yeah, I feel pretty crappy. Well look after yourself, it'll be alright." Make a joke or, you know. Try and have a laugh about something else. It's pretty supportive. (AC)

Acknowledging challenging situations and difficult outcomes may be an important part of interpersonal support.

Celebrate successes

It's nice to hear [positive feedback] from the team. I think it's an important part of keeping things going and keeping people motivated. (AC)

Engaging in informal or formal celebrations of success is important for providing cohesion within a team as well as providing points for reflection to help formulate future practice.

Ongoing development of effective collaborative practice in teams is an important aspect of quality client care. Attention to role clarity and flexibility, good communication and a positive teamwork climate promote the development of effective collaboration in health teams.

SUMMARY

Collaboration in health teams involves team members interacting through formal and informal communication processes to develop shared understandings of purpose, establish goals of treatment and deliver effective client care. During their careers physiotherapists are likely to work in a range of teams in different organisational contexts. They will experience varying degrees of collaboration, team integration and clarity of team processes. The ability to transform teamwork practices to suit different contexts is an important component of professional practice. An understanding of the complexities of health teams and the factors influencing effective teamwork and collaboration enables physiotherapists to further adapt and develop their professional practice to suit the range of team contexts they encounter during their careers.

Reflective questions

- What do you think constitutes effective collaboration in a team?
- What skills do you need to be an effective member of a health team?
- Think about a team you have experienced. What information about that team might new members find useful?
- How could collaborative practice in that team be improved?

References

Abramson J, Mizahi T 2003 Understanding collaboration between social workers and physicians: application of a typology. Social Work in Health Care 37(2):71–100

Barr H 1998 Competent to collaborate: towards a competency-based model for interprofessional education. Journal of Interprofessional Care 12(2):181–187

Belbin M 1993 Team roles at work. Butterworth-Heinemann, Oxford

Choi B, Pak A 2006 Multidisciplinary, interdisciplinary and transdisciplinary in health research, services, education and policy: 1. Definitions, objectives, and evidence of effectiveness. Clinical Investigative Medicine 29(6):351–364

Coyle J, 2008, Unpublished PhD Thesis, Charles Sturt University, Albury, Australia

Croker A, Higgs J, Trede F 2007a What do we mean by 'collaboration' and when is a 'team' not a 'team'?: A qualitative unbundling of terms and meanings. Paper presented at the AQR Conference: Research and the professions, Melbourne, November

Croker A, Higgs J, Trede F 2007b Identifying 'collaborative stepping stones': helping new and existing team members learn to reframe collaborative practice. Paper presented at ANZAME Conference: Linking learners and leaders, Canberra, September

D'Amour D, Ferrada-Videla M, Martin-Rodriguez et al 2005 The conceptual basis for interprofessional collaboration: Core concepts and theoretical frameworks. Journal of Interprofessional Care 19 (Suppl 1):116–131

Ellingson L 2003 Interdisciplinary health care teamwork in the clinic backstage. Journal of Applied Communication Research 31(2):93–117

Fried B, Rundall T 1994 Managing groups and teams. In: Shortell S, Kallunzy A (eds), Health care management: organization design and behaviour. Delmar, New York, pp137–163

Gibbon B 1999 An investigation of interprofessional collaboration in stroke rehabilitation team conferences. Journal of Clinical Nursing 8(3):246–252

Hall P 2005 Interprofessional teamwork: professional cultures as barriers. Journal of Interprofessional Care May(Suppl 1):188–196

Lawrence P, Lorsch J 1967 Differentiation and integration in complex organisations. Administrative Science Quarterly 12:1–47

Martin-Rodriguez L, Beaulieu M, D'Amour D et al 2005 The determinants of successful collaboration: a review of theoretical and empirical studies. Journal of Interprofessional Care 19(Suppl 1), 132–147

McKinnon S 1998 Team play: strategies for successful people management. Lothian Books, Melbourne

Mickan S 2005 Evaluating the effectiveness of health care teams. Australian Health Review 29(2): 211–217

Molyneux J 2001 Interprofessional teamworking: what makes a team work well? Journal of Interprofessional Care 15(1):29–35

Rehling L 2004 Improving teamwork through awareness of conversational styles. Business Communication Quarterly 67(4):475–482

Sicotte C, D'Amour D, Moreault M 2002 Interdisciplinary collaboration within Quebec community health care centres. Social Science and Medicine 55:991–1003

Tuckman B W 1965 Developmental sequences in small groups. Psychological Bulletin 63:384–399

Tuckman B W, Jensen M A C 1977 Stages of small group development revisited. Group and Organizational Studies 2:419–427

WORKING WITH PHYSIOTHERAPY ASSISTANTS

Martin Chadwick and Megan Smith

twenty-one

Key content

- The history of physiotherapy assistants in Australia and New Zealand
- Issues of utilisation of physiotherapy assistants
- Therapeutic relationship between the physiotherapist, assistant and client

INTRODUCTION: WHY ASSISTANTS?

Before we begin a chapter on physiotherapy aides and assistants, a valid question that could be asked is, 'Is there any need for physiotherapy aides or assistants in the provision of physiotherapy services?' This question could be elaborated with 'Can the profession of physiotherapy meet the requirements of the communities it serves with the workforce resources available?' The simple answer to the second question is 'No'. Demand for services provided by the physiotherapy profession in Australia and New Zealand is increasing with the growing populations and changing demographics of both countries (for example, the increased proportion of the aged in our communities). The profession finds itself in a situation where there is an inability to fully meet demand with current resources and the current methods of using those resources.

This situation of unmet current and future demand creates a tension, particularly amid growing acknowledgement of the potential expansion of non-traditional roles for physiotherapy (for example, physiotherapists in emergency departments or acting in 'gatekeeper' roles for specialty services; see also Croft 2006, Kennedy 2006, McClellan et al 2006, Oldemeadow et al 2007). Implementation of such expanded roles for physiotherapists has not lessened the demand for traditional roles of physiotherapy with acknowledgement of the positive impacts of intensive traditional physiotherapy on key indicators such as length of hospital stay (Hauer et al 2002, Jette et al 2005, Kahn et al 2002).

This brings us back to the question posed above: is there a need for physiotherapy aides or assistants in the provision of physiotherapy services? An answer in the affirmative implies that incorporating physiotherapy assistant roles would enhance the provision of physiotherapy services to the community. To approach future physiotherapy service provision with complete dependency on qualified physiotherapists might result in the community being unable to access optimal physiotherapy services. In the short term this might result in a gap in services. In the long term, however, there might be diminution in the scope of physiotherapy practice or encroachment by other professions into what has traditionally been the domain of physiotherapy. Further, there could be the loss of professional opportunities to explore non-traditional roles.

Physiotherapy is not alone in facing this dilemma. There is an acknowledged change in how health care is being delivered within other professions. Cooper (2001) and colleagues (Cooper, Henderson & Dietrich 1998; Cooper, Loud & Dietrich 1998) have examined how the skill mix of health service providers is changing, in particular the increased use of what they termed non-physician clinicians (NPCs). McKinley and Marceau (2006) investigated the future role of the primary care doctor or GP in health care provision and found services currently provided just by GPs can be provided just as effectively and, in most cases, more cheaply by NPCs. Richardson et al (1998) reinforced that a large proportion of GP work could also be delegated to other health professionals.

So there is an understanding that many traditional medical practitioner tasks could be carried out by other professional groupings. Can a similar pattern be identified within physiotherapy and, if so, how should we deal with it? Smith and Roberts (2005) examined the issue of skill mix from multiple perspectives, one of which was the perspective of the end users, patients – how they perceived the care they received and whether they could identify differences among those who provided services to them in a community setting. The authors reported that service users were not always able to distinguish among those providing the services. Does this mean that services could be provided just as effectively in alternative ways? As with doctors, it is appropriate to examine whether alternative skill mixes might be employed when providing physiotherapy services. A way forward is to look at a skill mix that consists of qualified physiotherapists working collaboratively with suitably trained physiotherapy assistants or aides.

The concept of having physiotherapy assistants provide elements of physiotherapy services is not new, having been applied in various forms over the years. Physiotherapy assistants and aides have long been employed in Australia and New Zealand in health care facilities and private practices. However, there has been a lack of consistency in the roles and education of assistants, particularly in relation to the provision of clinical services. The first documentation in New Zealand is from 1981, when the then Department of Health issued a publication titled 'Rules and conduct and training for hospital physiotherapy aides'. Reference was made to this publication in the 1988 'Physiotherapy code of safe practice' (Department of Health 1988). Both documents were referenced by the Ministry of Health in 1989 when a revised document 'Roles and functions of the physiotherapist' included 'Section IV: The physiotherapy assistant'. In these documents attempts were made to clarify how assistants should be employed, trained and utilised. However, concerns persisted about these very points, with concern being minuted at the annual Physiotherapy Hospital Managers' Conference about the training that was in place for physiotherapy assistants. This appeared to be a theme through the 1990s; in 1999 the same group commissioned a survey to more clearly understand how assistants were being utilised in various settings across the country.

These reviews illustrate the continued acknowledgement of the value of assistants in providing physiotherapy services, but it is often not clear how this is managed practically and consistently by the physiotherapy profession. The most recent attempt to address this issue occurred in 2005 when the New Zealand Society of Physiotherapists (NZSP) ratified the document *The physiotherapy assistant*, which attempted to provide some guidance as to expectations of the role and suggested competencies. Australia has followed a similar path, but the outcome has been greater uniformity, with the Australian Physiotherapy Council (APC) providing *Guidelines for physiotherapists working with assistants in physiotherapy practices/services* (APC 2007).

BENEFITS OF A PHYSIOTHERAPIST–ASSISTANT THERAPEUTIC PARTNERSHIP

The attention in recent times to the role of assistants reflects the recognition that there is benefit to be gained from having them as an integral part of physiotherapy service provision. One of these benefits is improved efficiencies in the services that can be provided with a combination of qualified physiotherapists and assistant staff (Saunders 1997a). However, there is a need to examine the nature of physiotherapy services in a given clinical setting, and to consider the optimal skill mix for physiotherapists and assistant staff to provide these services. This matter has received some attention in the literature (Alkinson 1993, Hunter 1999, Richardson 1999, Squires & Hastings 1997, Williams 1991). In some circumstances a shift may occur from a model of clinical service provision by physiotherapists only, with aides and assistants perhaps traditionally engaged in nonclinical activities, to one of physiotherapy service provision by collaboration between physiotherapists and assistant staff. Such a shift may require a revision in the mindset of the parties involved.

ISSUES ASSOCIATED WITH THE USE OF PHYSIOTHERAPY ASSISTANTS

There are a number of issues related to implementing the use of assistants to provide part of clinical care. The physiotherapy profession has documented a number of issues to be considered when implementing and utilising assistant roles, and also offers guidance as to addressing these issues.

Similar themes that need to be considered with regard to utilisation of assistants are:

- relationships between assistants and physiotherapists
- contribution to client-centred service delivery
- contribution to nonclient-centred service delivery.

The relationship between qualified physiotherapists and assistants involves delegation of tasks and supervision of their implementation. The American Physical Therapy Association (APTA) provides clear definitions for supervision, giving three specific levels of increasingly closer liaison between assistants and physiotherapists in providing services:

- general, where the qualified physiotherapist is not required to be on site, but is available for telecommunication at a minimum (e.g. an exercise class in an aged-care facility is devised by a visiting physiotherapist and then implemented by assistants)
- direct, where the qualified physiotherapist is available for direction and supervision, having contact with the client on each visit (e.g. the physiotherapy assistant independently mobilises a patient postsurgery after an assessment has been conducted by a physiotherapist)
- direct and personal, where the qualified physiotherapist is available to continuously direct and supervise any clinical care being performed by the assistant (Cohn 2006)

(e.g. physiotherapists and assistants work collaboratively in a rehabilitation facility to guide patients in their rehabilitation activities, or share tasks such as mobilising patients requiring the assistance of more than one person).

Competency standards for physiotherapy assistants have been addressed internationally. It has been suggested that, as professional staff are held to account to a set of competency standards, so too should assistant staff (Cohn 2006, Mackey & Nancarrow 2005). In 2002 the (UK) Chartered Society of Physiotherapy (CSP) published the 'Physiotherapy assistant code of conduct'. In 2005 the NZSP ratified the document *The physiotherapy assistant*, which includes definitions, roles and responsibilities of all parties, and suggested physiotherapy assistant competencies. Similarly in 2005 the APA board of directors issued a position statement detailing the educational and competency requirements of assistants. Table 21.1 summarises these standards.

Table 21.1 Standards for physiotherapy assistants

NZSP	APA	CSP
Definition: A physiotherapy assistant is a person employed to assist a physiotherapist to provide physiotherapy services in a safe, effective and efficient manner. This assistance may be in the form of patient contact and/or non-clinical activities and in any setting where physiotherapy is provided	**Definition:** A skilled technical health worker who, under the supervision of a physiotherapist, assists in delivering a patient's treatment program. The extent to which the physiotherapy assistant is involved in treatment depends upon the relevant physiotherapists registration act, the policies of the health facility, the direction of the supervising physiotherapist, the needs of the patient, and the capacity of the physiotherapist assistant	**Definition:** Physiotherapy assistants shall only practice to the extent that they have established, maintained and developed their ability to work safely and competently to the tasks delegated to them by chartered physiotherapists
Aspects covered: ■ Roles and responsibilities of the employer ■ Role and responsibilities of the physiotherapy assistant ■ Role and responsibility of the supervising physiotherapist ■ Provision of safe and effective clinical care ■ Effective communication ■ Contribution to a safe working environment ■ Demonstration of individual responsibility and accountability	**Aspects covered:** ■ Education ■ Role and conduct of physiotherapist assistants ■ Supervision ■ Guidelines for their employment	**Aspects covered:** ■ Relationship with physiotherapists ■ Relationship with patients ■ Confidentiality ■ Relationship with professional staff and carers ■ Duty of report ■ Advertising ■ Sales of services and goods ■ Standards of conduct

NZSP: New Zealand Society of Physiotherapists; APA: Australian Physiotherapy Association; CSP: Chartered Society of Physiotherapy, UK.

The APC (2007) made the distinction between a physiotherapy assistant and physiotherapy aide on the basis of education and supervision. An assistant was defined as 'a person who has completed a Certificate IV level qualification in Physiotherapy Assistance, or equivalent training in the vocational sector that is specified and assessed in accordance with the National Health Training Package'. A physiotherapy aide was defined as 'a person who is vocationally trained to perform designated routine tasks related to the operation of a physiotherapy service. A physiotherapy aide will work under the direct supervision of a responsible physiotherapist at all times' (APC 2007, p 1).

Physiotherapists need to be educated as to how to involve assistants effectively, and may need to change their clinical approach from one of providing all portions of the clinical care episode to one where they are managing the care being provided and working in partnership with the assistant (Chadwick 2007, Plack 2006). Effective mechanisms and mutual understanding are needed to determine how care is to be delegated between qualified physiotherapists and assistants (Saunders 1997b). For this to occur safely, it needs to be understood that assistants have not completed the education of physiotherapists, and do not have the clinical reasoning skills that are at the heart of physiotherapy practice (Doumanov & Rugg 2003). Therefore adequate and ongoing supervision is required from professional staff, who must monitor the care being provided, adjust it as necessary, and respond to questions or concerns of assistant staff (Ellis et al 1998, Russell & Kanny 1997).

To provide safe practice, however, requires that assistants monitor the client and understand the expected response to physiotherapy intervention. They will need to make decisions about how to modify their actions and liaise appropriately with the qualified physiotherapist (for example, if mobilising a patient they need to be able to recognise signs of exercise intolerance and to act appropriately). These expectations of assistants are necessarily underpinned by appropriate education and periods of clinical experience gained under the supervision of experienced physiotherapists or assistants. As noted previously the education or training of assistants has been inconsistent, often involving on-the-job training. In Australia the processes of formal education of assistants have progressed with the development of the Vocational Educational and Training Sector Certificate III and IV training and qualifications for physiotherapy and allied health assistants (details of the Australian National Health Training Package for allied health assistants are available at http://www.cshisc.com.au/load_page.asp?ID=234).

Where formal education processes do not exist it has been noted that utilisation of assistants to provide portions of clinical care without sufficient induction into the role, ongoing support and training can lead to dissatisfaction and problems of staff retention. Therefore it has been recommended that initial and ongoing training be considered an integral part of the assistant role (Ellis et al 1998). It would be beneficial if competencies also reflected the need for ongoing learning. It is also suggested that clear definition of task delegation can improve effective utilisation of assistants.

SCOPE OF PRACTICE OF THE ASSISTANT

The scope of practice of physiotherapy assistants is dependent on how they are used to provide services. In traditional models of service where assistants are not used physiotherapists provide the whole episode of care. Having assistants provide portions of clinical care entails a shift to a model where physiotherapists manage rather than directly provide all client care. The importance of a collaborative relationship between clients and physiotherapists is increasingly being recognised. A shift in practice incorporating assistants into a client's management requires that collaboration be expanded to include all parties involved in the client's care. Clients need to provide informed consent for the involvement of assistants in their care and, where payment for services is involved, the impact of care provided by assistants on the cost of services should be discussed.

The components of care potentially provided by a therapeutic partnership between a registered physiotherapist and an assistant can be divided roughly into those that are *skilled* in nature and those that are *prescriptive* in nature (Chadwick 2007). Skilled aspects of care are underpinned by clinical reasoning and judgement. It is this clinical judgement that is at the core of physiotherapists' professional education. Providing care that is skilled in nature, without the necessary underpinning education, is beyond the scope of physiotherapy assistants and would place clients at risk of adverse outcomes. Conversely, elements of care that are prescriptive in nature are necessary to the treatment episode but do not require skills in clinical reasoning. For example, prescriptive tasks may include mobilising a medically stable patient, providing postoperative exercises after total joint replacement, or running a pulmonary rehabilitation class. The scope of practice of assistants could be to provide support tasks and aspects of clinical care that are prescriptive in nature. The distinction between skilled and prescriptive work used here is not meant to imply that the work of assistants is unskilled in nature; rather that physiotherapists are required to retain the overall responsibility for decision making that encompasses a more highly skilled ability to assess and determine optimal interventions. This distinction between the work of physiotherapists and assistants is illustrated in Figure 21.1.

The assistant's responsibilities as an employee

Assistants' responsibilities reflect that they function in a therapeutic relationship with physiotherapists and clients. They provide services delegated by qualified physiotherapists who maintain ongoing supervision. Communication between physiotherapists and assistants is essential, and responsibility lies with assistants to inform physiotherapists of a client's status to allow any necessary changes in the plan of care. There must be clear understanding that physiotherapists retain overall management of the client's care, and any change in the client's status must be notified to the physiotherapist to inform further clinical decisions.

The physiotherapist's responsibilities as a supervisor

The therapeutic partnership between physiotherapist and assistant requires that the delegation of tasks is clear, and that appropriate supervision and professional oversight are occurring. A training program for assistants needs to be in place, to initiate assistants into the role and to provide ongoing training and skill development. Training is also warranted for physiotherapists if they have not had previous experience of working with assistants. This preparation helps to ensure a smooth transition to the alternative model of service delivery and allows services to be maximised.

Professional oversight

Physiotherapists remain ethically and legally responsible for all aspects of the care being provided. The onus remains on physiotherapists to interact frequently with their client and the assistant to determine the client's status and to adjust the care plan as necessary. Professional oversight also requires physiotherapists to ensure that assistants

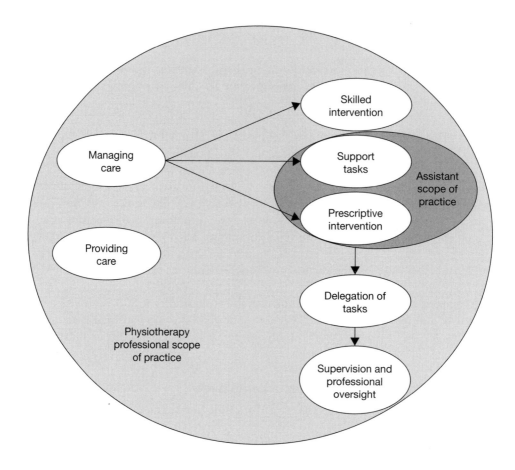

Fig. 21.1 Scope of practice of physiotherapists and physiotherapy assistants

act in a manner that protects the safety of clients and themselves. Any observed breach requires immediate intervention by the physiotherapist.

Prescriptive intervention

Managing client care includes determining which components of clinical care do not require a physiotherapist's clinical judgement and can be provided safely and effectively by an assistant. Clinical judgement is central to physiotherapy practice. It would be expected that assistants report frequently to physiotherapists about client status, to assist the physiotherapist to make judgements about progressing any established plan of care. The provision of prescriptive portions of clinical care should not be seen as a substitute for the evaluation or assessment of clients that is usually undertaken by physiotherapists.

Physiotherapists' decisions about which tasks are prescriptive in nature and appropriate to be carried out by assistants are influenced by factors that include the skill and experience of the assistant, the physiotherapist's knowledge of the client, and the physiotherapist's knowledge of the relative skill level of the assistant. These aspects contribute to the ongoing clinical judgements made by physiotherapists to determine what can be considered prescriptive and delegated safely to the assistant.

Delegation

Specific delegation of tasks to an assistant cannot occur until a decision has been made by the physiotherapist as to what are the prescriptive aspects of care. Delegation implies clear communication between physiotherapists and assistants about what is being delegated, and within which parameters the care is being delegated. The process could involve verbal review of clients and their problems and tasks that the assistant is to perform. This verbal review should also be reinforced with written documentation that provides sufficient information to inform and guide the assistant about the specific tasks to be performed. Information should include detail of the specific tasks to be carried out and their intensity, frequency and duration. Any delegation needs to be done with full knowledge of appropriate legislation and cognisance of any potential limitations in services that may be provided by a registered physiotherapist versus a nonregistered assistant.

Supervision

Once tasks have been delegated, ongoing supervision needs to be in place. The definitions of supervision provided by APTA (general, direct, and direct and personal) highlight that general supervision may be the only practicable expectation on an ongoing basis if tasks are within the scope of the assistant. This should not negate the need for communication between physiotherapists and assistants to be frequent and planned. Because physiotherapists retain overall responsibility for the care provided it is reasonable to expect daily interaction between physiotherapists and assistants about client status, to allow for adjustments to the care plan. Face-to-face interactions between physiotherapists and assistants should not negate the need for appropriate documentation to occur, detailing the tasks performed by assistants. This provides a record for physiotherapists about tasks carried out by assistants and also reinforces adjustments in the care plan communicated to assistants.

Support tasks

Support tasks do not involve direct clinical contact with clients, but still assist implementation of the clinical care episode. Examples include administrative tasks, preparation tasks, and tasks following the clinical encounter. Preparation for the clinical encounter is often time-consuming and may not be skilled in nature. Using assistants for these tasks can unburden physiotherapists to be more focused on the clinical encounter. This is also true for tasks following the clinical encounter and administrative tasks.

IMPLEMENTING A PHYSIOTHERAPIST–ASSISTANT MODEL TO PROVIDE CLINICAL SERVICES

The remaining section of this chapter examines frameworks that need to be in place for clinical services using physiotherapist–assistant partnerships to provide an acceptable standard of client care.

Induction of physiotherapists

Induction must include appropriate education for physiotherapists as to the roles and responsibilities of both parties. This should include the points raised in the previous section, with a particular focus on the concept of professional oversight, insofar as the physiotherapist remains ultimately responsible for care provided to clients and assistants cannot be used as substitutes. As noted, physiotherapists' education has at its core the concept of clinical reasoning; assistants do not have this skill as part of their training, and this is a primary factor distinguishing aspects of care that can and cannot be provided by assistants. It is important for physiotherapists and assistants to discuss their levels of education and competency during the induction process, as it forms the basis of developing understanding and trust between physiotherapists and assistants.

Induction of assistants

The primary difference between the induction of physiotherapists and that of assistants is that assistants may come to the role without any previous training. In Australia this may become less likely, as expectations of completion of level III and IV certificate courses become increasingly mandated. Where formal education has not been completed the onus is on employers to employ individuals who possess an appropriate skill set for likely success in the role, and then to provide training that lays the foundation for success in the conduct of their duties. Training of assistants must cover the points raised in the previous section, such as the basis of the therapeutic relationship and trust between physiotherapist and assistant. The focus of this initial training is to convey that the physiotherapist retains ultimate responsibility for the care provided, and any care provided is done on that basis.

Maximising the therapeutic partnership

Although there is no definitive guide as to the ideal ratio of physiotherapists to assistants, it has been suggested that a model of three physiotherapists to one assistant maximises efficiency (Saunders 1997a). This ratio provides sufficient professional staff to generate the prescriptive and supportive tasks needed for an appropriate workload for an assistant. The challenge of this model is for physiotherapists to communicate clearly to assistants and for different physiotherapists not to provide contradictory instructions.

Details of prescriptive care allocated to assistants should be communicated in multiple formats. There should be in place a system for a verbal handover to occur about each client, a brief history and description of the prescribed tasks that the physiotherapist is requesting the assistant to perform. This handover should include precautions the assistant should be aware of, as well as guidelines as to when the assistant should contact the physiotherapist should the client's status fall outside accepted parameters. This verbal handover should be further reinforced with entries in the client's notes detailing the prescriptive tasks as well as these acceptable parameters. A necessary legal requirement would also be that both parties, physiotherapists and assistants, record the client's consent to the use of an assistant and their subsequent actions in the client's notes.

Physiotherapists should implement an appropriate system that establishes the relationship between client, assistant and themselves. They also need a system for maintaining oversight of clients and the care being provided. The system for maintaining oversight varies according to the location in which care is provided, and may be as simple as a daily catch-up with the assistant in an inpatient setting, or involve establishing a formal client review meeting between physiotherapist and assistant on a regular basis, with time allocated to review all relevant clients and examine their progress. A process for communicating with the client directly also needs to be determined in advance, to enable the client to be actively engaged in the management provided by the physiotherapist–assistant partnership. A dedicated time for meeting is opportune for reviewing established plans of care and adjusting them appropriately. Any adjustments to care must be communicated and recorded to provide adequate guidance for assistants.

Initial and ongoing evaluation of clients requires clinical reasoning skills and it is important that these tasks be carried out by physiotherapists. It may be appropriate for assistants to undertake collation of data, which should be done in a way that assists but does not substitute for the physiotherapist.

Building and maintaining the therapeutic partnership

Once a therapeutic partnership has been established between physiotherapists and assistants, continuation of this relationship requires ongoing maintenance strategies. Although physiotherapists in Australia and New Zealand are under regulatory requirements to maintain their competence through continuing professional development, there is currently no such requirement for assistants. It is, however, in the best interests of all that effort is put into maintaining the skill set of assistants. Although the degree of formal training of assistants varies, there is much that can be learned via on-the-job training, and appropriate training schemes should be established. Similarly, it should not be assumed that physiotherapists can maintain high levels of efficiency in a physiotherapist–assistant therapeutic relationship, and time and training should be dedicated to maintaining efficiency on an ongoing basis.

PREPAREDNESS FOR THE FUTURE

The primary premise in writing this chapter is that the immediate future of the physiotherapy profession in Australia and New Zealand is inextricably linked to the promotion and increased usage of physiotherapy assistants. Concerns with this process have been detailed in this chapter, but there are further concerns that need to be monitored should this continue to be the path taken by the physiotherapy profession. In the USA the role of the 'physical therapy assistant' (PTA) has been formalised into a two-year diploma program from which assistants graduate with an 'associate degree'. This has led to a quandary of licensure, with some states requiring licensure and others not, and concerns have arisen as to where professional boundaries between physiotherapists and PTAs begin and end. The result has been creation of the term 'paraprofessional' to refer to PTAs (Packard 1997). Simplistically, a body of people has been created who exhibit many of the hallmarks of a profession but who are not considered to have a profession in their own right, instead falling under the umbrella of the physical therapy profession. This is an issue that APTA continues to grapple with. Although there is an identified need for a degree of standardisation in the education of assistants, it needs to be done in a way that avoids confusion about the roles of physiotherapist and assistant.

As already stated, moving to a therapeutic partnership model between physiotherapists and assistants requires in many instances a change in culture as to the way care is provided. Perhaps the greatest potential for culture change to occur is in the education of the next generation of physiotherapists. In New Zealand, undergraduate programs do not readily educate students about the concept and skills of delegation (Chadwick 2007). Adjusting curricula to include such concepts would place graduates in a better position to operate in an environment where physiotherapists are managers of the care provided. Doing so in the initial stages of education would create the groundwork that could be carried through future graduates' professional careers.

Lastly, if the described therapeutic partnership becomes an integral component of the provision of physiotherapy services, there is a need to sustain this new arrangement. Training for both physiotherapists and assistants in how to maintain the efficiency of this partnership should be ongoing, especially for those who have had to undergo a change process to integrate assistants into the provision of the supportive and prescriptive components of care. This has been detailed in the section on building and maintaining the therapeutic partnership, but is emphasised here as an important component of preparing the profession for the future.

SUMMARY

The profession of physiotherapy in both Australia and New Zealand is facing a health care environment where the potential demand for services may well outstrip the ability to provide them. In both countries the role of assistants has varied over time, but more recently there has been a concerted effort to consolidate it and clarify what a physiotherapist–assistant–client collaboration might look like. There is a need for clear understanding of components of the relationship such as delegation, supervision and professional oversight, as well as of the concepts of supportive and prescriptive tasks. Operating within the bounds of these concepts offers much potential for the partnership to meet the need for physiotherapy services.

Reflective questions

- Why is it important to examine the role of assistants in providing services?
- What are the potential issues around utilisation of assistants?
- Describe the key concepts required for a successful therapeutic relationship between physiotherapist, assistant and client.
- What are potential issues around increased utilisation of assistants in providing clinical care?

References

Alkinson K 1993 Reprofiling and skill mix: our next challenge. British Journal of Occupational Therapy 56(2):67–69.

APA 2005 Physiotherapy assistant competency development. Available: http://apa.advsol.com.au/independent/documents/submissions/Lawson May05.pdf 13 Nov 2007

APC 2007 Guidelines for physiotherapists working with assistants in physiotherapy practices/services. Available: http://www.physiocouncil.com.au/file_folder/APCGUIDELINESFORASSISTANTS 18 February 2008.

Chadwick M 2007 The feasibility of the role of the allied health assistant in the rural health delivery model. Available: https://www.nzirh.org.nz/content/682c98be-789c-4891-aa09-b1c803e557a3.html 13 Nov 2007

Chartered Society of Physiotherapy 2002 Physiotherapy Assistants Code of Conduct. Chartered Society of Physiotherapy (UK) Available: http://www.csp.org.uk/uploads/documents/csp_assistants_code_conduct.pdf

Cohn R 2006 Supervision and use of physical therapy personnel. PT Magazine January:60–62

Cooper R A, Henderson T, Dietrich C L 1998 Roles of non-physician clinicians as autonomous providers of patient care. JAMA 280(9):795–802

Cooper R A, Loud P, Dietrich C L 1998 Current and projected workforce of non-physician clinicians. JAMA 280(9):788–794

Cooper R A 2001 Healthcare workforce for the 21st century: the impact of non-physician clinicians. Annual Review of Medicine 52:51–61

Croft K L 2006 How does a full time physiotherapy service in the emergency department influence patient flow? New Zealand Society of Physiotherapists Conference free paper presentation, Auckland

Department of Health 1988 Physiotherapy code of safe practice. Wellington, NZ

Doumanov P, Rugg S 2003 Clinical reasoning skills of occupational therapists and support staff: a comparison. International Journal of Therapy and Rehabilitation 10(5):195–203

Ellis B, Cornell M A D, Ellis-Hill C 1998 Role, training and job satisfaction of physiotherapy assistants. Physiotherapy 84(12):608–616

Hauer K, Specht N, Schuler M et al 2002 Intensive physical training in geriatric patients after severe falls and hip surgery. Age and Ageing 31:49–57

Hunter A 1999 Skill mix for the millennium. Physiotherapy 85(1):4–5

Jette D U, Latham N K, Smout R J et al 2005 Physical therapy interventions for patients with stroke in inpatient rehabilitation facilities. Physical Therapy 85(3):238–248

Kahn S, Kahn A, Feyz M 2002 Decreased length of stay, cost savings and descriptive findings of enhanced patient care resulting from an integrated traumatic brain injury programme. Brain Injury 16(6):537–554

Kennedy M 2006 Role redesign in the emergency department. Australian Physiotherapy Association National Congress invited speaker address, Melbourne, May

Mackey H 2004 An extended role for support workers: the views of occupational therapists. International Journal of Therapy and Rehabilitation 11(6):259–266

Mackey H, Nancarrow S 2005 Assistant practitioners: issues of accountability, delegation and competence. International Journal of Therapy and Rehabilitation 12(8):331–338

McClellan C M, Greenwood R, Benger J R 2006 Effect of an extended scope physiotherapy service on patient satisfaction and outcome in an adult emergency department. Emergency Medical Journal 23:384–387

McKinley J B, Marceau L 2006 When there is no doctor: reasons for the disappearance of primary care in the US during the early 21st century. Unpublished paper

Ministry of Health 1989 Roles and functions of the physiotherapist. Wellington, NZ

NZSP 2005 The physiotherapy assistant. Wellington, NZ

Oldemeadow L B, Bedi H S, Burch H T et al 2007 Experienced physiotherapists as gatekeepers to hospital orthopedic outpatient care. Medical Journal of Australia 186(12):625–628

Packard B J 1997 A course correction: reconsidering the role of the PTA. PT Magazine 12:46–54

Plack M M 2006 Collaboration between physical therapists and physical therapists assistants: fostering the development of the preferred relationship within a classroom setting. Journal of Physical Therapy Education 20(1):3–13

Richardson G, Maynard A, Cullum, N et al 1998 Skill-mix changes: substitution or service development? Health Policy 45(2):119–132

Richardson G 1999 Identifying, auditing and implementing cost-effective skill-mix. Journal of Nursing Management 7:265–270

Russell K V, Kanny E M 1997 Use of aides in occupational therapy practice. American Journal of Occupational Therapy 52(2):118–124

Saunders L 1997a A systematic approach to delegation in outpatient physiotherapy. Physiotherapy 83(11):582–589

Saunders L 1997b Issues involved in delegation to assistants. Physiotherapy 83(3):141–147

Smith S, Roberts P 2005 An investigation of occupational therapy and physiotherapy roles in a community setting. International Journal of Therapy and Rehabilitation 12(1):21–29

Squires A, Hastings M 1997 Physiotherapy and older people: calculating staffing need. Physiotherapy 83(2):58–64

Williams J 1991 Calculating staffing levels in physiotherapy services. PAMPAS, Rotherham, Yorkshire

EVALUATION AND MANAGEMENT

SELF-MANAGEMENT: MANAGING YOURSELF AS A PHYSIOTHERAPIST

Anne Croker, Miriam Grotowski and Megan Smith

twenty-two

Key concepts

- Importance of self-care for physiotherapists
- Importance of balancing professional and personal life
- Strategies for self-determination at work
- Ways to nourish sustainable professional practice

INTRODUCTION

Physiotherapy is a rewarding profession that requires ongoing development of professional skills and self-management. Approaches to self-management include applying principles of self-care, establishing an appropriate equilibrium between work and personal life, and avoiding the harmful effects of stress. In this chapter we explore ways in which physiotherapists can manage the dynamic balance between professional life and personal life, and we discuss strategies for nourishing sustainable physiotherapy practice.

PHYSIOTHERAPIST: A PROFESSIONAL AND A PERSON

Self-care and self-determination are important aspects of self-management. Self-care facilitates the promotion of wellbeing in all aspects of professional and personal life. Self-determination enables physiotherapists to manage and shape their professional circumstances and to make decisions that facilitate alignment of personal needs with employment requirements.

Self-care as a basis for looking after self

By being aware of *self*, the physiotherapist is well placed to look after others and develop a model of sustainable professional practice that is responsive to changes occurring in professional and personal situations. *Self* refers broadly to the *whole of what makes up the entity called 'me'* (Longman 2007) and incorporates physical, emotional, social, intellectual and spiritual components; as follows:

- **Physical.** Physiotherapists are familiar with many aspects of optimising physical wellbeing, including physical fitness, adequate nutrition, sleep hygiene, workplace safety and avoidance of substance abuse. Although the need for attention to physical fitness, adequate nutrition and sufficient sleep may seem self-evident, in busy times these are often neglected as much by physiotherapists as by others. Adequate sleep is an important aspect of self-management, as work overload is associated with poor sleep quality (Knudsen et al 2007) and inadequate sleep affects concentration and can lead to poor decision making and errors on the job (Dawson & Reid 1997). For those whose job requires long working hours, catch-up sleep, as well as leisure and time-out from work, are important (van Hooff et al 2007).

- **Emotional**. Self-reflection, time-out and relaxation are important aspects of emotional wellbeing. There are also benefits in developing the ability to acknowledge and manage personal emotions, recognise emotions in others and handle relationships well (Goleman 1996).
- **Social**. People who identify with social groups of family, friends or workmates tend to have a higher self-esteem and reduced stress (Haslam et al 2005). Such groups can provide a supportive network. They may be based around sport, work, community, craft or religion. Being nurtured and rejuvenated by interactions with a range of people, both within and outside the profession, are beneficial ways of dealing with stress.
- **Intellectual**. Attention to professional development is an important component of being a physiotherapist, and physiotherapists have many opportunities for intellectual development within their profession. However it is also important to recognise that a range of other opportunities exists for intellectual development, such as music and literature.
- **Spiritual**. The meaning and nature of spirituality are inherently individual. For many people, time to reflect is an important aspect of maintaining work, personal and social balance: 'Above all give yourself time for reflection and consideration of the broader issues of life. The ultimate aim must be to live with yourself and the values which are eternal' (Connor 1998, p 81).

Self-determination as an approach to professional lives

Self-determination refers to the concept of individuals having the ability to shape their situation and direction through the choices they make. Self-determination underpins many aspects of how physiotherapists function as professionals at work.

Thriving at work

The notion of thriving at work provides a conceptualisation of self-determination in the workplace. This notion was described by Spreitzer et al (2005, p 538) as 'the joint action of vitality and learning, which communicates a sense of progress or forward movement in one's self development'. Thriving at work is facilitated by organisational components and individual attributes: organisational components incorporate structures that support agency in decision making, broad information sharing, and a climate of respect and trust; individual attributes include the abilities to explore new ideas and strategies, relate to others, and understand personal roles as well as the roles of others (Spreitzer et al 2005). Facilitation of organisational change, together with improvement of personal capacities for innovation and interpersonal interactions, enable physiotherapists to develop and thrive at work.

Assertiveness

Assertiveness is also related to the concept of self-determination. Skills in assertiveness may contribute to effective work relationships by facilitating greater control over challenging interpersonal situations. The following points (based on Ali et al 2002) provide examples of the use of assertive statements in communication:

- Factual statement – a straightforward statement that provides facts and makes wishes, needs, wants and opinions clear (e.g. 'I'd like to request a roster change.')
- Empathetic statement – a statement demonstrating sensitivity (e.g. 'Although I can see you are busy … ') that can be used to pre-empt an antagonistic person, followed by a straightforward statement (e.g. '… there is something I'd like to discuss …')
- Divergent statement – a statement establishing a difference between what was agreed and what is happening (e.g. 'We said we would schedule client appointments on a half-hourly basis. They appear to be scheduled every 15 minutes. We need to establish them as we agreed.')
- Expressive statement – A statement expressing negative feelings that lets people know the effect of their behaviour (e.g. 'When you arrive late I feel annoyed that you aren't available to assist.')
- Consequent statement – A statement that warns of a consequence of behaviour (e.g. 'I won't be able to implement this new treatment method unless I can attend the workshop.')
- Responsive statement – A statement or question that elicits others' views to make sure there is clear understanding (e.g. 'I'd like to know what you think about that.')

Change

Advocating for change and implementing change also relate to self-determination. Whether change is chosen or imposed, an understanding of change management processes can enable physiotherapists to be involved and assist in a smooth transition for themselves and those around them. Important behaviours for those advocating change include recognising the 'core' issue that needs to be tackled, being clear in direction and purpose, working creatively with key people who can assist with implementation of change, communicating with and involving all stakeholders, and using the ability to implement change wisely so that the cost does not outweigh the benefit.

Physiotherapists can develop the ability to advocate and implement change through experience and reflection on processes and outcomes. The following principles provide a useful guideline for implementing change (Fisher 2005):

- Position the change in relation to the past – recognise the good and bad elements of the past; understand what needs to be 'let go of'; mourn the loss; recognise the need for change; move towards closure; and then start to establish the new future.
- Use the present to lay the building blocks for the future – encourage discussion of the current situation; establish the need for change; identify the way forward; and develop a plan to move forward.
- Create an achievable, meaningful vision for the future – allow people the chance to internalise the vision; explore new ways of working within the new vision; understand the new situation and where people will fit.

- Centre implementation strategies around the people who will be affected by the change – communicate the nature, reasons, implications, timeline and roadmap for the change; involve all people affected by the change; encourage ownership of the change; ensure adequate infrastructure and resources; and celebrate success along the way.

APPLYING SELF-MANAGEMENT SKILLS TO DAY-TO-DAY WORK

Efficient management of daily tasks and situations in the workplace enables physiotherapists to spend more time with clients. Generic self-management skills provide a useful guide for developing and maintaining efficiency and a positive attitude to people and to paperwork. Such skills involve sorting and prioritising tasks, managing information, utilising others' strengths, developing skills to deal with difficult people or challenging situations, and managing your career. Hints for how to manage day-to-day tasks and situations are outlined in Table 22.1. Although these hints are relevant for all times, they may be particularly useful in situations when physiotherapists are overwhelmed by daily tasks and challenged by high workloads and limited resources.

Table 22.1 Self-management hints. Based on *Successful manager's handbook*, 2002, by M Ali et al, Dorling Kindersley	
Sort tasks	■ Separate important tasks from less important ones ■ Decide which can be put on hold or delegated ■ Prioritise accordingly
Manage information	■ Develop systems – have a good way (for you) to organise your paperwork and electronic information ■ Remember that different systems suit different people ■ Aim to handle correspondence once
Utilise others' strengths	■ Identify others who can guide and support you in situations that are outside your current professional capabilities ■ Share insights with others ■ Form productive relationships
Develop skills to deal with difficult people	■ Be objective, recognise your own biases and assumptions ■ Prepare by brainstorming their objections and planning responses ■ Listen before responding ■ Know when to stop ■ Take the emotion out of the issue ■ Explore and negotiate and agree on solutions ■ Deal with conflict or use mediation ■ Seek professional mediation to resolve conflict (if necessary)
Manage your career	■ Assess your current career position and explore options ■ Identify the need for change and know when to move on ■ Broaden your skills and knowledge base ■ Develop and maintain a network of contacts and connections, including mentors ■ Monitor scope and opportunities within physiotherapy

Self-management also requires physiotherapists to consider the physical nature of their work. Although physiotherapists are trained to prevent injury, the nature of physiotherapy practice leads to increased risk of musculoskeletal injury to oneself. For example, in a study of physiotherapists from Victoria, Australia, Cromie et al (2001) found that 91% experienced a work-related musculoskeletal disorder. Of those experiencing problems, one out of six was forced to make career changes as a result.

Cromie et al noted that the majority of the disorders related to the low back, neck, upper back, thumb, shoulder, wrist and hand. The workplace factors that were associated with these problems were the performance of repetitive tasks, sustained and awkward postures, insufficient rest breaks and performing manipulation and mobilisation techniques. Cromie et al devised guidelines for practice based on their review of the literature and their own work. These guidelines emphasise the importance of adopting proactive self-management approaches rather than waiting for problems to arrive (see the box below).

Guidelines for physiotherapy practice to reduce work-related musculoskeletal disorders

Adapted from Cromie et al (2001)

1. Familiarise yourself with the requirements of the legislation governing occupational health and safety (and in particular manual handling). Know and apply the principles of risk management and be able to apply hazard identification, risk assessment, control and review procedures in your workplace.
2. Identify factors in your workplace and away from work that increase your risk of injury.
3. Evaluate the design of your workplace and facilitate the implementation of established ergonomic guidelines for space, equipment, furniture and environmental conditions.
4. Organise your daily work to ensure variety in the physical demands of work. This may be done by:
   - scheduling different activities throughout the working day and week, and including a variety of techniques and treatment options into therapy sessions
   - scheduling adequate and regular rest breaks and involving a change in posture as well as activity level
   - seeing a range of clients with various conditions
   - participating in policy development in health care to ensure reasonable workloads and adequate work environments
   - increasing the range of treatment techniques at your disposal, aiming for variety in physical demands.
5. Be aware of the types and location of mechanical aids and equipment relevant to your work. Ensure that you have been trained in their correct use and promote their use in your daily work.
6. Access training in injury prevention that contains the risk management model of controlling risk and includes 'in principle' preventive measures rather than training in specific methods or techniques.
7. Engage in ongoing risk assessment and control. Review these for their effectiveness and modify risk control strategies when necessary, either through your actions or by promoting changes at an institutional level.
8. Recognise the physical demands and constraints of the job. Choose career paths that are congruent with your physical ability. Maintain an appropriate level of personal fitness for your work.

ALIGNING PERSONAL NEEDS AND EXPECTATIONS WITH EMPLOYMENT PARAMETERS

A sound understanding of employment parameters and one's personal situation provides guidance for physiotherapists in their choice of suitable employment. Identification of workplace parameters can be considered in terms of articulated and unarticulated aspects of work, such as those shown in Table 22.2. These parameters can then be balanced against personal employment needs and the expectations of employers.

The broad nature of these employment parameters may result in situations where the needs and expectations of employers are inconsistent with the personal needs of employees. Maintaining congruence between personal and employer needs may require ongoing consideration. When employer parameters and employee needs begin to diverge, action is required. Depending on the nature of the divergence such action may proceed in a variety of ways and may involve various levels of complexity. At one end of the spectrum, simple clarification of expectations may be all that is required, whereas at the other end of the spectrum a solution may require ongoing negotiation and mediation. Ideally a mutually beneficial solution will be reached. However, when this is not possible alternative employment may be considered. The following scenarios are examples of different employment situations with different outcomes.

Scenario 1

Requiring clarification and negotiation

Whispers of impending reductions in staffing levels throughout the hospital left physiotherapists concerned about the implication for physiotherapy services. They clarified the situation with management and were told that holiday relief positions were being abolished. However, on further questioning it was revealed that funding would be made available for allied health locum positions. The physiotherapists planned their holidays in advance and applied for this source of funding.

Scenario 2

Requiring change

A physiotherapist found that increasing workloads required him to continually stay behind to do paperwork. This situation created a problem with childcare pick-up times. Following clarification and discussion with his practice manager the physiotherapist realised that such overtime had become an unarticulated, though non-negotiable, expectation of his employer. Reviewing his situation the physiotherapist decided that his current situation was not compatible with family life and he sought alternative employment.

At times physiotherapists may encounter situations in the workplace that challenge personal, moral and ethical viewpoints. Such challenges need to be acknowledged. Consideration of attitudes, biases and cultural perspectives may be a good starting point for such acknowledgement. Further reflection and discussion with colleagues can provide greater insight, acceptance of a situation or, if appropriate, alternative action.

NOURISHING SUSTAINABLE PRACTICE

One of the primary aims of self-management for physiotherapists is to nourish sustainable practice. This includes managing stress and avoiding burnout.

Table 22.2 What physiotherapists need to know about where they work		
	Articulated	**Unarticulated**
Organisation	■ Aim of service provision ■ Management structure ■ Lines of reporting ■ Practice philosophy of employers	■ Problems within the system ■ How to 'get around' the system ■ Pressure for efficient/speedy patient management and discharge
Working conditions	■ Hours and conditions of work ■ Roster obligations ■ Annual leave ■ Staff replacement for leave	■ Expectations regarding finishing work and overtime ■ Attitudes to taking holidays
Service provision	■ Job description ■ Expectations of role ■ Time available for patient consultations ■ Expectations of number of consultations per day ■ Expectations of roles of others ■ After hours service ■ Referrals	■ Gaps and overlaps in roles ■ Prioritising of patients ■ Informal referral networks
Communication	■ Patient records ■ Meetings ■ Administration requirements ■ Lines of communication within the organisation ■ Lines of communication with external agencies	■ Opportunistic opportunities for communication ■ Networks (for service provision or support) ■ Priority of meetings versus patient care
Colleagues	■ Department or unit staff ■ Communication networks ■ Line management	■ Individual characteristics of staff ■ Preferences for communication methods ■ Availability of experienced and knowledgeable staff who are willing to provide guidance
Professional development	■ Regular events ■ Assistance with expenses ■ Access to off-site opportunities	■ Attitudes to time-out for professional development ■ Expectations for covering expenses ■ Expectations for professional development in own time

Stress and burnout

Burnout is a stress syndrome common in people-related professions. Burnout usually results from prolonged stress and is commonly conceptualised in terms of emotional exhaustion, dehumanisation of clients, and perceptions of diminished personal accomplishment (Cordes and Dougherty 1993). Cordes and Dougherty explained that people experiencing emotional exhaustion described feeling that their emotional resources were used up. They dreaded the thought of having to turn up to work, and they were unable to keep being responsible for others and giving of themselves at the same time. Younger employees, particularly those with high expectations and high work involvement, who have work as a central life interest, may be more likely to experience emotional exhaustion than more experienced employees. People experiencing depersonalisation may treat their clients as objects rather than people, interact in a detached or callous manner, display cynicism towards others, and withdraw from engaging with co-workers (Cordes & Dougherty 1993). The component of diminished personal accomplishment is characterised by negative evaluations of one's own ability, and feelings of inadequacy and lack of achievement in work or interactions with others. Ongoing stress may also lead to a range of related conditions such as the inability to work, relationship breakdown or financial difficulties, and to illnesses such as anxiety, depression, alcohol and substance abuse, or even to suicide.

Strategies for managing stress

Stress in the workplace may be unavoidable. However, stress can usually be managed, and in this way burnout can be avoided. Active coping strategies commonly involve reflective practice, accessing mentoring, sharing experiences with others, being assertive, exploring options and being creative with solutions. In the following scenario, the emotional exhaustion apparent in the physiotherapist indicates that she is at risk of emotional exhaustion unless strategies to deal with the condition are implemented.

Scenario 3a

At risk of burnout

A physiotherapist works on a busy hospital ward. Her workload involves a long list of clients and most days she doesn't manage to get through the list or spend as much time with clients as she would like. She feels that the nursing and medical staff are both over-referring, but she has learned that if she does not see the clients who have been referred there will be complaints made about the amount of physiotherapy service being provided. The physiotherapist feels that her problems are compounded by her limited experience and knowledge in the clinical area. She is the only physiotherapist on the ward. She can ask for help from more senior staff but she knows they are also busy. Each day the physiotherapist leaves work feeling exhausted and demoralised. She no longer looks forward to work and has contemplated making a career change.

Examples of antecedents of stress or burnout (adapted from Cordes & Dougherty 1993) and coping strategies physiotherapists may find useful in dealing with these antecedents are now provided:

- **Work involves constant time pressure and pressure to perform**. Seek mentoring from wise, more experienced colleagues to help structure your day and prioritise jobs; take allocated meal breaks and holidays; discuss work pressures with supervisors; anticipate and plan for high pressure times; consider doing the 'worst' jobs first (e.g. treating a difficult client early, scheduling a confronting meeting or completing challenging paperwork) when your tolerance levels may be higher. Alternatively, consider completing three small tasks early to give yourself a sense of achievement and thus be motivated to tackle the more difficult jobs; be realistic about what you can achieve.

- **Work involves frequent and intense interpersonal contact with clients.** Schedule regular breaks between 'draining' clients; 'refresh your head space' (e.g. have a quick chat with a colleague, look at favourite photos, listen to a bar or two of a favourite song or just watch the clouds move past the window for a moment); be aware that you can leave your physiotherapist role when at home and it is not necessary to do free consultations in social situations (a useful phrase in this circumstance is: 'My head isn't in that space at the moment, I'd be happy to talk further in work time'); remember that none of us is indispensable, and if we burn out we won't be there.

- **Work involves interpersonal difficulties with staff.** Be aware that 'difficult' staff may be stressed and in need of support; try to understand their challenges and constraints; aim to find common ground; plan communication strategies; speak with your supervisor or others experienced with interpersonal conflict in the workplace; take care not to compromise yourself or your client care when accommodating difficult colleagues; be assertive about your needs.

- **Work involves requirements to deliver services with inadequate resources.** Understand the limitations of the system and have realistic expectations of yourself and what can be achieved; be creative in accessing monetary support from the community or through grants; form alliances with other professional groups to advocate for increased resources.

- **Family life and work need better balance.** Find mentors who have similar aspirations; plan child care in advance; seek flexible workplace hours; be aware of workplace rights relating to leave allocations; access paid home help; feel OK about living in less than perfect order; be reassured by this quote, 'Our brains evolved to function in a messy world, and sometimes when we insist on thinking in neat, orderly ways we're really holding back our minds from doing what they do best' (Abrahamson & Freedman 2006, p 246).

RESILIENCE AND HARDINESS

Resilience and hardiness relate to the capacities within individuals that enable life events to be handled without significant negative consequences for their mental health and wellbeing. In relation to self-management, physiotherapists' resilience and hardiness may guide their understanding of their responses to such situations. These concepts may also provide a useful rationale for understanding the differing capacities of others to handle stressful life events and challenging working conditions. Strategies for dealing with adversity include problem-solving, optimistic thinking and help-seeking behaviour (Commonwealth Department of Health and Aged Care 2000). Good communication and social skills enable people to develop and utilise support systems. Employing positive self-care strategies, as discussed throughout this chapter, enables physiotherapists to draw on their inherent resilience and hardiness. Also, perceiving events as opportunities and challenges provides a sense of control over events and dedication to a purpose (Fusilier & Manning 2005), and helps facilitate an objective attitude that emphasises what is realistic (Lambert et al 2003).

Although people have varying levels of resilience and hardiness, these capacities can be developed. Personal resilience and hardiness can be enhanced using self-guidance or professional programs. Reflective questions regarding individual situations and how they are handled may be a useful first step in developing a personal understanding of resilience and hardiness. Physiotherapists with well-developed styles of resilience and hardiness are well placed to implement a range of strategies for managing stress.

In the following scenario the physiotherapist described in Scenario 3a demonstrates qualities of resilience and hardiness. She takes action to improve her work situation and successfully implements a range of coping strategies.

Scenario 3b

Taking action

The physiotherapist in the busy hospital spent some time reflecting upon her decision to be a physiotherapist. She reaffirmed that this was her preferred career; she liked her colleagues, she liked her workplace and she liked the work. However, she realised that she needed to take action in order for her work to be sustainable. Following a discussion with her manager three key strategies were implemented. The first strategy involved establishing a mentor relationship with an experienced senior to help the physiotherapist a) recognise ways to make her work more efficient, b) identify strategies to deal with difficult clinical situations, and c) access professional development courses to up-skill in her area of practice. The second strategy involved developing an understanding of the medical and nursing staff's reasoning for referrals and the rationale for their referral patterns. On the basis of this understanding a gradual change process was developed to alter well-established workplace patterns. Finally, at home the physiotherapist talked to her partner about joining her on a regular evening walk, which she found allowed her to reflect on her day and then switch off. These strategies enabled her to re-evaluate her situation with less personal blame and led to an altered perspective as to what was achievable. She still became stressed on busy days but felt she was coping better with these stresses, and they were impacting less on her emotional wellbeing.

ACCESSING PROFESSIONAL HELP

Even after implementing stress management strategies there may still be times in physiotherapists' lives when coping with everyday events proves to be overwhelming, even for the most resilient and hardy. Significant changes in personal or work lives may impact on physiotherapists' normal ability to manage situations. In these situations, physiotherapists can find themselves overwhelmed when normal coping strategies do not work. Difficulty sleeping, trouble relaxing, poor concentration, reduced work performance, irritability, overreacting to small things, constant fatigue or substance abuse are all signs that significant action needs to be taken. This action could include taking a break, re-evaluating the situation, and perhaps seeking assistance from supportive family, friends, or professionals such as counsellors, GPs, a workplace employee assistance program or a professional advisory service. Suggestions from colleagues to seek assistance should also be heeded.

SUMMARY

There is no 'one size fits all' style for self-management. For physiotherapists, self-management involves recognising opportunities and constraints within their professional and personal lives and understanding how they may be maximised, altered or accepted. Other components of self-management include understanding employment contexts, handling change, being assertive, managing time and workload, being reflective, building resilience, and understanding changing self and circumstances. Sustained practice for physiotherapists requires consideration of opportunities and constraints in terms of their impact on physical, emotional, spiritual, social and intellectual components of self. Through a proactive approach to life and work, the capacity to achieve meaningful, sustained practice is more likely to be realised.

Reflective questions

- How do I attain balance in my professional and personal life?
- How do I nourish all components of myself?
- What does my *life story* tell me about my resilience?
- What strategies do I currently use to deal with stress?
- What other strategies could I consider to deal with stress?

Further reading

Ashfield J 2007 Taking care of yourself and your family: a resource book for good mental health. Peacock, Norwood, SA

Cromie J, Robertson V, Best M 2001 Occupational health and safety in physiotherapy: guidelines for practice. Australian Journal of Physiotherapy 47:43–51

O'Hagan J, Richards J (eds) 1998 In sickness and in health: a handbook for medical practitioners, other health professionals, their partners and families, 2nd edn. Doctors' Health Advisory Service, Wellington

References

Abrahamson E, Freedman D 2006 A perfect mess: the hidden benefits of disorder. Orion, London

Ali M, Boulden G, Brake T et al 2002 Successful manager's handbook. Dorling Kindersley, London

Commonwealth Department of Health and Aged Care 2000 National action plan for promotion, prevention and early intervention for mental health. Mental Health and Special Programs Branch, Commonwealth Department of Health and Aged Care, Canberra

Connor B 1998 A professional odyssey in general practice: a review of the processes and functions of general practice. McGraw-Hill, Roseville, NSW

Cordes C, Dougherty T 1993 A review and an integration of research on job burnout. Academy of Management Review 18(4):621–656

Cromie J, Robertson V, Best M 2001 Occupational health and safety in physiotherapy: guidelines for practice. Australian Journal of Physiotherapy 47:43–51

Dawson D, Reid K 1997 Fatigue, alcohol and performance impairment. Nature 388:235

Fisher J, 2005 A time for change? Human Resource Development International 8(2):257–263

Fusilier M, Manning M 2005 Psychosocial predictors of health status revisited. Journal of Behavioral Medicine 28(4):347–358

Goleman, D 1996 Emotional intelligence: why it can matter more than IQ. Bloomsbury, London

Haslam A, O'Brien A, Jetten J et al 2005 Taking the strain: Social identity, social support, and the experience of stress. British Journal of Social Psychology 44(3):355–370

Knudsen H, Ducharme L, Roman P 2007 Job stress and poor sleep quality: data from an American sample of full-time workers. Social Science and Medicine 64(10):1997–2007

Lambert V, Lambert C, Yamase H 2003 Psychological hardiness, workplace stress and related stress reduction strategies. Nursing and Health Sciences 5(2):181–184

Longman R 2007 Meanings for self, soul and spirit. Available: http://www.spirithome.com/defsoul.html 16 Oct 2007

Spreitzer G, Sutcliffe K, Dutton J et al 2005. A socially embedded model of thriving at work. Organization Science 16(5):537–549

van Hooff M, Guerts S, Kompier M et al 2007 Workdays, in-between workdays and the weekend: a diary on effort and recovery. International Archives of Occupational and Environmental Health, 80(7):599–613

MANAGING A PRACTICE

Gordon Waddington and Peter Larmer

twenty-three

Key concepts

- Key differences between management and leadership
- Risk management
- Core components of practice management when providing private and public physiotherapy services

INTRODUCTION

As in many areas of health education, physiotherapy entry-level programs provide little emphasis on introducing the processes involved in practice management and leadership. However with increasing numbers of physiotherapy practitioners becoming involved in management and leadership, either in public or private practice, there is a need for better understanding of the principles of practice management and leadership.

Like professionals in all walks of life physiotherapists may practise within a number of career structure formats requiring differing management skill sets. These structures range from self-employed sole practitioners to salaried professionals working as part of a large health care entity. Each of these career structures has potential advantages and disadvantages that practitioners might consider when determining which structure best suits their philosophy of practice and life stage. Some examples of these advantages and disadvantages are outlined in Table 23.1.

This chapter provides a brief summary of the differences between management and leadership and a broad overview of factors involved in the management of physiotherapy practice. We include both public and private practice within the sphere of practice management. This chapter is not intended to be an exhaustive management text; there are many reference materials available for readers who seek more detailed management knowledge. The online resources listed at the end of this chapter are suggested for more specific readings about management.

MANAGEMENT AND LEADERSHIP

Management and leadership are distinctly different terms. However, they are often used interchangeably, potentially resulting in confusion as to their meaning. Although a manager and a leader can be the same person, it is critical to understand that each position has distinct attributes and characteristics. Managers are generally appointed by the organisation and given direct controlling authority over those staff and duties

Table 23.1 Advantages and disadvantages of different models of physiotherapy practice		
Career stucture	Advantages	Disadvantages
Practice – sole owner, self-employed	Can determine and set the philosophy of the practice Can dictate work hours Can maximise tax advantages of a private business	Ultimately has full responsibility for the business In a small practice may work in isolation May experience difficulty having time off Is responsible for caseload and supplying own locum cover Has no security of tenure Must provide own superannuation
Practice – partner	Needs to ensure that a shared philosophy of the practice has been established Shares tax advantages of a private business Shares responsibility for the business	Needs to ensure that partners constantly review sharing of workload and whether the shared vision still holds
Associate	Gains some tax advantages of small business	Has limited input as to how the business is managed
Salaried position, employee	Has minimal management responsibility Has guaranteed holidays and sick leave cover Receives employer superannuation contribution	Works as directed Has less flexibility of hours Makes limited contribution to philosophy of practice

for which they are responsible. Managers are often selected for their ability to control. Leaders, on the other hand, have qualities of influence and motivation rather than control and are often chosen by or emerge from a group (Robbins et al 2005).

Within a business environment managers have key tasks to do to avoid risks, follow business plans, comply with set budgets, solve problems and deliver a profitable bottom line. Leaders, however, set future visions, motivate people to change, identify new ways of doing business and may actively pursue opportunities that have a known risk.

When planning a new physiotherapy practice, be it a private practice or a new physiotherapy health project, it is the key components of leadership that set the future direction of the initiative. Leadership attributes are needed to outline the vision and goals for the future development of the project. However, once the project has commenced it is the key management attributes that are needed to ensure its viability and success. A more detailed analysis of these important management characteristics follows.

RISK MANAGEMENT

An essential framework underlying competent practice management is the management of risk. Risk is defined by the Australia/New Zealand Standard for Risk Management (AS/NZS 4360 2004) as 'the possibility of something happening that impacts on your objectives. It is the chance to either make a gain or a loss. It is measured in terms of likelihood and consequence'.

Effective risk management helps to maximise opportunities and achieve practice goals. Managing risk ensures that your practice organisation, whether public or private, can achieve its potential with minimal disruption from a risk eventuating. Effective risk management also puts the practice organisation in a position to take advantage of opportunities as they arise.

Risk management involves a global approach to the practice environment in a series of well defined predetermined steps. The risk management process is outlined schematically in Figure 23.1.

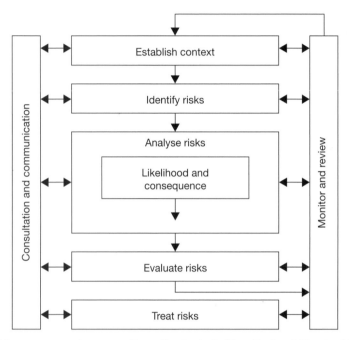

Fig. 23.1 The risk management process. From the Australia/New Zealand Standard for Risk Management, 2004, AS/NZS 4360

Establishing the practice goals and context is essential to develop and understand the environment within which you are practising. Risks and opportunities in public and private practice are many and varied and often unique to the practice entity. They can be as diverse as providing a new musculoskeletal physiotherapy triage service in an emergency department or identifying physiotherapy responses to public health issues such as obesity. Thorough analysis of these issues provides an understanding of the context within which the practice or department operates.

The Australia/New Zealand Standard for Risk Management (AS/NZS 4360 2004) describes the context of risk management as including strategic, organisational and risk management components. The strategic context entails the practice's relationship to its working environment. Mechanisms for analysing this relationship include SWOT analysis (practice **s**trengths, **w**eaknesses, **o**pportunities and **t**hreats) and PEST analysis (**p**olitical, **e**conomic, **s**ocietal and **t**echnological) (Robbins et al 2005). The organisational context refers to the practice organisation, its capability and goals, objectives and strategies. These obviously differ substantially between a single practitioner practice, a large tertiary hospital department and a multi-practitioner private practice. The risk management context describes the parts of the practice organisation, i.e. goals, objectives, or a specific project, to which the risk management processes are applied.

Identifying the risks requires a systematic determination of factors that may impact on the capacity of the practice to provide services. Careful and comprehensive evaluation of all potential sources of risk is important at this stage, as this process underlies the success of the risk management strategy. A structure for determining the global practice environment is outlined later in this chapter. Examples of different types of risk to physiotherapy practice include failure of computers or IT services causing loss of client records, changes in government policy reducing or removing Medicare rebates for Veterans Affairs clients or public hospital clients, changes in evidence to support treatment regimes, and inadequate insurance in the event of a claim against the practitioner.

Analysis of the risks involves an evaluation of the level of risk and its potential impact on the capacity of the practice to provide services. This involves analysis of controls already in place to deal with risks previously identified and identification of the need for new controls. Risks are then analysed on the basis of likelihood (what is the chance of occurrence?) and consequence (what impact will the risk have on the practice if it occurs?).

Evaluation of the risk is essentially the determination of whether the risk is acceptable or not. Risks that are assessed as acceptable will be monitored and risks that are determined to be unacceptable require a treatment strategy to be developed.

Treatment of the risk involves some level of either (a) avoiding the risk by not undertaking the activity, (b) undertaking some intervention to reduce the likelihood of the risk occurring, (c) reducing the consequences of any negative impact of the risk, (d) transferring or (e) retaining the risk.

Monitoring the risk involves putting in place a process to review the effectiveness of the treatments and recognising new risks as they arise.

THE PRACTICE MANAGEMENT ENVIRONMENT

Whether in the private or public sector physiotherapy practice management can be divided into three core components:

- strategic management
- financial management
- operational management.

Within each of the three core components, strategic, financial and operational management, are a number of sub-units of management practice.

Strategic management

Strategic management is the management of issues related to the environment within which the practice of physiotherapy exists. It embraces factors relating to the stakeholders of the practice, the overall governance processes of the practice and the impact of external economic factors, both national and international (see Fig 23.2).

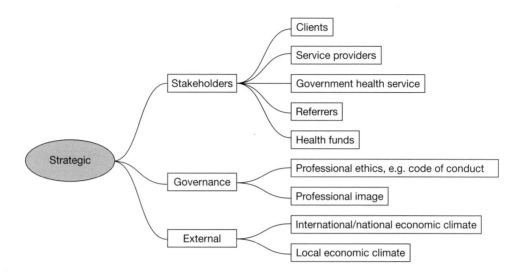

Fig. 23.2 Strategic management issues

Stakeholders

Stakeholders include all clients using the physiotherapy services provided by the practice. This includes those who use physiotherapy services in hospitals as part of a state or regional health service contract arrangement as well as those who attend a private practice on a fee-for-service basis. Clients also include corporate bodies such as health insurance entities, workers' compensation insurance and accident compensation insurance entities that purchase physiotherapy services directly on behalf of clients or employers.

Private health service providers such as private hospitals and private health clinics may also use physiotherapy services. Government health services may use private physiotherapy services through contracted arrangements for provision of service in public facilities. Referrers are significant stakeholders in that they are investing a component of their professional obligation to their own clients in the quality of the services provided by the health professional to whom they are referring the clients. Health funds are progressively becoming more involved in purchasing health services, including physiotherapy services, directly on their clients' behalf.

Governance

Effective practice governance requires the maintenance of high standards of professional ethics, in terms of both business and professional practice, and the application of professional codes of conduct. Maintaining high professional standards, on the part of the practitioner, enhances a climate of trust and professional integrity. In New Zealand it is common for both the service delivery and physiotherapists' continuing education to be audited by external agencies. For example Health and Disability Auditing New Zealand Limited (HDANZ 2008) may be contracted to audit the delivery of the service and the New Zealand College of Physiotherapy Inc. (NZCP 2008) may be contracted to accredit the in-service/continuing education program provided by the physiotherapy department or practice for its staff. Governance functions within the profession of physiotherapy at a number of levels.

International governance is led by the World Confederation for Physical Therapy (WCPT), an international body of more than 100 member organisations representing over 270,000 physiotherapists worldwide. The objectives of the WCPT are to (WCPT 2007):

- encourage high standards of physical therapy education and practice
- encourage communication and exchange of information
- encourage the development of associations of physical therapists and support the efforts of appropriate national organisations to improve the situation of physical therapists
- organise international congresses of physical therapists
- represent physical therapy internationally
- cooperate with appropriate national or international organisations
- comment on social and political issues affecting health
- do any and all lawful acts which may be necessary for the development of the Confederation.

In Australia, governance of the physiotherapy profession is overseen by the Australian Physiotherapy Council (APC), an organisation with members representing the Australian Physiotherapy Association (APA), universities teaching physiotherapy, and the state and territory registration boards. The role of the APC includes (APC 2007):

- accreditation of entry-level physiotherapy programs in Australian universities prior to registration of graduates to practice physiotherapy in Australia
- assessment of overseas qualified physiotherapists prior to registration to practise in Australia
- assessment of overseas and Australian qualified physiotherapists for the purpose of migration to Australia as a physiotherapist under the skilled visa categories
- provision of advice to government agencies and physiotherapists registration boards in Australia on legislative matters relevant to a consistent national approach to physiotherapy registration
- maintenance and regular review of the Australian Standards for physiotherapy.

In New Zealand, governance of the physiotherapy profession is guided by the *Health Practitioners Competence Assurance Act* 2003. The Physiotherapy Board of New Zealand is constituted under this Act. The board is appointed by the Minister of Health and consists of eight members, including two lay members. Its primary function is to protect the public of New Zealand. It manages this by (Physiotherapy Board of New Zealand 2007):

- registering physiotherapists who are safe to practise in New Zealand
- monitoring the practice of registered physiotherapists
- when necessary disciplining registered physiotherapists.

Most professional associations publish codes of conduct under which their members agree to practise (e.g. the APA Code of Conduct available at http://apa.advsol.com. au/ and the New Zealand Society of Physiotherapists Standards of Practice available at http://nzsp.org.nz).

Public and professional images of physiotherapy practice are determined by individual practitioners maintaining high standards of professional practice and by the profession as a whole embracing best quality practice, using frameworks such as evidence-based practice. The provision of services with clear clinical justification based on accepted outcome measures and in a cost effective manner is critical to maintaining high levels of public and referrer confidence.

External factors

The local economic climate impacts on the capacity of physiotherapy practices to provide services. In Australia, public health services are currently funded by the federal government through state and territory budget processes. The many competing demands on the public health dollar can mean substantial pressure on the financial support available for new or continuing physiotherapy services. The provision of fee-for-service physiotherapy (e.g. private services) may also be significantly affected by local economic factors. The majority of physiotherapy interventions in Australia are not funded under the Medicare system (a federally funded health service payment system) and, therefore, clients are usually expected to pay for the service at the consultation. Geographical areas of higher socioeconomic capacity are therefore more likely to support higher levels of private physiotherapy practice.

In New Zealand, funding of physiotherapy services comes primarily from one of three sources. The Ministry of Health, through district health boards, largely funds public physiotherapy services. The Accident Compensation Corporation (ACC) provides 24-hour no-fault personal injury insurance cover, and is the primary funder of private physiotherapy services. Thirdly, clients may fund their physiotherapy independently, with or without the costs being subsidised through private health insurance.

The national and international economic climate also impacts on the capacity of the practice entity to provide services. Downward trends in national and international economic activity may have substantial flow-on effects of reductions in funding or, more commonly, failure to maintain relative levels of funding to local health services and more indirectly to private practices. These factors can have an effect on aspects such as the timing of the introduction of new initiatives.

Financial management

Financial management involves an understanding of the market within which the practice of physiotherapy (both public and private) functions. It includes mechanisms to develop and manage a practice budget and cash flow, as well as processes for the maintenance of effective measures to comply with taxation and legislative processes

Understanding the market in which the service is operating

Features such as the nature of the client market and the capacity of the market to support physiotherapy services have been touched on previously. The availability of private health insurance impacts significantly on the capacity of clients to access physiotherapy services. In Australia there has been a significant shift in the last few years to electronic payment systems for those with private health insurance. The Australian Health Industry Claims and Payments Company (2007) lists at least 36 funds participating in electronic point-of-sale services to clients.

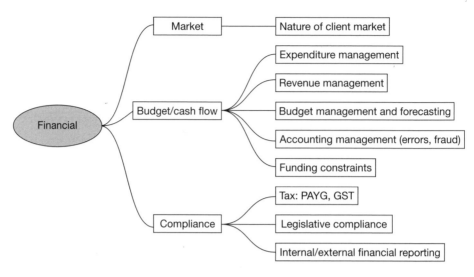

Fig. 23.3 Financial management issues

Providers servicing markets where financial support is provided by governments and where funding may be constrained by economic conditions (e.g. public providers) need mechanisms to ensure that service delivery and resources are directed to those most likely to benefit from the services available. Mechanisms for lobbying for additional resources need to be incorporated in management planning. Lobbying is often more effectively supported with documented evidence of cost effective outcomes.

Budget/cash flow management

Expenditure management is essential to any effective business structure. For small practices a budget mechanism for expenditure management is critical; many commercial software programs are available to provide this function. In larger entities and practice structures that are components of health services or hospitals, a clear understanding of the organisation's financial management system is necessary to ensure effective functioning within the larger service.

Revenue management is also critical to effective practice management. Efficient management of revenue and cash received into the practice ensures that adequate cash is available for effective day-to-day operation of the business. Mechanisms to manage client accounts and ensure timely payment are critical for business sustainability.

Budget management and forecasting are required for the day-to-day management of a physiotherapy practice and to effectively plan and develop extensions to services and new initiatives. Budget forecasting allows the provision of resources to be made in the most cost effective manner. For example, it allows for provision of replacement of plant and equipment in a planned and staged process to minimise disruption to service provision by breakdowns or equipment failure.

Effective accounting management is crucial to business best practice. It reduces the chance of errors and provides mechanisms to reduce the opportunities for fraud. A number of software programs are available that enhance effective accounting management for both sole practitioners and large multi-practitioner practices.

Funding constraints within governments and health services have a direct impact on the ability of public physiotherapy practices to provide client services. Funding constraints limit staff numbers and resources across all aspects of the service delivery. A lack of adequate funding also impacts on the capacity of the physiotherapy service, whether public or private, to participate in value-adding activities, such as research or clinical education placements for students.

Compliance with taxation and legislation requirements

Compliance with the requirements of taxation law is an essential component of all levels of practice management. Within Australia the minimum taxation requirements include income tax ('Pay As You Go' or PAYG) and compulsory superannuation, goods and services tax, and fringe benefits tax.

Legislative compliance includes compliance with regulations, such as local government requirements of business registration and procedures to satisfy infection control regulations. Legislation in both New Zealand and Australia requires physiotherapists to be registered with the relevant registration board prior to undertaking practice. Practices require a mechanism in place to ensure that all physiotherapy staff members maintain currency of registration. Increasingly there is a requirement for health care workers to have police probity checks prior to working in public facilities.

Public entities require both internal and external financial reporting. This involves a clear understanding on the part of the practice manager of the reporting requirements of the relevant responsible agencies.

Operational management

Operational management requires the development of skills and techniques to optimise and maintain the day-to-day procedural functions of the practice (see Fig 23.4). Examples of components of operational management are the development of basic policy and procedures, strategies for maintenance of plant and equipment, maintenance of adequate protection against potential disasters through disaster planning and provision of adequate insurance. This area also includes the management of information technology (IT).

Processes

Policy and procedures frameworks provide clear and readily accessible mechanisms to describe all aspects of the practice function. They describe the procedures and practices for the delivery of services and provide a structure from which the quality of management processes can be evaluated. Policy and procedure frameworks also provide a stepping-off point against which new initiatives or the development of new services can be benchmarked.

Planning for the management of potential business disruption and disaster management, such as physical disruption to IT services, is also critical. Provision of effective offsite back-up facilities for small practice IT services is often overlooked, but can be critical in the event of a major equipment failure.

Targeting of services to match the changing needs of client populations is necessary to ensure service viability. Client populations may change dramatically, for example with the introduction of (or loss of) new medical services at a hospital, or policy changes at a federal level. These may substantially alter access to certain types of physiotherapy services.

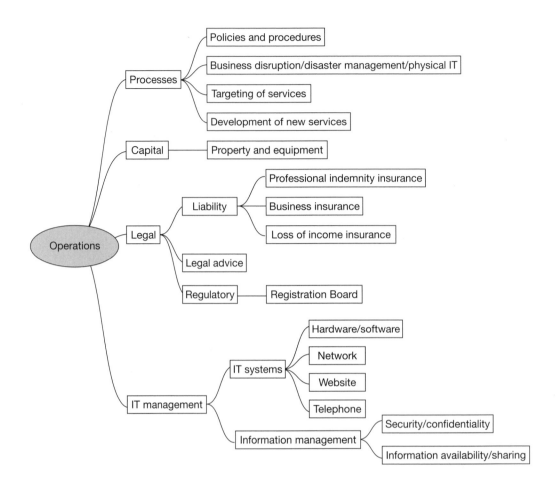

Fig. 23.4 Operational management issues

Development of new services is a core and continuing component of practice management. Meeting the needs of a progressively more sedentary and ageing population in a changing health care funding environment will continue to challenge physiotherapy practice managers.

Capital management

In any practice model, capital management (of property and services) requires a continuous process of maintenance, review of need and replacement. Failure to ensure satisfactory equipment maintenance may result in outcomes ranging from minor service disruption through to practitioner liability due to injury to a client. A formal process of management of property and services incorporated within the budget framework previously described is essential for effective practice management.

Legal advice and liability management

Liability management is undertaken by maintaining appropriate levels of insurance including:

- professional indemnity insurance, which is currently required by health practitioner registration boards in Australia so that practitioners maintain prescribed levels of insurance
- business insurance, which assists practitioners to manage the risks associated with different levels of business disruption or loss of assets
- loss of income insurance, which lessens the impact of an event causing individuals to be unable to earn an income.

Obtaining appropriate legal advice when managing contractual and compliance arrangements for a practice is an essential component of professional business practice. It is worth noting that legal advice obtained on behalf of a public or private entity by a practice manager is in the best interests of the public or private entity and not the practice manager. It may be appropriate for practice managers to obtain independent advice when there is any issue of their own liability involved.

Regulatory control of physiotherapy practice in Australia is overseen by the APC, with each state and territory registration board acting to implement the APC guidelines. Effective operational practice management requires that the practice manager be familiar with the regulatory requirements of physiotherapy practice as determined by the appropriate registration authority.

IT management

Effective contemporary practice management requires an understanding of the capability of effective IT systems to enhance physiotherapy practice. Adequate computer hardware systems (including offsite back-up, record scanning capability and electronic communication) and specialised practice management software significantly enhance communication and records management, potentially enhancing patient safety. Similarly, automated billing software and financial management mechanisms are available that allow efficient financial management.

Maintenance of adequate local networking of computer systems and effective linking across platforms in larger institutions enhance communication, information sharing and compliance capacity. Development and maintenance of an up-to-date internet presence is becoming more important for advertising and communicating information and services.

Effective telephone services and answering systems and processes are important to client satisfaction, as both are critical to client access, forming the first point of contact for clients. Efficient management of information within the practice environment and with outside entities is also critical to effective practice. All information management systems used must ensure that adequate security and confidentiality safeguards are in place, including appropriate firewalls and password-secured storage systems. Mechanisms for the effective sharing of necessary information between all members of the client management team, such as the capacity for current imaging technology to provide scans electronically, further enhance quality of care.

SUMMARY

The requirements of effective practice management may seem somewhat daunting to a practitioner new to the management area. However, the same concepts of management apply to any area of professional business practice. An understanding of these principles allows practitioners to make informed judgements about the requirements of providing physiotherapy as a component of health services, either public or private. These principles provide a guide to the skills necessary to understand what is involved in providing a cost effective physiotherapy service.

Reflective questions

- If you were considering setting up a physiotherapy practice what regulatory issues would you need to consider?
- How would you undertake an exercise to assess the risk management for a physiotherapy department or practice?
- What are the main income streams for a physiotherapist in your country?
- What ethical issues should be considered when setting up a new physiotherapy practice?

References

Accident Compensation Corporation of New Zealand 2007. Available: http://www.acc.co.nz/ 22 Oct 2007

Australia/New Zealand Standard for Risk Management (AS/NZS 4360) 2004, SAI Global Publishing. Available: http://www.saiglobal.com/shop/script/search.asp 1 Jul 2007

Australian Health Industry Claims and Payments Company 2007. Available: http://www.hicaps.com.au/ 19 Jul 2007

APC 2007. Available: http://www.physiocouncil.com.au/ 14 Oct 2007

Health and Disability Auditing New Zealand 2008. Available: http://www.healthaudit.co.nz/_physiotherapy 10 Feb 2008

New Zealand College of Physiotherapy Inc 2008. Available: http://www.physiotherapy.org.nz/Index02/COLLEGE/PDFs/In-Service_Guidelines_and_Forms_July_2006.pdf 10 Feb 2008

Physiotherapy Board of New Zealand 2007. Available: http://www.physioboard.org.nz/ 22 Oct 2007

Robbins S P, Bergman R, Stagg I et al 2005 Management, 4th edn. Pearson Education Australia, Sydney

WCPT 2007. Available: http://www.wcpt.org/about/whatis.php 14 Oct 2007

Further resources

Asia Pacific Management Forum: http://www.apmforum.com

Australian Human Resources Institute: http://www.ahri.com.au

Australian Institute of Management: http://www.aim.com.au

Human Resources Institute of New Zealand: http://www.hrinz.org.nz

New Zealand Institute of Management: http://www.nzim.co.nz

twenty-four

EVALUATION OF PHYSIOTHERAPY PRACTICE

Megan Davidson, Jenny Keating and Peter Hamer

Key concepts

- Understanding best practice
- Reasons for evaluating practice
- Areas of practice that can be evaluated
- Methods and tools to evaluate practice (e.g. clinical audit, accreditation)
- Outcomes of evaluation

INTRODUCTION

> If we don't continually evaluate and re-evaluate ourselves, we fall into patterns and believe that what we're doing is right. (Neil LaBute, http://www.brainyquote.com)

In this chapter we consider ways that physiotherapists can evaluate their clinical practice. We introduce the concepts of practice evaluation, reasons for evaluation, areas where evaluation is important and tools for evaluation. What do we mean by evaluation of physiotherapy practice? *Physiotherapy practice* encompasses all professional activities in physiotherapy, from delivering services to individual patients, to implementing a community program, to managing a hospital department or private practice. *To evaluate* means to appraise or assess something. When we evaluate physiotherapy practice, we make a judgement about the quality of some aspect of practice. Evaluation of what one does is a central aspect of what is expected of a health professional. Evaluation is the means by which we ask ourselves, 'Is this the right thing to do?' and 'Is this the best I can do?'

Evaluating practice serves the goals of achieving, maintaining and improving standards. We evaluate our practice whenever we take steps to answer questions such as:

- What does the evidence show to be the most effective intervention or management for this situation, condition or patient?
- What are the potential risks and benefits of this intervention or management for this situation or patient?
- Should I refer this patient to someone who has knowledge or skills I do not have?
- What measurable benefit is evident for this person or community after my intervention?
- Are patients satisfied with the service/treatment they have received?
- Is this practice consistent with the relevant clinical practice guideline?

- To what extent do the physiotherapy records kept in this practice meet accepted medico–legal standards?
- What manual handling risks are there in this situation, and how can those risks be controlled?

REASONS TO EVALUATE

> Facts do not cease to exist because they are ignored. (Attributed to Aldous Huxley, 1927, Proper Studies, http://www.quotationspage.com)

The overarching reason to evaluate practice is the professional responsibility to strive for excellence or best practice in the delivery of health services and to be accountable for what we do. This is part of our duty of care, which is an ethical as well as a legal responsibility demanded of professionals by society, our professional code of ethics and regulatory authorities.

As well as meeting these responsibilities, evaluation should be about learning. It involves learning about 'what', 'why' and 'how' the practice of physiotherapy influences our clients or patients, the community and ourselves. Evaluation allows us to make systematic improvements to our practice.

There are many specific reasons to evaluate practice, including to:

- ensure practice is evidence-based
- optimise outcomes for a particular patient
- improve care for all patients with a particular condition
- document the perceived benefits of a new program
- justify clinical services to third party payers
- provide an argument for funding a particular service
- ensure a safe workplace
- comply with medico–legal requirements
- improve client satisfaction
- improve practitioner/employee satisfaction and optimise staff retention
- improve the market share of the professional group concerned
- assess the costs and benefits of treatment options
- foster a culture of self-review and evaluation.

USING A QUALITY IMPROVEMENT CYCLE

The evaluator needs to plan the evaluation, monitor its stages, review the outcomes and make decisions about actions arising from the report. The quality improvement cycle (see Fig 24.1) depicts how evaluation can be used to continually improve practice. This process is predicated upon a cyclic process of action–inquiry. It involves:

- gathering feedback from patients/clients, staff and community about the health service provided, and information on developments in knowledge and understanding about physiotherapy interventions
- critically reflecting on the feedback and developed knowledge
- working towards best practice in service provision by responding to evaluation findings
- re-evaluating practice goals, capabilities, standards and actions.

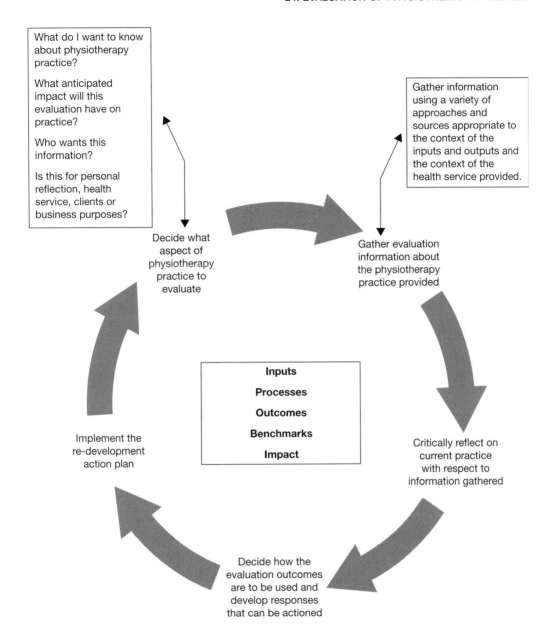

Fig. 24.1 The cyclic process of evaluation of practice. Adapted from Kemmis and McTaggart (1988) and McNiff (2000)

Note: It is possible to enter this cycle at any of the steps, as completion of the cycle begins the next cycle.

EVALUATION PRINCIPLES

Regardless of the methods that are used in the evaluation there are some important general principles in evaluation:

- When evaluation is undertaken as part of ongoing quality improvement, its purpose and anticipated benefits should be made explicit to key stakeholders.

- Evaluations are more likely to be successful if they include collaboration between evaluators, consumers and stakeholders.
- Evaluations that are seen as irrelevant are less likely to engage target users of the practices.
- Evaluations are conducted to improve decision making and need to be supported by those who are making the decisions.
- There should be a commitment to acting on the outcomes of evaluation to refine practice.
- A culture of engagement in evaluation may need to be developed before evaluation commences if the outcomes are to lead to positive change in practices.
- It would be inappropriate to use evaluation to justify decisions that have already been made or to delay quality improvement.
- The methods employed and the cost of practice evaluation should be considered in the context of the anticipated benefits.
- Evaluation involves setting standards to be achieved and identifying indicators that can be assessed to determine the extent to which a standard is achieved or progress toward a goal has occurred.
- Evaluation findings should be shared with those who have been evaluated, who should also be given the opportunity to discuss their reflections on the findings.
- Actions should focus on improving practices rather than criticism.
- Once an evaluation has occurred, it is important that the results be used to improve the aspect of practice that was evaluated.

Evaluation may be part of the everyday quality improvement processes of an organisation, or be a special project for which external funding is available.

Case study 1
Evaluation of a new role for physiotherapists in hospital orthopaedic outpatient departments

Patients with non-urgent musculoskeletal conditions referred by their GP to an orthopaedic surgeon at a public hospital may face a long wait (months or even years) before they are seen. Many of these patients do not require surgical or medical management, and can be appropriately managed by a qualified physiotherapist. If physiotherapists were able to screen patients first, to determine whether they need to see an orthopaedic surgeon or would benefit from conservative therapy, waiting times could be substantially reduced.

Funding from the Victorian Department of Human Services allowed this approach to be trialled and evaluated in 2005 at the Northern Hospital in Melbourne. Forty-five patient referrals were screened and the patients were assessed by one of two experienced physiotherapists with postgraduate qualifications in musculoskeletal physiotherapy and by the orthopaedic surgeon. Under these conditions, 63% of patients could be managed by non-surgical means. The physiotherapists and surgeon agreed on the patient management plan for 74% of patients, and patients and doctors were very satisfied with the physiotherapy-led style of service delivery (Oldmeadow et al 2007).

This evaluation of a new triage role for physiotherapists contributed to a system development that will endeavour to ensure that future patients at this facility receive the appropriate treatment early, thereby improving their health status sooner.

AREAS FOR EVALUATION

Evaluation can be made of any aspect of health care delivery, including inputs or infra-structure, process, outputs and outcomes. *Inputs* are the infrastructure that supports practice, the buildings and equipment, the service providers and the knowledge and skills of those service providers, as well as the patients and conditions to be managed. *Process* encompasses policies and procedures, modalities and techniques, management and discharge plans. *Outputs* are the service units produced by the process, for example, the number of patients treated or the number of treatments or occasions of service provided. *Outcomes* are the benefits to patients, providers and management systems derived from the processes. This approach repeats core foci of the classic CIPP (context, input, process, product) model of Stufflebeam (1983).

Process evaluation investigates aspects of program or service delivery. A process indicator might be the extent to which the service deliverers' care is consistent with desirable clinical practice. Inputs and outputs together might be investigated to determine efficiency – that is, how much is accomplished with the available resources.

Outcome evaluation investigates what outcomes have occurred, whether or not the program or service resulted in the expected benefits and whether positive or negative unexpected outcomes occurred. Cost effectiveness is the cost of the benefits derived and can be determined from the inputs and outcomes. Outcome evaluation is not the same as evaluation of the efficacy of a treatment. Treatment efficacy is best evaluated via research (rather than program evaluation) using quality randomised controlled trials. However, clinicians can use program evaluation methods to benchmark their intervention outcomes against research findings where similar treatments and patients were involved. They can ask, 'On average, am I getting the same kinds of results as those described in the literature?' Benchmarking is a type of evaluation in which the inputs, processes, outputs or outcomes of one program are compared with those of another program, or to a national average, or to 'best practice' target values.

Case study 2 provides examples of outcome evaluations for groups of patients at a major metropolitan hospital. Case study 3 demonstrates evaluation of the process of service delivery to a particular community.

Case study 2

Evaluating patient outcomes at Sir Charles Gairdner Hospital, Perth

1. For 179 patients attending a respiratory rehabilitation program (1,682 class attendances), scores on the Chronic Respiratory Disease Questionnaire (a disease-specific QoL scale) (Guyatt et al 1987) shifted from a mean of 81 to 97 points following participation in the program. Their 6-minute walk (6MWT) distances improved by 10% and their 20-minute walk distances increased by 19%.

2. 48 patients who completed a heart failure rehabilitation program were assessed for outcomes including a 6MWT. The mean increase was 54 m, which was a 14.7% increase on pre-program measures.

3. 106 patients who completed a cardiac rehabilitation program were assessed for outcomes including a 6MWT and a quality of life measure (Physical Functioning scale of the SF-36 Health Survey) (Ware 2000). The 6MWT improved by a mean of 62 m. The SF-36 physical functioning scale increased by a mean of 8.3 points.

4. Hospital admissions and length of stay were assessed in patients with chronic obstructive pulmonary disease referred to the outpatient pulmonary rehabilitation (PR) program. Before the PR program was introduced 42% of patients were admitted to hospital and had an average length of stay (LOS) of 8.1 days. After the PR program was introduced only 20% of patients had to be admitted and they had an average LOS of 7.7 days.

Case study 3
Evaluating service delivery to Indigenous clients

Physiotherapy appointments for paediatrics and general outpatients were being offered to Indigenous people at the hospital in an Australian town. After six months of offering appointments, the attendance rate was evaluated and the percentage of non-attendance was found to be 80%. Discussions with Aboriginal health workers and liaison officers at the local Aboriginal Health Service indicated that the patients were not comfortable attending the hospital and many did not have transport to get to their appointment. A different approach was taken, resulting in amalgamating physiotherapy clinics with the paediatrician's clinics when visiting the communities and also introducing a weekly afternoon physiotherapy outpatient clinic at the Aboriginal Health Service Centre. The Aboriginal Health Service assisted by informing patients of their appointments and providing transport. After six months, this approach was evaluated and non-attendance had halved, indicating a better utilisation of the services offered.

STANDARDS FOR PHYSIOTHERAPY

The Australian Physiotherapy Council (APC, http://www.physiocouncil.com.au/) is a national body comprised of representatives of state and territory Physiotherapists Registration Boards, the Australian Physiotherapy Association (APA) and representatives of physiotherapy programs in Australian universities. The main role of the APC is to work towards ensuring that standards of practice in the physiotherapy profession are maintained. In New Zealand, practice competencies are established by the Physiotherapy Board of New Zealand (http://www.physioboard.org.nz/docs/registration_requirements.pdf).

The APC promotes a safe and competent physiotherapy workforce. It evaluates and accredits entry-level physiotherapy programs in Australian universities prior to registration of graduates to practise physiotherapy in Australia. Program evaluation includes assessment of the views of students, the skills and qualifications of teachers, the content of curricula and the views of employers on the skills of new graduates. The Australian Standards for Physiotherapy (2006) (see Table 24.1) are targets for quality practice set by the APC. These provide a comprehensive framework of practice areas, which serve as the basis for the evaluation of professional practice and education programs. For instance, practitioners can ask, 'How do I and/or the environment within which I work satisfy each of these standards?' and use their evaluation findings as the basis for reviewing standards and quality of practice.

TOOLS FOR EVALUATION

We have discussed why one might want to evaluate physiotherapy practice and areas of practice that are important to monitor for quality. In this section we present three common tools used to evaluate aspects of physiotherapy practice: clinical audits, accreditation programs and the measurement of patient outcomes.

Table 24.1 Australian Standards for Physiotherapy (http://www.physiocouncil.com.au/)

Standards	Elements
1. Demonstrate professional behaviour appropriate to physiotherapy	1.1 Demonstrate practice that is ethical and in accordance with relevant legal and regulatory requirements 1.2 Demonstrate strategies to maintain and extend professional competence. 1.3 Operate within individual and professional strengths and limitations
2. Communicate effectively	2.1 Communicate effectively with the client 2.2 Adapt communication style recognising cultural safety, and cultural and linguistic diversity 2.3 Communicate effectively with other service providers 2.4 Prepare and deliver presentations to groups 2.5 Prepare and provide documentation according to legal requirements and accepted procedures and standards
3. Access, interpret and apply information to continuously improve practice	3.1 Demonstrate a working knowledge and understanding of theoretical concepts and principles relevant to physiotherapy practice 3.2 Apply contemporary forms of information management to relevant areas of practice 3.3 Acquire and apply new knowledge to continuously improve own practice 3.4 Apply an evidence-based approach to own practice
4. Assess the client	4.1 Collect client information 4.2 Form a preliminary hypothesis 4.3 Design and conduct an assessment 4.4 Conduct assessment safely
5. Interpret and analyse the assessment findings	5.1 Compare findings with 'normal' 5.2 Compare findings with what is expected for the condition, and include or exclude alternative diagnoses 5.3 Prioritise client needs and potential management 5.5 Re-evaluate as required, to develop a sustainable hypothesis 5.5 Identify areas that are outside skills and expertise and refer client appropriately
6. Develop a physiotherapy intervention	6.1 Develop a rationale for physiotherapy intervention 6.2 Set realistic short- and long-term goals with the client 6.3 Select an appropriate intervention 6.4 Plan for possible contingencies that may affect intervention plan 6.5 Prioritise the intervention plan in collaboration with the client 6.6 Determine a plan of evaluation that uses valid and reliable outcome measures
7. Implement safe and effective physiotherapy intervention(s)	7.1 Obtain informed consent for the intervention 7.2 Prepare equipment and treatment area appropriate to the intervention 7.3 Implement the intervention safely and effectively 7.4 Manage adverse events 7.5 Provide strategies for client self-management 7.6 Implement health promotion activities
8. Evaluate the effectiveness and efficacy of physiotherapy intervention(s)	8.1 Monitor the outcomes of the intervention 8.2 Evaluate the outcomes of the intervention 8.3 Determine modifications to the intervention

Table 24.1 Australian Standards for Physiotherapy (http://www.physiocouncil.com.au/) *continued*	
9. Operate effectively across a range of settings	9.1 Use a model of service delivery relevant to the practice setting 9.2 Work effectively within a team 9.3 Manage own work schedule to maximise safety, efficiency and effectiveness 9.4 Operate within own role and according to responsibilities 9.5 Participate in quality improvement processes

Clinical audits

A clinical audit is a process whereby an aspect of practice is critically analysed. Audits involve a cyclical process that generally has a number of stages (Redfern & Norman 1996, p 333):

1. Identify the issue to be audited.
2. Set the standard/identify the target.
3. Measure the variable of interest.
4. Compare results to the desired standard.
5. Identify whether change is needed.
6. Decide strategies for change.
7. Implement necessary changes.
8. Monitor the effect of change against the standards.

Case study 4 provides an example of how a clinical audit can be used to improve practice.

Case study 4
Audit of physiotherapy management of low back pain: are guidelines followed?

A physiotherapy outpatient department in the UK audited its patient records in 1996 and 2001 to determine the extent to which its practice was consistent with current guidelines relating to best practice management of patients with acute and chronic low back pain (Sparkes 2005). The audit process evaluated each patient record against a set of explicit standards for back pain management based on current clinical practice guidelines, for example 'all patients should receive advice to keep active', 'evidence of diagnostic triage following assessment including "red flags"', 'referral for rehabilitation for those not returned to ordinary activities by 6 weeks'.

In the 2001 audit 57% of records indicated that patients were advised to keep active, 100% showed evidence of diagnostic triage, and 60% were referred for rehabilitation. The physiotherapy department identified that some aspects of their practice had improved and some had deteriorated between the two audits. Changes that were put in place to improve practice included systems for new appointments and for referrals, and professional education for staff.

Accreditation programs

The accreditation of programs incorporates an evaluation process and an evaluation report. Awarding of 'accredited provider' status is valued by provider and consumer alike as an external evaluation that high standards of service provision are met by that organisation or practice.

Example 1: ACHS EQuIP Program

The majority of health care organisations in Australia are assessed and accredited as quality service providers by The Australian Council on Healthcare Standards (ACHS). Health care organisations participating in ACHS quality programs include teaching hospitals, corporate offices of private health companies, day surgeries, nursing agencies, community health centres and divisions of general practice. Accreditation is awarded to an organisation following external evaluation by a third party and determination that an organisation meets predetermined and transparent standards. Perhaps surprisingly, accreditation is not compulsory in Australia.

The ACHS has developed accreditation standards called the Evaluation and Quality Improvement Program (EQuIP). The EQuIP standards (http://www.achs.org.au/EQUIP4/) were developed and reviewed with reference to relevant literature and a comparison of the EQuIP standards and criteria developed in other countries (UK, Canada, USA, New Zealand, Ireland, France and Japan) (ACHS 2006).

When comparing an earlier version of the standards, EQuIP3, to EQuIP4 one can see how important it is to stay abreast of changing health service needs if we are to continue to deliver quality care. For example, the following criteria were added to the EQuIP standards in August 2006:

1.1.6 Systems for ongoing care of the consumer / patient are coordinated and effective.

1.1.7 Systems exist to ensure that the care of dying and deceased consumers / patients is managed with dignity and comfort.

1.3.1 Health care and services are appropriate and delivered in the most appropriate setting.

1.4.1 Care and services are planned, developed and delivered based on the best available evidence and in the most effective way.

1.5.4 The incidence of falls and fall injuries is minimised through a falls management program.

1.5.5 The system for prescription, sample collection, storage and transportation and administration of blood and blood components ensures safe and appropriate practice.

These new criteria reflect a growing understanding of the importance of sustained care and the move of services out of the acute hospital environment and into the community and home. Criterion 1.4.1 shows that respect for the role of evidence derived from quality research is increasing; 1.5.4 shows that programs for detecting and averting falls and falls related injuries have developed across time; 1.5.5 shows that increasing pressure to ensure that blood is safe has led to the inclusion of criteria that reflect the health service response to known dangers.

Let us take up the following evaluation challenge defined by EQuIP: *2.1.3 Health care incidents, complaints and feedback are managed to ensure improvements to the systems of care.*

Steps in the process might include the following:

1. Define what the organisation wants to provide, e.g. a method for ensuring that health care incidents, complaints and feedback are managed to ensure improvements to the systems of care.

2. Identify a project coordinator. This could be you.
3. Identify a project team. Who are the people who would benefit from this information? Draw together a team of key stakeholders.
4. Identify a local auditor. This person will need to be able to access or generate the data of interest.
5. Define the time scale.
6. Agree on inclusion criteria. What records or processes will you audit?
7. Agree on the sample size. How many records will you audit?
8. Agree on the method of sampling. How will you ensure a representative sample?
9. Brief project participants. Make sure everyone involved knows what the audit is about and why it matters.
10. Collect the records.
11. Collect data from the records.
12. Analyse the data and review practice.
13. Present and discuss results.
14. Formulate and agree on recommendations in collaboration with the team and interested stakeholders.
15. Implement the recommendations.
16. Re-audit.
17. Provide feedback.

Notice that the process is cyclical, with the results of the evaluation leading to recommendations for change so that compliance with the standard can be achieved.

Example 2: APA Quality Endorsement Program (QEP)

The APA offers a formal accreditation program for physiotherapy practices and departments. A set of standards (see Table 24.2) provides a benchmark against which a physiotherapy practice is judged (APA 2007). The standards are organised into categories. Each standard has specific criteria, and for each criterion there is an explanation and indicators for assessment.

Table 24.2 Summary of the Standards of the APA Quality Endorsement Program. APA standards for physiotherapy practices, 2007, APA

Category	Standards	Criteria
1. Rights and needs of clients	1.1 Human rights	1.1.1 Respect
		1.1.2 Privacy
		1.1.3 Informed consent
		1.1.4 Client communication
		1.1.5 Culturally appropriate care
	1.2 Client-centred care	1.2.1 Collaborative goal setting
		1.2.2 Health promotion
2. Practice services	2.1 Client health record	2.1.1 Compliance
	2.2 Coordination of care	2.2.1 Referral
		2.2.2 Communication
	2.3 Access to services	2.3.1 Responsive health care

Table 24.2 Summary of the Standards of the APA Quality Endorsement Program. APA standards for physiotherapy practices, 2007, APA *continued*		
3. Practice management	3.1 Business systems	3.1.1 Strategic plan
		3.1.2 Operations
		3.1.3 Practice communication
	3.2 Human resource management	3.2.1 Human resource management systems
		3.2.2 Credentials
	3.3 Health information systems	3.3.1 Confidentiality and privacy
		3.3.2 Collection
		3.3.3 Security
		3.3.4 Use and disclosure
		3.3.5 Access
	3.4 Risk management	3.4.1 Risk management
		3.4.2 Occupational health and safety
		3.4.3 Manual handling
		3.4.4 Emergency systems
	3.5 Improving practice management	3.5.1 Quality improvement
4. Physical environment	4.1 Facilities	4.1.1 Practice environment
		4.1.2 Compliance
		4.1.3 Practice access
	4.2 Equipment	4.2.1 Equipment safety and maintenance
	4.3 Infection control	4.3.1. Infection control standards
5. Quality physiotherapy	5.1 Clinical best practice	5.1.1 Recognised best practice
		5.1.2 Outcome measures
		5.1.3 Clinical risk management
	5.2 Professional standards	5.2.1 Professional conduct
		5.2.2 Continuing professional development
		5.2.3 Clinical supervision
	5.3 Quality improvement	5.3.1 Client feedback
		5.3.2 Improving clinical care

Outcome measurement tools

Measuring the outcomes of care for individual patients or groups of patients is a method of evaluating the health status and relevant characteristics of people who utilise our services. In 2003 the APA statement on 'Clinical justification and outcome measures' (APA 2003, p 1) included:

As part of a clinical justification for physiotherapy, outcome measures should be used to:

- evaluate and document the demonstrable benefits of physiotherapy in relation to treatment goals
- evaluate the need to continue physiotherapy to maintain or improve patient status
- help evaluate the cost benefits of physiotherapy in relation to treatment goals
- identify, document and act on factors that may compromise treatment outcomes or predict poor outcomes
- determine and document when physiotherapy treatment should cease or where relevant, to determine and document when the client should be referred to another professional within the multidisciplinary health care team.

An outcome measurement tool (or outcome measure) is a test or instrument used to measure some aspect of health, which may be impairment, activity limitation or participation restriction, or some broader construct such as quality of life. The particular aspects of health that are chosen to be measured are related to patients' goals and what one can reasonably expect to change with the treatment. Sometimes treatment is aimed at slowing an inevitable deterioration or maintaining rather than improving function. Treatment benefits can be difficult to infer in these cases. Usually treatment must be withdrawn for a period of time and measurements taken to determine whether or not the treatment appears to be having a measurable benefit. The box below provides some key databases and collections of outcome measurement tools. The choice of test used to measure outcomes is based on considerations of practicality, validity and reliability. A useful test is one that is sufficiently valid (measures what you want to measure) and reliable (has acceptable error) for the measurement task and is practical for the patients and circumstances in which the test will be administered.

People usually seek health services because they want to improve their health. It is important to identify which aspect of health they want to improve. Categories of health have been defined by the World Health Organization (WHO) International

---

Where to find standardised outcome measures

Websites:

Centre for Outcome Measurement in Brain Injury (COMBI), http://www.tbims.org/combi/ 2 Oct 2007

Chartered Society of Physiotherapy Searchable Database, http://www.csp.org.uk/director/effectivepractice/outcomemeasures/database.cfm 2 Oct 2007

Pulmonary Rehabilitation Toolkit, http://www.pulmonaryrehab.com.au/welcome.asp 2 Oct 2007

Transport Accident Commision, http://www.tac.vic.gov.au 2 Oct 2007

Victorian WorkCover Authority, http://www.workcover.vic.gov.au 2 Oct 2007

Manuals (available from the Australian Physiotherapy Association http://apa.advsol.com.au/ 2 Oct 2007):

Atlas of Clinical Tests and Outcome Measures for Low Back Pain

Hill K, Denisenko S, Miller K et al 2005 Clinical outcome measurement in adult neurological physiotherapy, 3rd edn. Australian Physiotherapy Association Neurology Special Group (Vic), St Kilda, VIC

Classification of Functioning, Disability and Health (ICF) (http://www.who.int/classifications/icf/en/ accessed 2 Oct 2007). The WHO recommends that we consider measuring outcomes across a number of domains: how the body functions (e.g. do the joints move fully, is there pain or weakness?) and what activities the person would like to be able to do or participate in (e.g. dress independently, do the housework or shopping, do usual work). A good reason for measuring health in a number of domains is that the relationship between outcomes in different domains is not necessarily strong. People can have high pain levels but be active and participate fully, or have minor movement limitation but be unable to get back to work. These anomalies are attributable partly to environmental factors, such as access to modifiable work duties, and partly to personal factors that are highly variable (such as a person's health beliefs and behaviours).

SUMMARY

Evaluation is part of being a professional health service provider. Many aspects of practice can benefit from evaluation that aims to achieve improvements in processes and outcomes. The methods used in evaluation will depend on the budget, the task and the importance of the issue. A successful evaluation needs to engage key stakeholders because, without the commitment of the stakeholders, change may not follow the evaluation. Having a culture of evaluation in an organisation or practice is healthy as it demonstrates a willingness to change and evolve practices. Although it is an important role of managers to implement an evaluation culture, everyone should engage in review of practice.

Reflective questions

- What are the possible dangers associated with not engaging in regular practice review?
- What are the advantages of having a national set of standards describing physiotherapy practice?

Further reading

Grembowski D E 2001 The practice of health program evaluation. Sage, Thousand Oaks, CA

Hammond R, Lennon S, Walker R et al 2005 Changing occupational therapy and physiotherapy practice through guidelines and audit in the United Kingdom. Clinical Rehabilitation 19(4):365–371

Hills R, Kitchen S 2007 Satisfaction with outpatient physiotherapy: a survey comparing the views of patients with acute and chronic musculoskeletal conditions. Physiotherapy Theory and Practice 23(1):21–36

McGregor A H, Dicken B, Jamrozik K 2006 National audit of post-operative management in spinal surgery. BMC Musculoskeletal Disorders 7:47

Pearse E O, Maclean A, Ricketts D M 2006 The extended scope physiotherapist in orthopaedic out-patients – an audit. Annals of the Royal College of Surgeons of England 88(7):653–655

Physiotherapy Board of New Zealand Registration requirements, competencies and learning objectives. Available: http://www.physioboard.org.nz/docs/registration_requirements.pdf 14 Feb 2008

Posavac E J, Carey R 2007 Program evaluation: methods and case studies. Prentice Hall, Pearson, NJ

References

Australian Council on Healthcare Standards 2006 The ACHS EQUIP 4 guide. ACHS, Sydney

APA 2003 APA position statement. Clinical justification and outcome measures. Australian Physiotherapy Association, Melbourne

APA 2007 APA standards for physiotherapy practices. Australian Physiotherapy Association, Melbourne

APC 2006 Australian standards for physiotherapy. Australian Physiotherapy Council, Canberra

Guyatt G H, Berman L B, Townsend M et al 1987 A measure of quality of life for clinical trials in chronic lung disease. Thorax 42:773–778

Kemmis S, McTaggart R 1988 The action research planner. Deakin University Press, Geelong

McNiff J 2000 Action research in organisations. Routledge, London

Oldmeadow L B, Bedi H S, Burch H T et al 2007 Experienced physiotherapists as gatekeepers to hospital orthopaedic outpatient care. Medical Journal of Australia 186(12):625–628

Redfern S J, Norman I J 1996 Clinical audit, related cycles and types of health care quality: a preliminary model. International Journal for Quality in Health Care 8(4):331–340

Sparkes V 2005 Treatment of low back pain: monitoring clinical practice through audit. Physiotherapy 91(3):171–177

Stufflebeam D L 1983 The CIPP model for program evaluation. In: Madaus G F, Scriven M S, Stufflebeam D L (eds) Evaluation models: viewpoints on educational and human services evaluation. Kluwer-Nijoff, Boston, pp 117–142

Ware J E 2000 SF-36 Health survey update. Spine 25(24):3130–3139 Available: http://www.qualitymetric.com/products/sfsurveys.aspx 24 September 2007

INDEX

Note: *c* denotes case study; *f* denotes figure; *t* denotes table